AF344413

The Management of Bladder Cancer

Consultant Adviser

Professor Michael J. Peckham MD, FRCP, FRCR

Director, British Postgraduate Medical Federation; Professor of Radiotherapy, University of London; and Honorary Consultant Radiotherapist, Royal Marsden Hospital London

Related titles

The Management of Terminal Malignant Disease, 2E
Edited by Cicely M. Saunders

Malignancies of the Ovary, Uterus and Cervix
Raymond S. Bush

The Management of Testicular Tumours
Edited by Michael J. Peckham

The Prevention of Cancer
Edited by Michael Alderson

Carcinoma of the Liver, Biliary Tract and Pancreas
Edited by J.-C. Gazet

The Management of Lung Cancer
Edited by John F. Smyth

Bone Tumours and Soft-Tissue Sarcomas
Edited by G.J. D'Angio and A.E. Evans

Malignant Tumours of the Oral Cavity
Edited by J.M. Henk and J.D. Langdon

Primary Management of Breast Cancer: alternatives to mastectomy
Edited by Jeffrey S. Tobias and Michael J. Peckham

The New Endocrinology of Cancer
Edited by Jonathan Waxman and R. Charles Coombes

Practical Radiotherapy Planning
Royal Marsden Hospital Practice
Jane Dobbs and Ann Barrett

The Management of Bladder Cancer

Edited by

Derek Raghavan, MB BS (Sydney), PhD, FRACP

Senior Oncologist, Department of Clinical Oncology,
and Research Director, Urological Cancer Research Unit
Royal Prince Alfred Hospital, and University of Sydney, Sydney,
Australia

Edward Arnold

© Edward Arnold (Publishers) Ltd 1988

First published in Great Britain 1988 by
Edward Arnold (Publishers) Ltd, 41 Bedford Square, London WC1B 3DQ

Edward Arnold (Australia) Pty Ltd, 80 Waverley Road, Caulfield East,
Victoria 3145, Australia

Edward Arnold, 3 East Read Street, Baltimore, Maryland 21202, U.S.A.

British Library Cataloguing in Publication Data

The Management of bladder cancer.
  1. Bladder ——— Cancer
  I. Raghavan, Derek
  616.99′462   RC280.B5

  ISBN 0–7131–4528–5

Text set in 9½ on 11pt Baskerville
by Wearside Tradespools, Fulwell, Sunderland

Printed and bound in Great Britain by
Biddles Ltd, Guildford and King's Lynn

Contributors

Numbers in square brackets identify the relevant chapter(s).

S.P. Ackland [10]
Oncology Unit, Newcastle Mater
Misericordiae Hospital, Newcastle,
NSW, Australia

C.L. Arteaga [3]
University of Texas, San Antonio,
Texas, USA

C. Bouffioux [14]
Hopital Baviere, Liege, Belgium

G.M. Clark [3]
University of Texas, San Antonio,
Texas, USA

F. Debruyne [14]
Radboud Hospital, Nijmegen, The
Netherlands

L. Denis [14]
A.Z. Middelheim, Antwerp,
Belgium

D. Eisinger [16]
Urological Cancer Research Unit
and Department of Urology, Royal
Prince Alfred Hospital, and
University of Sydney, NSW,
Australia

M. Garnick [12]
Dana Farber Cancer Institute,
Harvard Medical School, Boston,
Massachusetts, USA

R. Grundy [9]
Urological Cancer Research Unit
and Department of Clinical
Oncology, Royal Prince Alfred
Hospital, and University of Sydney,
NSW, Australia

W.F. Hendry [4]
Institute of Urology, and Royal
Marsden and St Bartholomew's
Hospitals, London, UK

J.E. Husband [5]
Royal Marsden Hospital, and
Institute of Cancer Research,
London and Sutton, UK

S.B. Kaye [13]
Department of Medical Oncology,
University of Glasgow, Scotland

K.H. Kurth [14]
Erasmus University, Rotterdam,
The Netherlands

P.H. Lange [2]
Urology Section, Veterans
Administration Medical Center, and
Department of Urologic Surgery,
University of Minnesota School of
Medicine, Minneapolis, USA

C. Limas [2]
Anatomical Pathology Section,
Veterans Administration Medical
Center, and Department of
Laboratory Medicine and Pathology,
University of Minnesota School of
Medicine, Minneapolis, USA

R.H. MacDougall [13]
Department of Clinical Oncology,
University of Edinburgh, Western
General Hospital, Edinburgh,
Scotland

L.T. Malden [9, 16]
Ludwig Institute for Cancer
Research, Royal Melbourne
Hospital, Parkville, Victoria,
Australia

vi Contributors

M. De Pauw and members of the
EORTC Genito-Urinary Group [14]
EORTC Data Center, Brussels,
Belgium

B.S. Pearson [16]
Urological Cancer Research Unit,
and Department of Urology, Royal
Prince Alfred Hospital, and
University of Sydney, NSW,
Australia

J. Philips [1]
Department of Morbid Anatomy,
Royal North Shore Hospital,
Sydney, NSW, Australia

D. Raghavan [1, 9, 15, 16, 17]
Urological Cancer Research Unit
and Department of Clinical
Oncology, Royal Prince Alfred
Hospital, and University of Sydney,
NSW, Australia

J.P. Richie [7]
Department of Urology, Brigham
and Women's Hospital, Harvard
Medical School, Boston,
Massachusetts, USA

M. Robinson [14]
Normanton and District Hospital,
Castleford, UK

M.A. Rose [8]
Harvard Medical School, and the
Joint Center for Radiation Therapy,
Boston, Massachusetts, USA

P.J. Russell [1]
Urological Cancer Research Unit,
Royal Prince Alfred Hospital,
Sydney, NSW, Australia

W.U. Shipley [8]
Harvard Medical School, and the
Department of Radiation Medicine
and Massachusetts General Hospital
Cancer Center, Boston,
Massachusetts, USA

M.S. Soloway [6]
Department of Urology, University
of Tennessee Center for the Health
Sciences, and the Veterans
Administration Medical Center,
Memphis, Tennessee, USA

G. Stoter [14]
Free University, Amsterdam, The
Netherlands

R. Sylvester [14]
EORTC Data Center, Brussels,
Belgium

R.P. Symonds [13]
Glasgow Institute of
Radiotherapeutics and Oncology,
Western Infirmary, Glasgow,
Scotland

I. Tannock [11]
Department of Medicine, Princess
Margaret Hospital, and University
of Toronto, Ontario, Canada

D.A. Tolley [13]
Department of Urology, Edinburgh
Royal Infirmary, Edinburgh,
Scotland

K. Tonkin [11]
Department of Medicine, Princess
Margaret Hospital, and University
of Toronto, Ontario, Canada

N.J. Vogelzang [10]
Section of Hematology/Oncology,
Department of Medicine, University
of Chicago Medical Center, and
Michael Reese Hospital, Chicago,
Illinois, USA

D.D. Von Hoff [3]
University of Texas, San Antonio,
Texas, USA

E.J. Wills [1]
Department of Anatomical
Pathology, Royal Prince Alfred
Hospital, Sydney, NSW, Australia

D.C. Young [12]
Dana Farber Cancer Institute, and
Harvard Medical School, Boston,
Massachusetts, USA

To my family with thanks for their
love and forebearance over many years

Preface

The management of bladder cancer is currently evolving through a renaissance. A greater understanding of the biology of the disease has been achieved with the use of new experimental models, through the demonstration of the oncogenes in bladder cancer and the elucidation of some of their functions, and the discovery of the wide range of functional heterogeneity that exists among populations of morphologically identical bladder cancer cells. The technological advances in flow cytometry, immunocytochemistry and non-invasive investigation allow more accurate determination of the prognosis for a patient at first presentation. A clearer definition of the end-points of treatment in the elderly patient, accompanied by more accurate measurement of the indices of 'quality of life', allow more appropriate tailoring of the treatment to fit the patient.

More recently, innovations in surgical technique, such as the use of the continent ileostomy and nerve-sparing pelvic dissection, have altered some of the concerns regarding the role of radical cystectomy. Furthermore, the introduction of more effective cytotoxic regimens may revolutionize the management of metastatic disease, analogous to the important progress made in testicular cancer. There is even evidence that these drugs may have a role earlier in the management of the patient with bladder cancer, either in combination with radiotherapy or as an adjunct before or after radiotherapy or surgery.

Nevertheless, the management of this disease remains highly controversial: surgeons, radiotherapists and oncologists appear to have substantially different perceptions of what constitutes 'optimal management'. In addition, patterns of practice differ substantially from one continent to another. This volume presents a broad perspective of the innovations and approaches to the practical management of urothelial malignancy, resolving some of these controversies, and providing the practising clinician with an overview to assist in the management of this complex group of neoplasms.

Many thanks to Ann Mills, Judy Hood, Patricia Raghavan and Betty Raghavan for assistance in the preparation of the manuscript.

1987   Derek Raghavan

Contents

1

The biology of urothelial cancer*

P.J. Russell, D. Raghavan, J. Philips and E.J. Wills

Introduction

Cancer of the urothelial tract has been the subject of great interest for clinicians and scientists alike, as it reflects many important aspects of the biology of neoplasia. As a model of carcinogenesis, both experimentally and clinically, the urinary tract perhaps is matched only by the skin and respiratory tract. The presence of a wide spectrum of differentiation, both with respect to degree and morphology, the availability of experimental models, and the accessibility of human tissue for clinical and experimental study, also contribute to the interest generated by this group of diseases. Finally, the apparent aetiology of bladder cancer, with smoking, industrial exposure and the role of some compound analgesics, and its prevalence in the community, are factors contributing to its importance.

Epidemiology

Cancer of the urinary bladder is the fifth commonest malignancy in males in occidental populations. In the USA, more than 35 000 cases are diagnosed each year, representing a prevalence of 16 new cases per 100 000 males per year. About five new cases per 100 000 females are diagnosed annually. The disease is one of older age groups, with a peak prevalence in the 60–70 year age group. It also appears that the incidence is rising (Davies, 1982).

The epidemiology of urothelial cancer has been reviewed extensively elsewhere (King and Bailar, 1966; Morrison and Cole, 1976; Wynder and Goldsmith, 1977; Davies, 1982; Bouffieux, 1984). However, in brief, several factors (some of them highly controversial) have been described in association with increased prevalence of the disease: industrial exposure (Doll *et al.*, 1970); urban environment (Clemmeson and Nielsen, 1956); tobacco intake (Holsti and Armala, 1955; Armstrong and Doll, 1974); dietary sweeteners (Friedman *et al.*, 1972); excessive exposure to motor vehicle exhaust fumes (Silverman *et al.*, 1986); schistosomiasis (Dimmette *et al.*, 1956) and possibly coffee drinking (Cole, 1971; Jensen *et al.*, 1986).

---

*The work reported in this chapter was supported by grants from the National Health and Medical Research Council of Australia and the New South Wales State Cancer Council.

However, the most compelling data relate to occupational carcinogens (Anthony and Thomas, 1970). Specific industries have been implicated, including dye works, the manufacture of leather, rubber, paint and heavy machinery, tailoring and hairdressing. Several specific occupational carcinogens have been identified, including aniline dyes, beta-naphthylamine, benzidine and nitrodiphenyl (Hueper *et al.*, 1938; Spitz *et al.*, 1950).

In Scandinavia and in Australia in particular, excessive intake of phenacetin-containing compound analgesics has been an unusual sociological feature, most notably in females in the lower socio-economic classes and particularly in process workers. This has been associated with the development of chronic renal failure (so called analgesic nephropathy), and more recently an increased prevalence of urinary tract neoplasia (Bengtsson *et al.*, 1968; Fokkens, 1979; McCredie *et al.*, 1983). However, the clear definition of risk levels and aetiological factors is hampered somewhat by such variables as multiple exposure, population drifts, latency of carcinogenic effect, etc.

Pathology

Macroscopic appearance

Tumours of the urothelium may be single or multiple, and may consist of fine or coarse papillary fronds, sessile or nodular lesions, regions of ulceration or merely areas of mucosal reddening or granularity. Depending on the extent to which a tumour penetrates into the bladder wall, there may be a variable amount of thickening in and around its base, a factor that will also be influenced by prior endoscopic surgical treatment (cautery).

Tumours may occur anywhere in the urothelium, but have a predeliction for the trigone, the region of the ureteric orifices and the postero-lateral walls. Tumours are not restricted only to the lower urinary tract, but may also be found in the renal pelves or ureters (see Chapter 16).

Histology

The urinary bladder is lined by a specialized epithelium, the urothelium. The surface of this epithelium is formed by a layer of 'umbrella cells', the structure of which is unique and integral to the barrier action of the epithelium (Koss, 1975; Pugh, 1973). The urothelium, composed predominantly of transitional epithelium, has the potential to undergo metaplasia to both glandular and squamous epithelium. Vascular and lymphatic channels are present in the connective tissue immediately deep to the basement membrane, which lies underneath the surface epithelium. The muscle coat consists of three interwoven layers of smooth muscle. The outer wall of the bladder is lined by an incomplete mesothelium, the remaining wall blending in continuity with the adjacent connective tissue.

Numerous attempts at classification of carcinoma arising in the urothelium have been made. The major indices in the systems of classification to date have been the pattern of growth (papillary versus solid), the presence or absence of invasion (stage) and the degree of differentiation (grade). Typical systems of classification are summarized in Table 1.1 and Chapters 2 and 4.

Table 1.1 Histology of tumours of the urinary tract

Transitional cell papilloma
Transitional cell papilloma (inverted)
Squamous cell papilloma
Transitional cell carcinoma (grades I–II–III)
Mixed carcinoma, including two or more of the following:
   transitional cell carcinoma
   squamous cell carcinoma
   adenocarcinoma
   undifferentiated carcinoma
Squamous cell carcinoma
Adenocarcinoma
Undifferentiated carcinoma

The clinical or prognostic significance of tumour heterogeneity has not been incorporated into the current systems of classification. Although pure squamous carcinoma or adenocarcinoma of the bladder may be associated with a different prognosis (Pugh, 1982; Chomette *et al.*, 1984), the presence of squamous or glandular elements within a predominantly transitional cell carcinoma has not been described as a specific prognostic factor (Pugh, 1973; Murphy, 1983). The histogenesis of the varied elements of bladder cancer (transitional, squamous, glandular) is the subject of ongoing research in our laboratories. We are attempting to assess whether these tumour patterns have a shared histogenesis from a common progenitor, or evolve independently (see the later section on experimental models).

An area of considerable controversy in the recognition and grading of urothelial malignancy has been the difficulty in distinguishing between a benign papilloma and a grade-I papillary carcinoma (Pugh, 1973). Other points of histological debate include the prognostic significance of papillary versus solid lesions (particularly in the non-invasive tumour), and the overlap between dysplasia, carcinoma-in-situ and papilloma. Central to this issue is the concept that urothelium, in the presence of carcinoma, may show a 'field' defect of unstable epithelium and that the flat precursor lesion may be prognostically more ominous than the papillary tumour with regard to subsequent invasion (Koss, 1975; Daly, 1976).

The prognostic significance of the histological demonstration of lymphatic or vascular invasion is uncertain. Although it has been suggested that these factors correlate with an adverse prognosis (Bittard, 1984), the data remain equivocal in view of the complicating independent variables of grade, stage and pattern of growth. As with other aspects of tumour pathology, the utility of pathological staging of urothelial cancer is often limited by the size of the available biopsies submitted and the presence of surgically induced artefacts (diathermy effect, etc.) or prior radiotherapy or chemotherapy. This is of particular importance when inadequate 'nip' biopsies fail to include muscle tissue, thus precluding the demonstration of possible muscle infiltration.

Ultrastructure

Compared with tumours arising in other sites, the ultrastructure of human bladder cancer has been explored relatively little. A major reason for this has been the difficulty in obtaining satisfactory specimens; standard cysto-scopy techniques involve filling the bladder with an unphysiological solution of low osmotic pressure which introduces considerable artefacts in the fine structure of the cells. It is also difficult to obtain truly normal control material, recourse usually being made to histologically normal areas of bladder mucosa in patients undergoing cystoscopy for non-neoplastic geni-tourinary disease. The large body of work in experimental bladder cancer, chiefly in rats, is beyond the scope of this review. Nevertheless many studies of the progression of changes from the earliest stages of hyperplasia to overt cancer, produced by carcinogenic agents, have given useful insights into the human disease.

Transmission electron microscopy (TEM) of transitional cell carcinomas

The superficial epithelial cells of the normal bladder are unique in posses-sing a rigid asymmetric plasma membrane with a thick outer leaflet. This membrane, which is restricted to the aspect of the cell facing the bladder lumen, is thrown up into a series of surface ridges and also forms fusiform vesicles in the subjacent cytoplasm (Fulker *et al.*, 1971; Koss, 1977; Tannen-baum, 1979a,b). As is usual in epithelia that form a permeability barrier, these are tripartite junction complexes that include a continuous belt of tight junctions between the lateral plasma membranes near the lumen. All these features may be retained in low-grade papillary transitional cell carcinomas (TCCs) but disappear with decreasing differentiation (Fulker *et al.*, 1971; Koss, 1977; Tannenbaum, 1979a,b; Fig. 1.1). It is unfortunate that the most characteristic features of urothelium are of little diagnostic help with

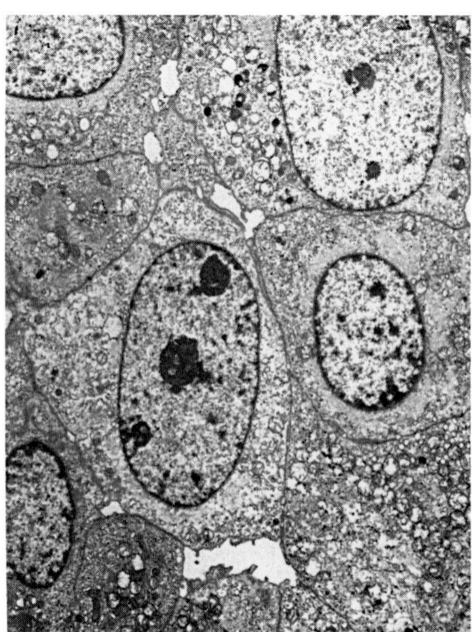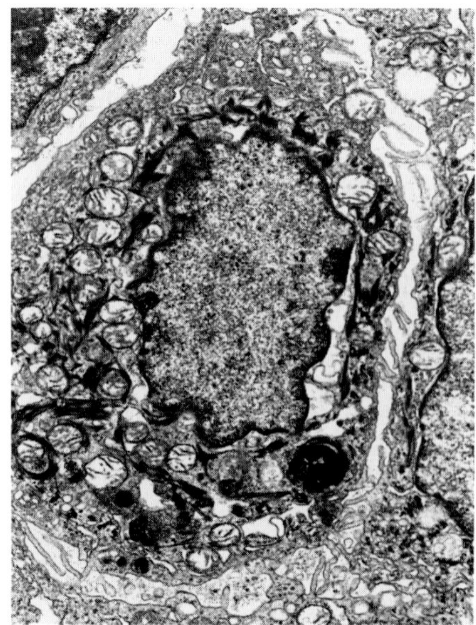

Fig. 1.1 Electron micrograph of xenografted TCC: (a) typical intermediary transitional cells; (b) focus of squamous differentiation. Reproduced with per-mission from Russell *et al.* (1986)

tumours that have spread beyond the confines of the bladder. In place of asymmetric membrane, the free surface becomes lined by symmetric unit membrane that may develop microvilli covered by glycocalyx. The other ultrastructural features of TCCs are not particularly distinctive but include comparatively wide intercellular spaces containing interdigitating plasma membranes, cytoplasmic intermediate filaments (particularly in high-grade tumours), plentiful free ribosomes and polyribosomes, glycogen, but rather sparse other organelles. Intracytoplasmic lumina are present in cells that have undergone glandular metaplasia (Alroy *et al.*, 1979), while squamous cells contain the usual cytoplasmic tonofilament bundles and well-formed desmosomes with tonofilament–desmosome complexes (Tannenbaum, 1979a).

The epithelial–stromal interface has provided interesting insights into the mechanism of tumour invasion (Alroy, 1979; Alroy and Gould, 1980; Tannenbaum, 1979a). 'Reversed polarity', where cells at the advancing edge show the greatest differentiation (including the presence of microvilli and junction complexes with tight junctions), has been described. The basal lamina, normally well-developed and often forming a lacy network, becomes attenuated or disappears and the tumour cells lie in direct contact with the elements of the lamina propria. The absence of the normal hemidesmosomal attachments to the basal lamina, the presence of microfilaments (? actin type) and lysosomes in the basal tumour cell cytoplasm provide a morphological basis for the mechanism of invasion. Whether the decrease in desmosomes in high-grade tumours is related to invasiveness is uncertain, but this (together with the high rate of cell turnover) doubtless contributes to their increased exfoliation (Alroy *et al.*, 1981).

Morphometric analysis has been applied in attempting to define the earliest recognizable features of neoplasia and to predict the biological potential of low-grade TCCs. The techniques are tedious and unlikely to find universal application, but have provided confirmation of what were sometimes subjective impressions (Alroy *et al.*, 1981; Fulker *et al.*, 1976; Moriyama *et al.*, 1984; Smith, 1981, 1982, 1985). From their evaluation of multiple factors in cells at different levels, Moriyama and coworkers (1984) concluded that the basal layer showed the greatest differences between neoplasia and inflammatory reactions, tumour cells being characterized by bulky irregular cytoplasm containing numerous vacuoles and enlarged Golgi areas. Smith (1981) found that of the morphological parameters examined, loss of asymmetric unit membranes with the formation of microvilli and the development of atypical junction complexes were the earliest recognizable abnormalities in preneoplastic cells. High-grade tumours were shown to have a greater nuclear volume and more spherical shape than low-grade tumours or normal bladder (Fulker *et al.*, 1976), while the basal lamina alterations previously mentioned seemed to distinguish invasive from non-invasive tumours (Smith 1981).

Scanning electron microscopy (SEM)
Considerable attention has been devoted to the urothelial luminal surface as revealed by SEM (Kjaergaard *et al.*, 1977; Newman and Hicks, 1977; Nelson *et al.*, 1979; Tannenbaum, 1979a,b; Jacobs *et al.*, 1981; Moriyama *et al.*, 1984). Considerably greater areas can be surveyed by this technique than by

TEM and there has been particular interest in the changes found in 'normal' mucosa adjacent to tumours or from other areas of tumour-bearing bladders.

Dysplasia, carcinoma-in-situ and TCCs all lose the normal surface microridges and develop a cobblestone pattern of cells with microvilli. Whether or not these microvilli are sufficiently pleomorphic in neoplasia to permit distinction from hyperplastic cells (which may also develop microvilli) is contentious, as also is the question of whether the surface structure of TCCs varies with their grade. 'Umbrella cells' may still be seen in well-differentiated papillary TCCs but are lacking in grade II–III tumours.

Macroscopically 'normal' mucosa from tumour-bearing bladder may possess pleomorphic microvilli, although there is some question as to whether they can develop in histologically normal epithelium (Newman and Hicks, 1977) or only in severe hyperplasia and carcinoma-in-situ (Nelson *et al.*, 1979). One investigation (Kjaergaard *et al.*, 1977) concluded that such areas were no different from the mucosa of bladders without tumours so that the use of SEM as a predictor for subsequent biological behaviour of the urothelium in a particular individual remains to be established.

Hyperplasia, dysplasia, carcinoma-in-situ
In general, a progression through the stages of development of carcinoma can be traced at the ultrastructural level (Koss, 1977; Tannenbaum, 1979a; Smith, 1985). The surface of hyperplastic cells is lined partly by asymmetric membrane, partly by symmetric membrane with microvilli. Nuclear and nucleolar enlargement is seen in dysplasia, together with decreased numbers of desmosomes, attenuation of tight junctions, increased polyribosomes and intermediate filaments. There may be defects in the basal lamina through which the epithelial cells send down pseudopods or large cytoplasmic extensions, so that some of these lesions can be regarded as already ultrastructurally microinvasive.

Uncommon forms of bladder cancer
The bladder has only recently been added to the large list of extrapulmonary sites in which small-cell neuroendocrine carcinomas (oat cell carcinomas) may arise. Recognition of these tumours which, in the lung, demonstrate a propensity for early metastasis and response to specific chemotherapy, has important clinical implications. However, to date there are too few reported cases to know whether bladder tumours of this type behave in a similar fashion. Demonstration of the characteristic ultrastructure with the usual sparse, small-sized, dense-core neurosecretory granules (Davis *et al.*, 1983; Reyes and Sonera, 1985) may be the most effective means of diagnosis and will distinguish these tumours from others that are small-celled but not neuroendocrine in type.

Spindle celled tumours may present a diagnostic problem in the bladder, as in other sites. Electron microscopy allows the separation of squamous carcinomas with pseudosarcomatous stroma, which contains reactive fibroblasts (Jao *et al.*, 1975), from sarcomatoid squamous carcinomas in which the cells, though elongated, retain their epidermoid features. These can be differentiated from carcinosarcomas or mixed mesodermal tumours (Duong *et al.*, 1981) in which the mesenchymal elements are genuinely neoplastic.

Electron microscopy in exfoliative cytology
The interpretation of cytology smears containing cells that have been
exfoliated in urine is difficult (see Chapter 2) and there have been attempts
to determine whether scanning electron microscopy could improve diagnostic accuracy. Prominent pleomorphic microvilli, partially and completely
covering the surface, were considered sufficiently characteristic by Croft *et
al.*, (1979) to distinguish tumour cells from those in inflammatory and other
conditions that also develop microvilli. However, although cells become
more numerous with increasing grade and invasiveness, the surface features
do not help determine grade. Others (Kjaergaard *et al.*, 1977) were unable to
distinguish tumour cells from normal intermediate basal cells, or found that
many of the cancer cells that were most typical by light microscopy lacked
any distinguishing features by SEM (Donagala *et al.*, 1979). Thus this
approach remains controversial and its diagnostic potential has not been
borne out in practice.

Functional pathology

As noted above, urothelial cancer is a heterogeneous, multicentric neoplasm
with two dominant patterns of natural history: 'low-risk', low-grade, frequently recurring superficial cancer, and 'high-risk', high-grade, invasive
cancer with a great metastatic potential (see also Chapter 2). The prediction
of likely natural history on the basis of light or electron microscopy remains
inexact. Thus alternative approaches to the identification of tumours with
low or high potential for metastasis and recurrence are required.

Tumour markers
To date, the most useful additional prognostic determinant for bladder
cancer has been the measurement of expression of blood group antigens, as
reviewed in detail in Chapter 2. In brief, the expression of the blood group
iso-antigens (A, B and H substances) by urothelial tissue is usually associated
with an improved prognosis. Conversely, loss of expression of these substances is associated with a worse prognosis (Chapter 2). By contrast, bladder
cancers express the peanut lectin binding substance, T-antigen or Thomsen–Friedenreich antigen, whereas in normal bladder tissue, the antigen is
masked. However, as discussed by Limas and Lange, these substances have
major limitations of specificity and sensitivity as tumour markers or as
prognostic determinants.
   Some of the limitations of this system may be overcome by studies using
multiparametric flow cytometry to study ABH expression and DNA staining
simultaneously (Devonec *et al.*, 1985). This approach will be important for
two reasons: the potential predictive value of tumour ploidy (see below); and
the possible variation in antigenic expression throughout the cell cycle (for
example, the expression of the Ca antigen on T24 bladder cancer lines *in
vitro* is higher during the G2 plus M phase than in G1, which in turn is
higher than in the S phase; Czerniak *et al.*, 1984). Similar data have been
produced for other tumour antigens (Burk and Drewinko, 1976).
   The biological implications of the changes in the expression of blood
group and T-antigens in tumour cells versus those seen in normal cells are
not understood. Each suggests a role for glycosyl transferases or glycosidases

which are commonly located at the cell surface, and may be involved in the cell–cell interactions. The recent observation of microheterogeneity of spatial expression of peanut agglutinin (PNA) binding sites in the extra cellular matrix of cultured T24 cells and fibroblasts has led to the suggestion that the modulation of galactose expression in this matrix may provide a spatial signal for cell recognition and interaction (Trejdosiewicz *et al.*, 1985).

Epithelial cell markers
Several antigens associated with epithelial tissue have been evaluated as potentially specific markers of bladder cancer. Epithelial membrane antigen (EMA) and carcinoembryonic antigen (CEA) are both expressed by bladder cancer, but also may be found in other malignancies and even in non-malignant states. Although controversial, it is generally agreed that CEA has only limited value as a tumour marker of transitional cell cancer because of its variable expression with stage, grade and histological subtypes, and a poor correlation with tumour progression (Murphy *et al.*, 1977; Zimmerman, 1979; Wahren *et al.*, 1982). In our experience, patchy positive staining for CEA is found in human and xenografted TCC, correlating predominantly with squamous differentiation (Russell *et al.*, 1986). However, the presence of this antigen is inconstant and we believe it to be of only limited value. In a series of 50 patients with invasive non-metastatic TCC, only 20 per cent had raised levels of CEA in the blood at presentation (Raghavan, unpublished).

The anti-cytokeratin antibodies constitute another potential tumour marker for this disease. For example, Feitz *et al.*, (1985) have studied ploidy (DNA content), tumour invasiveness and the expression of cytokeratins as prognostic determinants. In low-grade low-stage TCC, only a small proportion of tumour cells express cytokeratin 18, whereas in metastatic deposits this antigen is expressed by the majority of tumour cells (Ramaekers *et al.*, 1985; Feitz *et al.*, 1985).

Similarly, tissue polypeptide antigen (TPA), a cytoskeletal protein synthesized during the S phase of the cell cycle and released from rapidly growing cells, may be expressed in serum and urine from patients with bladder cancer (Kumar *et al.*, 1981) and has been demonstrated in tumour biopsy specimens. However, TPA also lacks specificity for the presence and type of malignancy.

Recently it has been shown that most invasive bladder carcinomas express receptors for epidermal growth factor (EGF) (Neal *et al.*, 1985). More of the poorly differentiated (18/21) than moderately differentiated (10/27) tumours express these receptors, whereas they are only occasionally found in non-invasive tumours and have not been reported to occur in normal urothelium. This finding may be of considerable importance as EGF is found in the urine, and may thus constitute a useful marker for invasive bladder cancer.

A detailed discussion of all putative tumour antigens is beyond the scope of this chapter, but has been reviewed elsewhere (see Chapter 2).

Lectin binding
The changes of surface carbohydrates in normal versus neoplastic bladder cells, as outlined previously, suggest that other surface properties may also be altered—for example, other lectin binding sites. Changes have been

reported in concanavalin-A binding of rat bladder cells treated with carcinogens (Kakizoe *et al.*, 1979). Lectins that bind increasingly to bladder tumours of increasing stage and grade include *Trichosantos Kinlowi*, soybean agglutinin, concanavalin-A (Takayama, 1984; Rubben and Lutzeyer, 1985) and wheatgerm agglutinin (Dus *et al.*, 1985). A leucoagglutinin-binding glycoprotein of molecular weight 115 kilodaltons has been demonstrated on cell lines of transformed bladder TCC and on a melanoma cell line, but not on normal urothelium nor in squamous carcinoma of the bladder (Paulie *et al.*, 1983). Using flow cytometry, we have demonstrated heterogeneity in binding of a series of lectins, including peanut lectin. *Ulex europaeus*, soybean lectin, concanavalin-A and wheatgerm agglutinin by a bladder cell line, UCRU-B1-17CL (Russell, Wotherspoon, Jelbart and Raghavan, unpublished). Soybean agglutinin binds to fixed cells but not to unfixed cells, suggesting involvement of components of the cell membrane.

Antibodies to membrane components of urothelial cells

Attempts have been made to raise polyclonal (heterologous) or monoclonal antibodies (MoAb's) specific to determinants expressed in neoplastic but not in normal urothelium in mice and in humans (Bloom, 1978; Lee *et al.*, 1985; Masuko *et al.*, 1985). Although these reagents have been used extensively in experimental systems, as indices of differentiation and for radio-immunolocalization, their clinical role has not yet been defined.

Schneider *et al.*, (1980a,b) have raised rabbit antibodies against the T24 bladder cancer line and against a 110 kilodalton surface protein expressed by urothelial tumour lines. After appropriate adsorptions with normal tissue, both antisera lyse target tumour cells more than normal cells in a cytotoxic assay, but subsequently neither has found wide clinical use.

MoAb's have been produced by immunization with a human prostatic cancer line DU145 (Starling *et al.*, 1982) and with bladder cancer lines, including EJ (Nadakavukaren *et al.*, 1984), RT112 (Trejdosiewicz *et al.*, 1985b) and KU1 (Masuko *et al.*, 1984). The MoAb's against DU145 cross-react with several cell lines of bladder TCC, the antibodies against EJ recognizing keratin filaments and the antisera against RT112 yielding a spectrum of determinants associated with epithelial and urothelial differentiation. The MoAb raised against KU1 appears to recognize glycopeptide complexes which are found in sialo-glycoproteins on bladder cancer cells but not on normal human cells. These antibodies may provide useful probes for the study of normal differentiation and malignant transformation in human urothelial tissue, and may also have diagnostic applications.

Other factors produced by bladder cancer cells

Bladder cancer grown *in vitro* has been shown to secrete a variety of factors which may have relevance *in vivo*. These include polypeptides, such as transforming growth factor and colony stimulating factors, and angiogenic activity. The production of these proteins *in vitro* is discussed in the section on experimental models.

We have observed that several bladder tumours, when cultured on rat-tail collagen, erode the collagen layer to plate down on the underlying plastic surface. Testing of the supernatants from some of these cell preparations has revealed collagenolytic activity in a fluorescence assay. Although these observations are preliminary, the production of collagenase may constitute a marker of the ability of bladder cancer to invade or possibly of superficial bladder cancer to recur after transurethral resection (Russell, O'Grady, Jelbart and Raghavan, unpublished) (see Table 1.2).

Table 1.2 Collagenase production by bladder tumours *in vitro*

Patient	*TCC grade*	*Stage*	*Erosion of collagen I*	*Collagenolytic activity (fluorescence assay)*	*Type of cell**
1	II	Ta	±	–	E
2	II	Ta	–		
3	I–II	Ta	+	+	E and F
4	II–III	Ta	–		
5	II	T2	+	NT	E
6	III	T2	+	+	E and F
7	II	T3	+	NT	E
8	III	T4	+	NT	E and F
9	II–III	Tx	+	NT	E

*E: epithelial; F: fibroblast; NT: not tested.

Flow cytometric analysis of bladder cancer cells

Flow cytometric (FCM) analysis relies on the interaction of various dyes or fluorochromes with DNA, resulting in light emission on exposure to high-intensity light (see, for example, Fig. 1.2). There is no FCM staining procedure which is universally accepted; the various methods have been reviewed elsewhere (Frankfurt and Huben, 1984). Studies of flow cytometry of bladder cancer have been used to characterize tumour cell populations and to predict progression or response to treatment. Two parameters are predictive: the cellular DNA content or 'ploidy', which reflects the total amount of chromosome material based on a normal diploid or $2n$ content; and the percentage of cells in the synthetic (S) phase of the cell cycle, which reflects the proliferative rate of these cells. Correlation between FCM and chromosomal changes has been observed (Wijkstrom *et al.*, 1984a). By using acridine orange which binds to single- or double-stranded nucleic acids, resulting in red or green fluorescence respectively, and by measuring the length of the fluorescence pulse which is related to the diameter of the nucleus, additional measurements of RNA content and nuclear dimensions can also be assessed (Melamed, 1984). Bladder specimens for such studies have been obtained by irrigation (Melamed, 1984; Devonec *et al.*, 1982) or from biopsy specimens (Tribukait *et al.*, 1982). In low-stage bladder tumours, aneuploidy is most frequently detected in biopsies from the deep part of the tumour, whereas for carcinoma-in-situ most information is gained from flow cytometry of bladder washings. For invasive tumours (stages T2–T4), both bladder washings and biopsy specimens are suitable for these studies (Tribukait *et al.*, 1982). FCM analyses have also been successfully performed on paraffin-embedded tissues (Hedley *et al.*, 1983) and on post mortem tissues (Raber *et al.*, 1984).

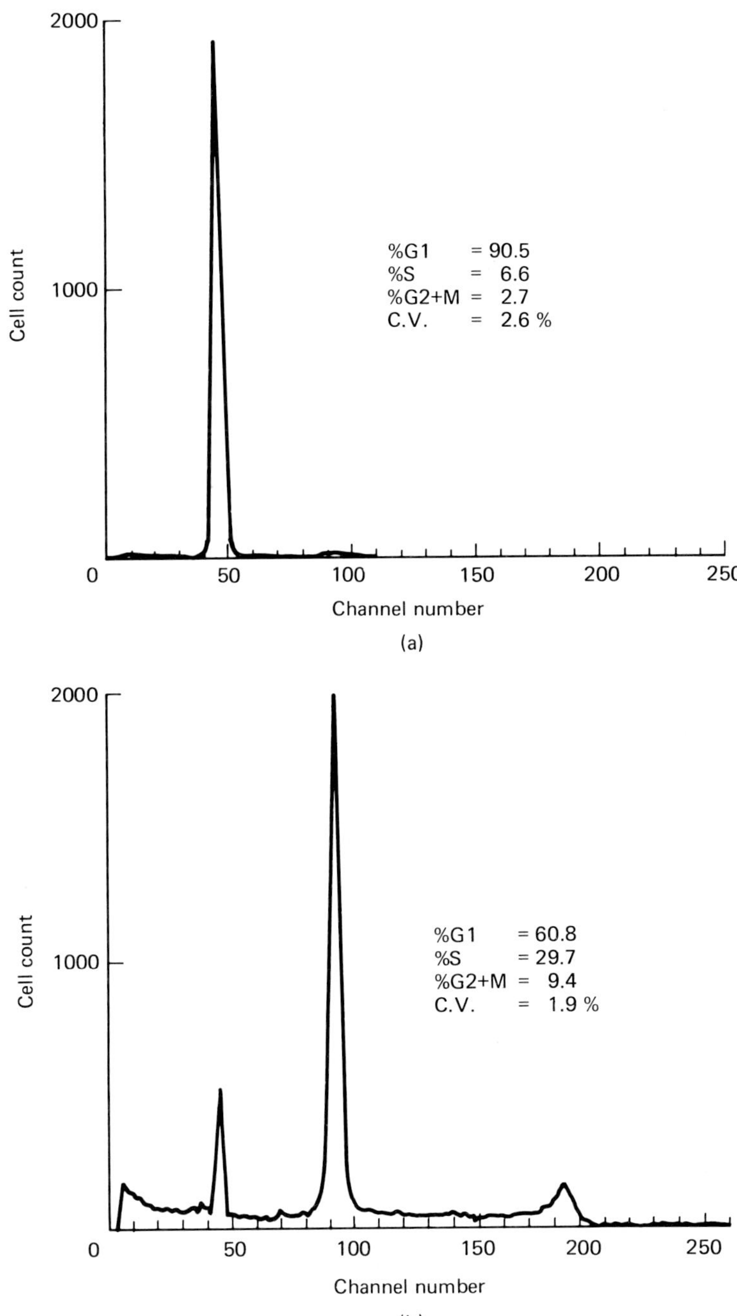

Fig. 1.2 DNA histograms of (a) diploid tumour; (b) aneuploid DNA content—note the additional peak

Relationship between flow cytometric profile and stage and grade of disease

In general, there are two major flow cytometric patterns seen in bladder tumours: diploid or near diploid; and gross changes in DNA levels (Tribukait *et al.*, 1982; Farsund *et al.*, 1984). There appears to be a strong correlation between ploidy and both the level of differentiation of the tumours (grade) and their depth of invasion (stage). A grade-I TCC is usually diploid with a low proliferative rate (<10% S-phase); whereas grade-III tumours are usually aneuploid with a high proliferative rate (>20% S-phase). Many of the aneuploid tumours contain multiple populations of cells with various degrees of chromosomal change (multiple aneuploidy), a feature which may correlate with increasing tumour aggression (with the possible exception of tetraploidy).

Ploidy versus prognosis

Similarly, tumour progression and recurrence appear to correlate with aneuploidy and a high proliferative rate for superficial tumours (Gustafson *et al.*, 1982b) and with multiple aneuploidy, a high proliferative rate and a high proportion of exfoliated cells for carcinoma-in-situ (Gustafson *et al.*, 1982a).

Measurement of ploidy appears to be of less value as a prognostic determinant in patients with invasive tumours, most of which are aneuploid with a high S-phase proportion (Wijkstrom *et al.*, 1984b).

FCM in 'normal looking' bladder mucosa

Of particular interest has been the demonstration of aneuploidy and high proliferative rates in cells taken from (apparently) histologically normal bladder mucosa in patients with bladder tumours. In some instances, identical changes in ploidy and proliferative rates have been found in tumours and in apparently normal mucosa (Farsund *et al.*, 1983, 1984). This is consistent with the concept of a field defect, perhaps initiated by a carcinogen, with changes in DNA preceding those of tumour development.

One important technical limitation that should not be forgotten is the impact of 'passenger' leucocytes with normal ploidy—a constituent of normal bladder tissue which is increased in the presence of inflammation. The technology to overcome this problem is being developed (Ramaekers *et al.*, 1984).

Cytogenetics of bladder cancer

Much of the available information regarding the chromosomal composition of bladder cancer has been derived from the direct study of human biopsy specimens (Falor and Ward, 1976; Gibas *et al.*, 1984). Studies of this type have demonstrated the relationship between abnormal chromosome complement and prognosis. However, detailed studies have been restricted somewhat owing to the technical difficulties encountered. For example, detailed analysis of karyotype was hampered by features such as a low mitotic index and difficulty in banding metaphase spreads (which tend to show contracted and 'fuzzy' chromosomes). In general, non-invasive TCCs (grades I and II) are associated with a diploid karyotype with occasional marker chromosomes, whereas grade-III tumours are often grossly aneuploid with multiple and varied markers. Similarly, invasive tumours show a greater level of chromosomal aberrations.

Considerable effort has been expended in attempts to karyotype bladder cancer cell lines *in vitro* (Moore *et al.*, 1978; Sandford *et al.*, 1978). However, work carried out on cell lines is difficult to interpret because of the possibility of cross-contamination between these lines (O'Toole, 1983; Gibas and Sandberg, 1984). Furthermore, detailed study of long-term cell lines will often reveal a complex pattern of secondary changes which may, in fact, be a characteristic of long-term survival *in vitro* rather than a measure of the behaviour of the tumour in the patient (Gibas *et al.*, 1984). These secondary changes include extreme hyperploidy and the presence of multiple marker chromosomes. It has been suggested that some of the markers may be linked to the ability of tumour cells to form colonies *in vitro* (Hastings and Franks, 1981), although we have demonstrated colony formation without the presence of these markers.

More recent approaches have included the use of short-term culture techniques, with exposure to methotrexate and colcemid, yielding high-resolution karyotypes (Gibas *et al.*, 1984, 1986). In this fashion, detailed chromosome maps have been produced, including the demonstration of putatively specific markers of transitional cell carcinoma, such as an isochromosome of the short arm of chromosome 5, a deletion from chromosome 13, trisomy of chromosome 7, monosomy of chromosome 9, and major changes in chromosomes 1 and 11 (Gibas *et al.*, 1984, 1986; Atkin and Baker, 1985; Fearon *et al.*, 1985). We have observed changes in chromosome 5 in two bladder cell lines (Russell *et al.*, 1987; Russell, Garson and Raghavan, unpublished), UCRU-BL-17CL and UCRU-BL-13CL. In both cases the changes were consistent with an iso-chromosome of the short arm of 5, but could have been 5q−. It is necessary to use C-banding to discriminate between these two possibilities. These specific changes may suggest different aetiologies of bladder cancer, or perhaps the involvement of different types of cells (which may be morphologically similar but different at a functional or molecular level). The definition of the primary chromosomal change in bladder carcinogenesis may help to define the exact gene(s) involved in this process. Secondary chromosomal changes, on the other hand, may play a major role in the biology of the disease—invasion, metastasis and response to treatment. Further studies may help to clarify these issues.

The role of oncogenes in bladder cancer

The conversion of normal cells to malignant tissue appears to be a multistage process (Land *et al.*, 1983), and it appears that several mutational events are required for the development of carcinomas (Klein and Klein, 1985). The development of cancer appears to be determined at the molecular level by the complex interactions of three major groups of genes—the oncogenes, tumour suppressors (anti-oncogenes), and modulating genes (Klein and Klein, 1985).

Cellular oncogenes

Cellular oncogenes have been discovered recently through the convergence of two lines of work: the study of oncogenic RNA viruses (retroviruses) which can transform cells, inducing tumours; and the use of gene transfer technology to investigate the difference between normal and transformed cells at the molecular level (Land *et al.*, 1983). The cellular oncogenes are a small class of normal cellular genes similar to, and most probably the source of, the transforming genes of retroviruses. They appear to be critically involved in the regulation of normal cell growth and differentiation, since they are highly conserved and expressed in normal cells at various stages of the cell cycle and in the process of cellular maturation. When activated, the oncogenes have the potential to transform cells to a malignant form, either by expression of an altered form of a normal cellular protein or by over-expression of an otherwise normal gene. The existence of more than 20 different transforming genes (oncogenes) in a variety of human tumours has been well-documented (Cooper, 1982; Barbacid, 1985). In particular, oncogenes of the *ras* gene family have been implicated in tumours of the bladder, as discussed below.

Tumour suppressors (anti-oncogenes)

Tumour suppressors are a group of genes which can counteract the transforming effects of different retroviral oncogenes (Noda *et al.*, 1983), and which may have to be deleted or functionally incapacitated before a tumour can develop. This mechanism may also account for the suppression of tumourigenic behaviour in hybrids derived from the fusion of malignant and normal cells (Green and Wyte, 1985). Cytogenetic analysis of these hybrids suggests that different suppressor genes can occur on different chromosomes.

Modulating genes

Modulating genes do not themselves induce transformation, but they modify the spread of neoplastic cells within the organism—for example, by influencing the display of major histocompatability antigens (Taniguchi *et al.*, 1985) or by controlling the expression of proteolytic enzymes (Dano *et al.*, 1985).

Transforming genes in bladder tumours

The techniques for studying gene transfer have been widely used to study the activation of oncogenes in bladder tumours. For example, transfection experiments rely on the capacity of cultured cell lines (such as the mouse fibroblast line, NIH3T3) to take up and express purified DNA added as a co-precipitate with calcium phosphate to the tissue culture medium (Graham and van der Eb, 1973). Transfection with DNA-containing activated oncogenes can lead to malignancy in the recipient cells (Kronteris and Cooper, 1981). Using this technique, DNA from some 10–20 per cent of randomly selected tumour cell lines or solid tumours, but not from equivalent normal tissues, has been shown to contain transforming genes (Santos *et al.*, 1984). In some bladder tumours, the transforming genes are of the *ras* gene family (Der *et al.*, 1982; Parada *et al.*, 1982; Santos *et al.*, 1982). Three different *ras* oncogenes (H-, K- and N-*ras*) have been characterized to date. K-*ras*, which is most commonly found in human tumours, is located on chromosome 12 and is a cellular homologue of a transforming gene found in Kirsten sarcoma virus. H-*ras* (a homologue of a transforming gene initially found in the genome of Harvey sarcoma virus) is located on the short arm of chromosome 11 and N-*ras* is found on chromosome 1. Each of these codes for structurally and immunologically related proteins of 21 000 daltons (known as p21), comprising 189 amino acid residues (Shih *et al.*, 1979). These genes have been found to acquire transforming potential by single point mutations. However, it has been calculated that the number of potential mutations which can give rise to transforming *ras* gene products is 42, based on three *ras* genes, each with possible mutations at positions 12 and 61 (Santos *et al.*, 1984).

There is evidence that exposure to carcinogens can induce point mutations in the cellular *ras* genes (Guerrero *et al.*, 1985). These effects of carcinogens on the *ras* genes, as well as the frequent finding of activated *ras* genes in human and animal tumours of clonal origin, strongly support the possible role of these genes in neoplasia.

When attempting to demonstrate the role of altered *ras* genes in the genesis of malignancy, the function of p21 protein becomes important. Normal p21 can hydrolyse guanine triphosphate to diphosphate, whereas this function is impaired in the oncogenic protein (McGrath *et al.*, 1984). The p21 proteins from normal and activated *ras* genes are located on the inner face of the plasma membrane, where they have the capacity to bind a single guanine nucleotide with high affinity (Newbold, 1984). The p21 protein may thus behave like one of the G-proteins, guanine nucleotide binding proteins responsible for stimulation and inhibition of adenylate cyclase following attachment of polypeptide hormones to cell surface receptors (Newbold, 1984). By regulating the levels of c-AMP, these G-proteins (and perhaps p21 which shares sequence homology) can transduce signals from growth factors at the cell surface to the rest of the cell to initiate cell division. The loss of GTPase activity in the mutant p21 could result in a permanent signal in the presence of low levels of growth factor which are insufficient otherwise to make normal cells divide (Marshall, 1984; Newbold, 1984).

Future studies

In addition to the methods for transfection and gene cloning, three techniques may be useful for studying the involvement of activated oncogenes in bladder cancer. Some of the mutations of the *ras* gene result in polymorphism (Santos *et al.*, 1984), with predictable changes in restriction enzyme cutting of the resultant DNA (Barbacid, 1985). The isolation of DNA from bladder tumours followed by endonuclease cutting and Southern blot analysis should give insights into the presence of particular mutations of these genes.

The technique of differential hybridization of gene probes can detect a single mismatch (i.e. a point mutation) in the *ras* gene, without the need for transfection assays (Guerrero *et al.*, 1985).

Mutations in the p21 protein result in different physicochemical properties (Seeburg *et al.*, 1984). These can be exploited in the production of different monoclonal antibodies which can recognize the different mutants. For example, a monoclonal to a synthetic peptide reflecting amino acid positions 10 to 17 of H-*ras* gene of the T24 cell line has been prepared and indicates increased *ras* p21 expression in epithelial cells of colonic and mammary tumours (Hand *et al.*, 1984). Using this monoclonal, we have found increased *ras* p21 expression in the UCRU-BL-13 xenograft line and its parent human tumour, but not in another line studied (UCRU-B1-14) (Russell *et al.*, unpublished).

Experimental models

An important restriction in the study of human urothelial malignancy is the lack of available tumour tissue for experimental purposes. Potential sources of bladder cancer tissue for study include fragments obtained from routine biopsies, but these are often damaged by intraoperative handling and are also frequently of only small volume. Material is occasionally available from cystectomy specimens, but these are often damaged by previous treatment (e.g. radiotherapy). Finally, tissue can sometimes be obtained from autopsy specimens, and in this instance post mortem necrosis or autolysis may preclude adequate biological study.

To overcome some of these problems, experimental models have been assessed, including the use of spontaneous or induced animal tumours, the growth of murine or human bladder cancer in tissue culture, and the use of xenografted human tumours in immunodeficient hosts.

Animal tumours

The major types of animal tumours include those which arise spontaneously, tumours induced by carcinogens and those that arise after viral induction. The main source of spontaneous tumours for experimental purposes has been the inbred mouse or rat. The use of inbred strains has facilitated the characterization of such tumours as they can often be transplanted without rejection in these species. An important benefit of such a system is that it provides a large supply of animals with virtually identical tumours at the same stage of growth. However, a major concern remains the degree to which tumour heterogeneity may be lost through serial transplantation. Spontaneous tumours usually take longer to develop than those that are induced, and often have a more variable morphology and pattern of growth. Although spontaneous urothelial tumours are uncommon in rodents, a high incidence of tumours of the bladder and ureter has been documented in brown/Norway rats and other selected strains (Boorman *et al.*, 1977). These multifocal tumours are usually papillary in type, and are often associated with carcinoma-in-situ.

2-naphthylamine was the first agent shown to cause tumours of the bladder. A variety of agents have had application to this model, and in particular, the nitrosamine group of chemicals, which have been shown to be specific carcinogens for rodent urothelium (Druckrey *et al.*, 1964; Ito *et al.*, 1969; Okajima *et al.*, 1971). Histologically the tumours are transitional cell carcinomas, resembling those found in man. In rats, these agents induce multiple papillary lesions with low-grade cellular atypia. By contrast, the tumours induced in mice may sometimes be sessile, high-grade and invasive. It has thus been suggested that the rat model is more suited to the study of superficial bladder cancer, whereas the murine model reflects invasive disease (Okajima, personal communication, 1986). N-butyl-N-(4-hydroxybutyl) nitrosamine (BBN) also induces urothelial tumours in dogs (Okajima *et al.*, 1981). In this instance the dosage of BBN correlates with the nature of the disease—low dosages are associated with superficial transitional cell carcinomas, whereas high doses yield high-grade, high-stage invasive tumours in a shorter period of time. Extensive studies have been carried out with N-(4-[5-nitro-2-furyl]-2-thiazoyl formamide (FANFT), a bladder carcinogen in mice, rats and dogs (Erturk *et al.*, 1967, 1969). The tumours formed are malignant and show invasion, metastasis and transplantability (Tiltman and Friedell, 1971; Soloway *et al.*, 1973). They constitute predominantly transitional cell carcinomas, but with a spectrum from hyperplasia through dysplasia, carcinoma-in-situ and frank malignancy. This model has been used extensively for the study of chemosensitivity testing and to investigate the development of bladder cancer from hyperplasia through other stages of the disease (Soloway and Murphy, 1979).

It should not be forgotten that tumours in rodents often grow more rapidly than in the equivalent human setting, and drug metabolism may vary markedly from the human situation. It is thus important to validate the data obtained from rodent tumours in models that more closely resemble the human disease, or directly in human tumours.

Growth of urothelium in tissue culture

The establishment *in vitro* of continuous cell lines derived from human urothelium is useful, to provide sufficient numbers of cells for detailed studies of such indices as light and electron-microscopy, the expression of tumour antigens and hormone receptors, DNA flow cytometry, karyotype, sensitivity to treatment and specific requirements for cellular growth. The tissue culture system suffers from the lack of a truly physiological environment and its 'two-dimensional' nature, although this does allow the analysis of individual 'clones' of cells. To some extent, this problem can be overcome by parallel studies of animal models or xenografted tissue.

To date, considerable difficulty has been experienced in establishing continuous urothelial cell lines (cultures that can repeatedly be transferred), whereas primary, short-term cultures are relatively easy to grow (Hepburn and Masters, 1983).

Normal bladder epithelium in culture

The characterization of 'normal' urothelial tissues *in vitro* has been reviewed in detail (Franks, 1983). Several problems have been encountered in the growth of normal urothelium in this environment:

1. Epithelial cells appear to require some mesenchymal cells for growth in

culture, yet it is these mesenchymal cells that tend to overgrow the primary urothelium.

2. Once in culture, the urothelial cells have a finite life span of only 6–8 weeks—differentiated normal cells, in particular, fail to survive *in vitro* and the usual cell markers are often lost.

3. The less 'differentiated' state of normal urothelium grown *in vitro*, compared with *in vivo*, mandates the use of such tools as electron microscopy and immunocytochemistry for the characterization of the cells—morphology is not sufficient as stromal cells are invariably present and are difficult to distinguish by their morphology alone.

4. The growth of normal cells in culture appears to show more stringent requirements than that of tumour cells and a variety of growth factors may be needed.

Furthermore, whether the longer-term cell populations are truly 'normal' is open to debate, in view of the adaptation required for their growth in such an artificial environment, and the risks of laboratory contamination (Franks, 1983).

Transformed cell lines

A variety of agents may be used to initiate the transformation from 'normal' to pre-neoplastic or neoplastic urothelium. After exposure to agents such as SV40 virus (Elliott *et al.*, 1974) or nitrosamines (Hashimoto and Kitagawa, 1974), the changes in the target cells can be observed serially in tissue culture. The morphology of the cells becomes increasingly bizzare, cell transfer is facilitated and the doubling time decreases. Electron-microscopy often reveals increased nucleoli and variable spectra of morphological differentiation. In this setting, abnormal chromosome patterns evolve, accompanied by the presence of markers (Cowell, 1979).

Several markers of transformation (and perhaps of neoplasia) have been studied in these cells. Enzyme production may, for example, alter with transformation (production of alkaline phosphatase (Herz *et al.*, 1974) or adenyl cyclase activity (Droller, 1976)). Changes in surface binding of the cells have also been reported (Kakizoe *et al.*, 1979). Changes in reactivity to monoclonal antibodies raised against normal and neoplastic urothelium can also be used to monitor the evolution of transformation (Grossman, 1983; Fradet *et al.*, 1984).

It is possible that such approaches will be too crude to distinguish between benign and malignant cell populations. The ability to transfect genes into normal urothelial cells provides a potential model for the study of the genes that are important in malignant transformation, as discussed previously. It is thus possible that single mutations may cause stepwise changes from 'normal' through to cancer of the urothelium, and a subtle gradation may exist within such a spectrum. Further studies will clarify the steps involved in the genesis of malignancy.

Growth of tumour cells in tissue culture

The growth of cells derived from malignant tissue is beset by many of the problems outlined above. As yet, one cannot predict which cells will grow *in vitro* and no relationship has been defined between pathological grade and stage versus the ability to grow in artificial environments. Non-specific factors, such as the degree of necrosis within a specimen and the release of toxins from dying cells, may be of importance. Other considerations include the physical preparation of tissues, the substrate for cell growth and environmental conditions such as gas tensions and pH. We have found that individual lines derived from different tumours often require different conditions for optimal growth. For example, the addition of insulin, hydrocortisone, 2-mercapto-ethanol, or growth factors, in addition to serum, facilitates growth in some lines, but appears to be unnecessary in others. As yet, the role of the mesenchymal or supporting cells has not specifically been defined. Growth of tumour cells on extracellular matrix overcomes the requirement for stromal tissue in some cases.

Despite these problems, more than 40 lines have now been reported, in most cases being derived from bladder transitional cell carcinomas, and occasionally from ureter or renal pelvis (see reviews by Williams, 1980; Hepburn and Masters, 1983). Some of the characteristics of these bladder tumour cell lines have been summarized, listing the pathological grade and stage of the donor tumours, the medium used for maintenance of the cell lines, the karyotypes of the cultured cells and their doubling times *in vitro*, the ability of the cells to grow in soft agar (anchorage independent growth) and to form tumours after xenografting into immunosuppressed host animals (Hepburn and Masters, 1983). Most of the lines described were derived from transitional cell carcinomas: nine from grade-I and grade-II tumours, ten from grade-III, eight from undifferentiated (grade-IV) tumours, and ten from tumours whose grade was not reported. One tumour, SCaBER, was derived from a squamous cell carcinoma of the bladder, stage T3 (O'Toole *et al.*, 1976). The characteristics of more recently established human bladder tumour cell lines are summarized in Table 1.3. In addition, several tissue culture lines derived from FANFT-induced rate bladder carcinomas have been described (Cohen *et al.*, 1981; Harn *et al.*, 1980).

The cell lines were heterogeneous with respect to morphology, varying between 'anaplastic' cells, whose features are somewhat difficult to discriminate from fibroblastic cells, and epithelial cells, which generally have more recognizable growth patterns (Nayak *et al.*,1977). These include growth in sheets of polyhedral cells with one or more nuclei, non-adherent growth in islands of smaller squamous epithelioid cells, or growth as single cells. We have also observed 'dome' formation in bladder tumour cells grown *in vitro* from UCRU-BL-18, a TCC, grade-II, stage T3 (see Fig. 1.3). This is apparently a consequence of transepithelial transport of water and ions which result in fluid accumulation between the culture dish and the cell layer (Bologna *et al.*, 1984).

Ultrastructural studies have demonstrated many cellular organelles, including numerous microvilli, mitochondria, free ribosomes and polyribosomes (Elliott *et al.*, 1974, 1977) or inclusions such a glycogen (Rigby and Franks, 1970) but the presence of desmosomes and bundles of tonofibrils or tight junction complexes has rarely been reported (Elliott *et al.*, 1974; Nayak *et al.*, 1977; Russell *et al.*, 1987), apart from the SCaBER (O'Toole *et al.*, 1976) and Gibb lines (Pontes *et al.*, 1984). We have observed typical transitional cell carcinoma cells, squamous carcinoma cells and mucin-producing cells in the cell lines UCRU-BL-13CL and UCRU-BL-17CL, and

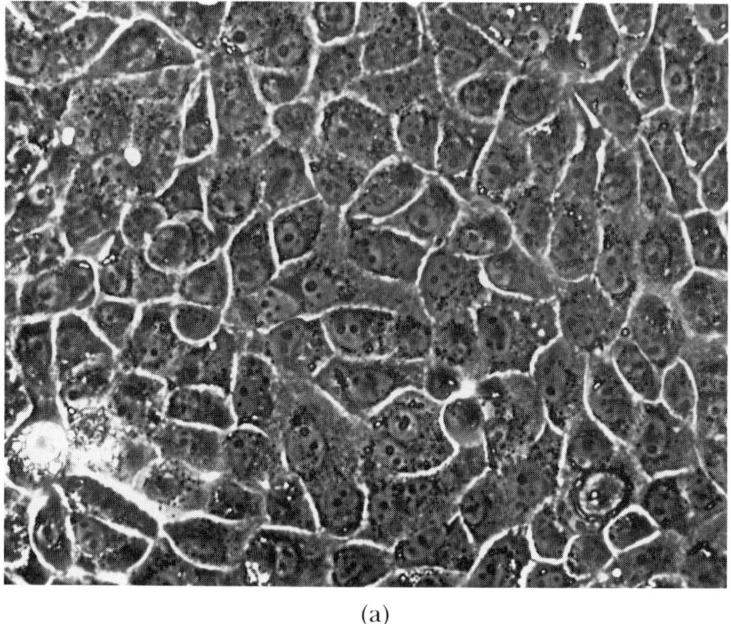

(a)

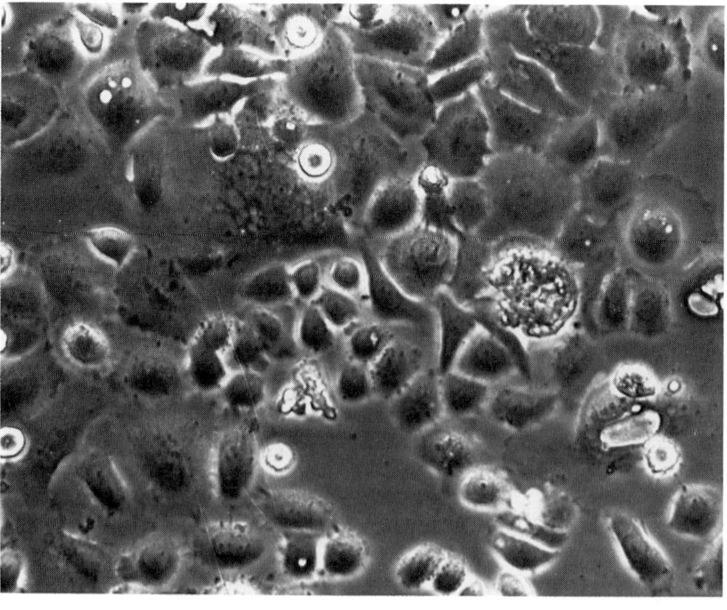

(b)

Fig. 1.3 (a) Typical morphology of TCC cells *in vitro*: the epithelial cells characteristically grow in a mosaic pattern with well-defined borders. Note the multiple nucleoli. (b) Cell line derived from a TCC, showing predominant glandular differentiation *in vitro*

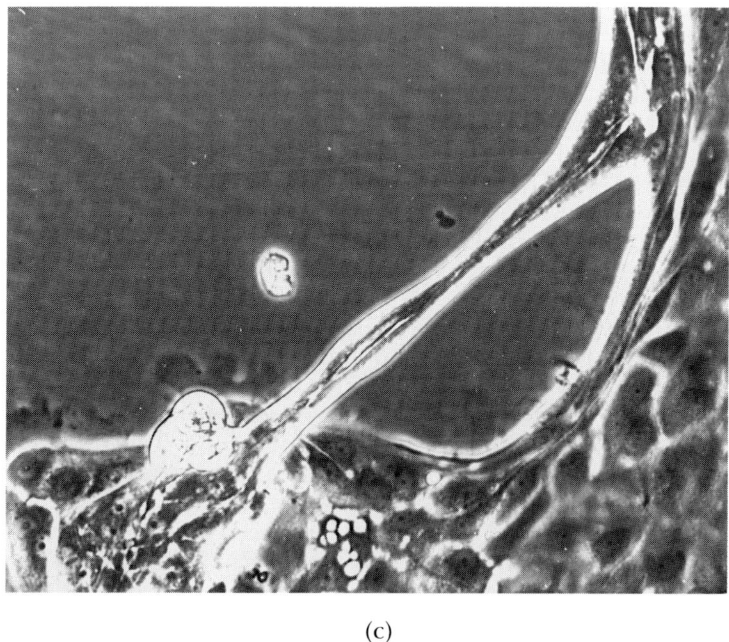

(c)

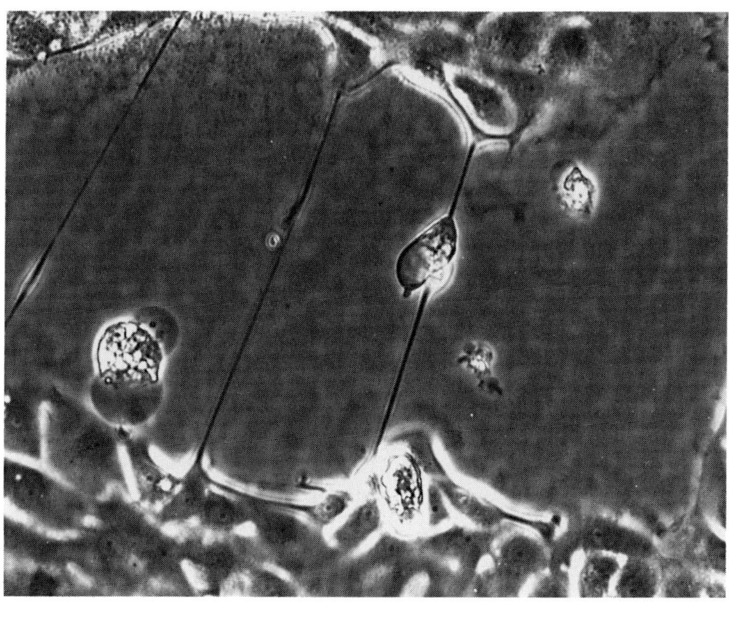

(d)

Fig. 1.3 (c) and (d) Epithelial cells derived from bladder cancer. Cells often form intercellular bridges, of unknown significance

have found features suggestive of both squamous differentiation and adenocarcinoma within the one cell in UCRU-BL-17CL (Russell *et al.*, 1987). This suggests a common histogenesis for these two cell types.

Unfortunately, there are few reports of immunocytochemical marker studies which would greatly assist in a more defined classification of cell types. Such studies have been carried out on our lines (see Table 1.4). Recently, Christensen *et al.*, (1984) devised a classification scheme for urothelial tumour cells grown *in vitro*, based on the ability of the cells to grow in the absence of fibroblasts, prolonged survival, increasing chromosomal abnormalities, antigenic modulations and the ability to form tumours in nude mice.

In addition to cultures of single cells as monolayers, we have attempted to grow fragments of bladder tumours as organ cultures, for example, on millipore membranes on a support matrix such as gelfoam (Russell *et al.*, unpublished). A recently described model for cancer propagation is the histophysiological gradient culture system (Leighton and Tchao, 1984). These systems have the advantage of a three-dimensional structure, which may more closely mimic the *in vivo* situation.

Preparations of bladder cancer cells *in vitro* have been used to determine the kinetic characteristics of bladder cancer (Elliott *et al.*, 1977; Hastings and Franks, 1981, 1983). A wide range of doubling times from 20 to more than 50 hours have been reported. Similarly, indices such as plating efficiency and percentage increase in cell number vary substantially, depending on the tumour of origin and the techniques used. The application of tissue culture for drug sensitivity testing has been reviewed in detail (see Chapter 3).

For many years, cell lines of TCC have been studied biochemically and immunologically to define possible prognostic indicators and to develop reagents for diagnostic and therapeutic use. Several specific proteins have been elaborated by bladder cancer *in vitro*, including alkaline phosphatase (Benham *et al.*, 1977), HCG (Rosen *et al.*, 1980), fibrinolytic proteins (Kinjo *et al.*, 1979), angiogenic factor (Chodiak and Summerhayes, 1984) and prosta-glandins (Droller *et al.*, 1979). Furthermore, a variety of granulocyte and macrophage colony stimulating factors have been produced *in vitro* (Welte *et al.*, 1985; Zinzar *et al.*, 1985). Similarly, transforming growth factor (TGF), a polypeptide which can confer a transformed phenotype on cells in soft agar, has been demonstrated in supernatants from bladder cancers grown *in vitro* (Heckl *et al.*, 1985).

However, of particular concern is the potential for cell lines *in vitro* to become contaminated—for example by other tumour lines, the presence of mycoplasma or viral particles, or overgrowth of stromal elements. Cell lines established from tissues grown in nude mice or other immunosuppressed hosts must regularly be karyotyped to demonstrate that the material is of human and not host origin. Heterokaryons, thought to be derived from hybridization *in vitro* of host stromal tissue and tumour cells, have been described in cultures established in this fashion (Goldenberg and Pavia 1981). Further confusion is sometimes added by the multiple naming of cell lines, the change of name occurring with transfer from one laboratory to another; for example, examination of the identity of a series of extensively published urothelial cell lines (EJ, MGH-U1 and T24) by HLA-ABC typing and isoenzyme analysis revealed that cultures of EJ (MGH-U1) and some

Table 1.3 Long-term human bladder TCC lines *in vitro**

Line	Race, sex	Histol. grade	Site	Medium with FCS (10–20%)	Morphology	Chromosomes Modal no.	Markers (M)	Cloni-genic	Tumouri-genic	Reference
KU-7	?	I	?	RPMI 1640	Spindle cells	?	?	−	?	Tachibana (1982)
KU-1	?	II	?	RPMI	Ep	?	?	−	?	Tachibana (1982)
UM-UC-1	N, M	II	BL	MEM	Ep	68(−Y)	4m	?	+	Grossman (1984)
UM-UC-2	C, M	TIS	UR	MEM	?Ep	48(−Y)	3m	?	+	Grossman (1984)
Gibb	C, M	?	BL	RPMI or MEM+	EP(+EM)	48–52 (−Y)	13m	?	+	Pontes (1984)
MGH-U2	?		BL	McCoy's 5A	Ep			+	+	Lin (1985)
MGH-U3	C, M	I	BL	McCoy's 5A	Ep	40–50	Several	+	+	Lin (1985)
MGH-U4	C, M	TIS	BL	McCoy's 5A	Ep			−	−	Lin (1985)
UCRU-BL-13	C, M	II	BL	RPMI†	Ep(+EM)	63	Several (+dm)	+	+	Russell (unpublished)
UCRU-BL-17	C, F	III	BL	RPMI†	Ep(+EM)	70	Several (+dm)	+	+	Russell (1987)

*See Hepburn and Masters (1983) for lines up to 1982.
†Plus insulin, hydrocortisone and 2-mercapto-ethanol.

Abbreviations: TCC—transitional cell carcinoma; C—Caucasian; N—Negro; BL—Bladder; U—Ureter; RPMI—Roswell Park Memorial Institute; MEM—Minimal essential medium; FCS—fetal calf serum; Ep—epithelial cells; EM—electron-microscopy; dm—double minute chromosomes.

Table 1.4 Tumour markers *in vitro*

	Cytochemistry					Growth in agar/MC	Tumouri-genecity in nudes	DNA flow cytometry*
Tumour	EMA	Keratin	CEA	PNA	BHCG			
UCRU-BL-13								
Patient biopsy	ND	ND	+(Sq)	++	−			$2n(30)$, 2.3–$2.9n$
Xenograft X0	ND	ND	+(Sq)	+	−			$2n$, $2.5n$, $2.9n$
Cell line	+	+	+	+	±	+	+	$2.3n$, $4.6n$, $5.1n$(P5); $4.4n$, $5n$(P26)
UCRU-BL-17								
Patient biopsy	ND	ND	++	+	−			$2n(90)4n$
Xenograft X0	ND	ND	++	+	−			$2n(90)4n$
Cell line	+++	++	++	++	ND	+	+	$2n(9)$, $4n(91)$, $3n$(P25)

* Note: In parentheses, percentage of G1 cells with ploidy shown; P=passage number *in vitro*.

cultures of J82 were, in fact, T24 cells (O'Toole *et al.*, 1983). Similar contamination of cell lines has also been observed by others (Gibas *et al.*, 1984; Lin *et al.*, 1985). These findings indicate that it is essential to determine either HLA typing or isoenzymic patterns or both, before publication of work concerning newly established cells lines. Furthermore, multiple naming of identical lines should be avoided.

Xenografts

During the past century, many approaches have been used in an attempt to transplant neoplastic tissues from one species to another. Several privileged sites have been demonstrated in which heterologous tissue can survive, including the anterior chamber of the eye, kidney, salivary glands, sub-cutaneous tissues, jugular vein, hamster cheek pouch and brain. However, the utility of these sites is limited by excessive morbidity in the recipient animals and difficulties of physical access to the growing tumours. An alternative approach has been provided by systemic immunosuppression of the recipient animal through whole-body irradiation, neonatal thymectomy, treatment with anti-lymphocyte globulin, or combinations of these, as reviewed elsewhere (Steel and Peckham, 1980). More recently, an important advance was the introduction of priming techniques, in which cytosine arabinoside is administered 24–48 hours before whole-body irradiation, protecting the normal tissues from the lethal effects of radiotherapy (Steel *et al.*, 1978).

Nearly twenty years ago, the congenitally athymic 'nude' mouse mutant was introduced into cancer research (Rygaard and Povlsen, 1969). An extensive literature has evolved characterizing the use of these models for the study of a wide variety of tumour types, as reviewed previously (Fogh and Giovanella, 1978; Steel and Peckham, 1980; Raghavan, 1983).

In general, good correlations have been demonstrated between the original tumours and their corresponding xenografts for light morphology, ultrastructure, cellular kinetics, DNA content and tumour marker production (Fogh and Giovanella, 1978; Povlsen, 1980; Raghavan, 1983). The utility of the xenograft model as an index of treatment sensitivity (Bailey *et al.*, 1984) and as a model of metastasis (Sharkey and Fogh, 1979) is less well defined.

This model has some advantages when compared against animal tumours or cell culture *in vitro*: provision of a physiological milieu, reproducible growth of large amounts of 'human' tumour tissue for study, perhaps a greater similarity to the human disease state than in animal tumours, and the potential for demonstration of new tumour antigens because of a high tumour:host mass ratio. However, important drawbacks should not be forgotten, including the differences between host and human metabolism, risks of contamination by transformed host cells, cross-species immunologic-al interactions, low 'take' rates, low rates of spontaneous metastasis, abnor-mal sites of growth and a potential biological hazard to laboratory personnel.

Xenografts of bladder cancer

Many of the models discussed above have been applied to the study of bladder cancer (see Table 1.5). Tumours have been grown in the hamster

Table 1.5 Xenografted human TCC*

| | Human tumour | | | Xenografts | | 'Take' rate | | | | |
	Dominant histology	Grade	Dominant histology	Grade	Initial	Serial	Host	Applications	Reference
1°/2°									
2°	TCC	III	TCC	III	3/7	2/7	Hamster	Kinetics, drugs	Burt *et al.* (1966) Kaufmann *et al.* (1969)
1°	TCC	I–III	TCC	I–III	8/20	0/20	Nude	—	Sufrin *et al.* (1979)
1°	TCC	II–III	TCC		8/31	8/31	Nude	Fibrinolysis	Naito *et al.* (1980a)
1°†	TCC	III	TCC	III	3/8	3/8	Nude	Fibrinolysis	Naito *et al.* (1980b)
1°	TCC	I–III	TCC	I–III	7/18	4/18	Nude	—	Matthews (1982)
1° and 2°	TCC	I–III	TCC		20/53	9/53	Thym-X	Kinetics, treatment	Kovnat *et al.* (1984)
1°	TCC	I–III	TCC		—	—	Nude	Treatment	Huland *et al.* (1985)
1°	TCC	I–III	TCC adeno CA	II–III	11/20	7+/20	Nude	Cachexia, treatment, markers, differentiation	Russell *et al.* (1986), and in press

*Lines derived directly by implantation of human material.
†Upper-tract tumours.

cheek pouch (Kaufmann *et al.*, 1969), in artificially immunosuppressed mice (Kovnat *et al.*, 1982, 1984) and in nude mice (Sufrin *et al.*, 1979; Kyriazis *et al.*, 1983; Russell *et al.*, 1986) and have retained the dominant features of the original human bladder cancers. Xenografts have been established from primary and metastatic tumours, both from previously treated and un-treated patients. In some instances, cell lines *in vitro* have been tested for tumourigenicity by xenografting, thus giving rise to transplantable lines.

Most established xenograft lines have the morphological characteristics of grade II-III transitional cell carcinoma (Table 1.5), with occasional foci of squamous or glandular differentiation (Kovnat *et al.*, 1982; Russell *et al.*, 1986). Grade and histology do not appear to correlate with success of xenografting (Kovnat *et al.*, 1982, 1984; Russell *et al.*, 1986), and as yet, successful xenografting has not been shown to be an index of stage or prognosis in the patients from whom the biopsies are taken.

Using a combination of xenograft lines and the growth of bladder cancer in tissue culture, we have explored the histogenetic relationships between the subtypes of bladder cancer. It appears that transitional cell carcinoma and at least some forms of adenocarcinoma of the bladder arise from a common 'stem' cell, and furthermore that elements of squamous or glandu-lar differentiation may coexist within the one cell (Russell *et al.*, 1986, 1987). Clearly this factor would make histological classification more difficult, and provides a possible explanation for the apparent changes in light morpholo-gy of bladder cancer in individual patients over a period of time.

The use of the xenograft model has allowed a more detailed characteriza-tion of bladder cancer at the ultrastructural level because of the availability of more controlled conditions for fixation, greater amounts of tissue for study, and the absence of artefact due to diathermy or intraoperative handling. Our results from the electron-microscopy study of xenografted bladder cancer, in combination with data obtained from growth *in vitro*, were summarized in the foregoing section on ultrastructure.

The xenograft model has also been useful in the search for new tumour markers. The production of carcinoembryonic antigen, alphafetoprotein and human chorionic gonadotrophin has been studied in other tumour types, relating the production of these proteins to histology, tumour mass and response to treatment (Raghavan *et al.*, 1980; Raghavan, 1983). To date, specific bladder cancer antigens have not been revealed from xenograft studies. However, carcinoembryonic antigen, epithelial membrane antigen, blood-group substances and lectin-binding activity have been documented in these studies (Russell *et al.*, 1986, 1987). It is of interest to note the demonstration of human prostatic acid phosphatase in xenograft lines derived respectively from a male and a female with bladder cancer (Reid *et al.*, 1984; Russell *et al.*, 1987).

Preliminary data are available from studies of the treatment options for bladder cancer. The radiobiology of xenografted bladder cancer has been studied, yielding Do values of 1.1–1.5 Gy for a series of xenograft and cell lines and showing the presence of a large hypoxic fraction (Tannock *et al.*, 1984). After studying the interaction of cisplatin and radiation in a variety of schedules and sequences, Kyriazis *et al.* (1983) concluded that optimal tumour kill is achieved when the administration of cisplatin follows the

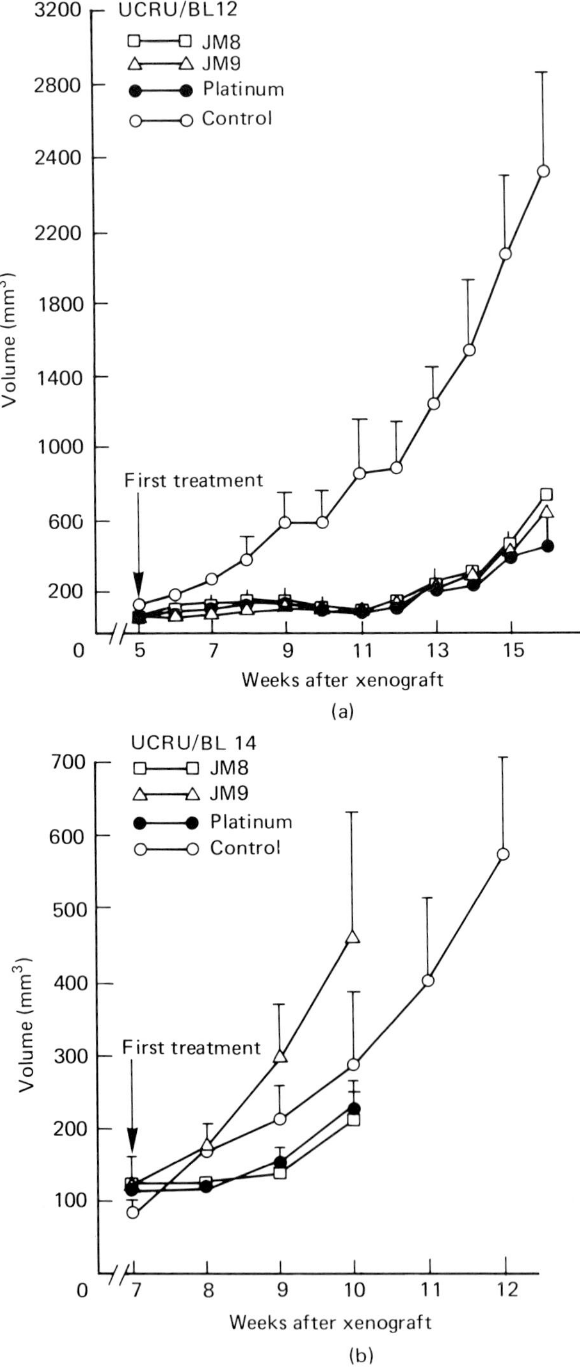

Fig. 1.4 Xenograft chemosensitivity testing. (a) UCRU-BL-12, a TCC sensitive to cisplatin and its analogues, carboplatin and isopropyl platinum. Reproduced with permission from Russell *et al.* (1986). (b) UCRU-BL-14, a morphologically similar TCC which is resistant to cisplatin and analogues

conclusion of radiotherapy. However, these data have not been supported in clinical studies.

We have used xenografts to compare the use of cytotoxic agents (e.g. cisplatin) and novel analogue compounds (carboplatin, isopropyl platinum), and have shown common sensitivity or resistance to each compound in a series of three lines (Russell *et al.*, 1986; Fig. 1.4). We have also demonstrated common patterns of resistance to the doxorubicin analogues, mitoxantrone and 4'-epidoxorubicin (Fig. 1.5). From a small series of experiments, it has also been suggested that there are differences in chemosensitivity between early (slowly growing) and late (rapidly growing) xenograft passages, and that the latter should be used specifically as models for chemotherapy of metastases (Huland *et al.*, 1985). As yet, it is not clear whether treatment sensitivity testing in animal models (Soloway and Murphy, 1979), *in vitro* (see Chapter 3), or in xenografts provides the most useful results. Perhaps the optimal approach at this time may be afforded by the use of the three models in parallel, validating each by comparison with the others and with the available clinical data.

Of particular concern with regard to the use of the xenograft model is the potential for contamination of human material by host stromal cells, the implications of a different metabolic system in the host animal, and the potential for loss of tumour heterogeneity through the selection processes that allow growth in an artificial environment. We have resolved these issues to some extent: it is clear that tumour heterogeneity is preserved somewhat in the xenografts that we have studied, at least with respect to morphology, the expression of tumour antigens and variability of DNA flow cytometric profiles (Russell *et al.*, 1986). Furthermore, careful karyotyping and serial DNA flow cytometry can demonstrate that predominantly human material remains within the xenografted tissue, although, as discussed elsewhere, there remains the potential for the formation of heterokaryons (Goldenberg and Pavia, 1981). However, the impact of the admixture of human and host cells on the metabolism of cytotoxic drugs is not known, and these issues will be resolved as more information becomes available, allowing the definition of the sensitivity and specificity of this model as a predictor of response to treatment.

Summary

In this brief overview we have summarized the available knowledge of the biology of bladder cancer. There is a great need for continued interaction between the basic scientist and the clinician in order to unravel further the complexities of urothelial malignancy: the tools of epidemiology, identifying populations at increased risk, combined with the probes of molecular biology and cytogenetics, and the use of the methods for studying carcinogenesis in experimental models may define the origins of the disease. Similarly the interfaces between biochemistry, molecular biology, clinical and experimental pathology and clinical medicine will eventually identify reliable prognostic determinants and methods of prevention and cure.

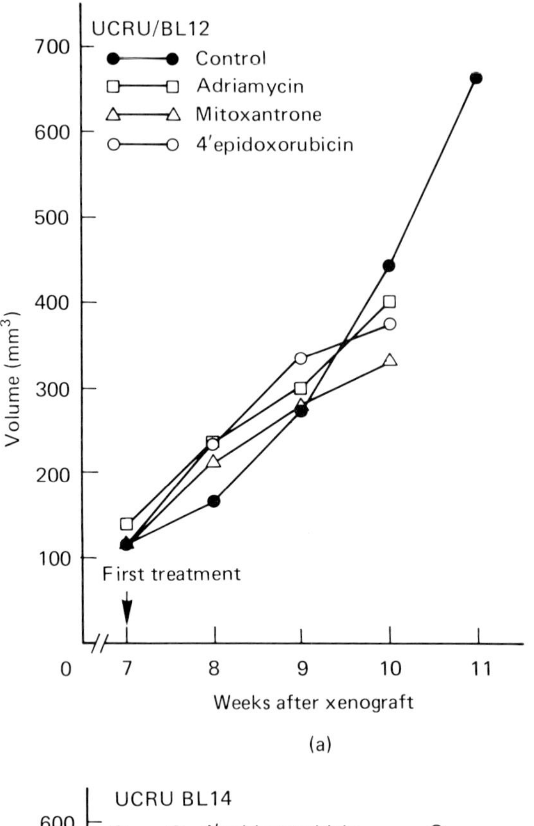

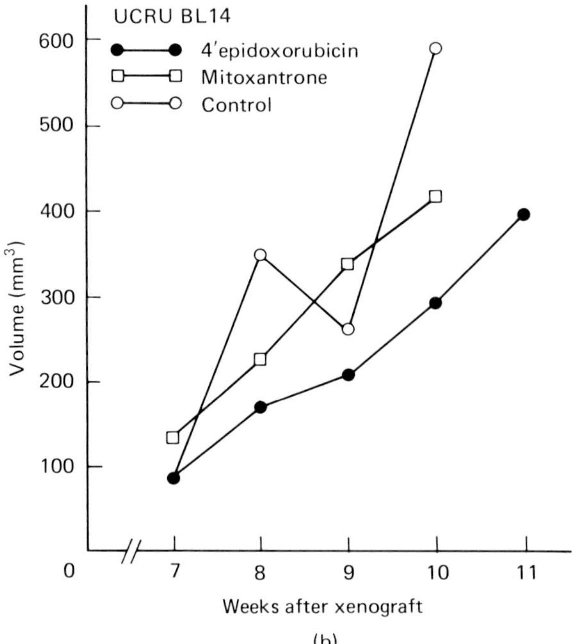

Fig. 1.5 Xenograft chemosensitivity testing of doxorubicin analogues. Note the common resistance to mitoxantrone and 4'-epidoxorubicin in two lines, UCRU-BL-12 and UCRU-BL-14

References

Alroy, J. (1979). Tight junctions adjacent to tumor stromal interface in human invasive transitional cell carcinomas. *Virchows Archives of Cell Pathology (B)* **30**: 289–96.

Alroy, J. and Gould, V.E. (1980). Epithelial–stromal interface in normal and neoplastic human bladder epithelium. *Ultrastructural Pathology* **1**: 201–10.

Alroy, J., Pauli, B.U., Hayden, J.E. and Gould, V.E. (1979). Intracytoplasmic lumina in bladder carcinomas. *Human Pathology* **10**: 549–55.

Alroy, J., Pauli, B.U. and Weinstein, R.S. (1981). Correlation between numbers of desmosomes and the aggressiveness of transitional cell carcinoma in human urinary bladder. *Cancer* **47**: 104–12.

Anthony, H.M. and Thomas, G.M. (1970). Tumors of the urinary bladder: an analysis of the occupation of 1030 patients in Leeds, England. *Journal of the National Cancer Institute* **45**: 879–95.

Armstrong, B. and Doll, R. (1974). Bladder cancer mortality in England and Wales in relation to cigarette smoking and saccharin consumption. *British Journal of Preventative and Social Medicine* **23**: 233–40.

Atkin, N.B. and Baker, M.C. (1985). Cytogenetic study of ten carcinomas of the bladder: involvement of chromosomes 1 and 11. *Cancer Genetics and Cytogenetics* **15**: 253–68.

Bailey, M.J., Jones, A.C., Shorthouse, A.J., Raghavan, D., Selby, P.J. and Peckham, M.J. (1984). Limitations of the human tumour xenograft system in individual patient drug sensitivity testing. *British Journal of Cancer* **50**: 721–4.

Barbacid, M. (1985). Oncogenes in human cancers and in chemically induced animal tumors. *Progress in Medical Virology* **32**: 86–100.

Bengtsson, U., Angervall, L., Eckman, H. and Lehmann, L. (1968). Transitional cell tumours of the renal pelvis in analgesic abusers. *Scandinavian Journal of Urology and Nephrology* **2**: 145–76.

Benham, F., Cottell, D.C., Franks, L.M. *et al.* (1977). Alkaline phosphatase activity in human bladder tumor cell lines. *Journal of Histochemistry and Cytochemistry* **25**: 266–74.

Bittard, M. (1984). Defining prognostic parameters for urothelial tumors of the bladder. *Progress in Clinical and Biological Research* **162A**: 161–76.

Bloom, E.T. (1978). Detection of antigens on transitional cell carcinomas with a xenogeneic antiserum. *National Cancer Institute Monographs* **49**: 57–8.

Bologna, M., Festuccia, C., Napolitano, T. and Angeletti, P.U. (1984). Dimethylsulphoxide stimulation of dome formation in cultured rat prostate epithelial cells. *The Prostate* **5**: 269–75.

Boorman, G.A., Burek, J.D. and Hollander, C.F. (1977). Animal model: spontaneous urothelial tumors in BN/BiRij rats. *American Journal of Pathology* **88**: 251–4.

Bouffieux, C.R.A. (1984). Epidemiology of bladder cancer. *Progress in Clinical and Biological Research* **162A**: 11–25.

Burk, K.H. and Drewinko, B. (1976). Cell cycle dependency of tumor antigens. *Cancer Research* **36**: 3535–8.

Burt, F.P., Pavone-Macaluso, M., Horn, J. and Kauffman, J.J. (1966). Heterotransplantation of bladder cancer in the hamster cheek pouch: *in vivo* testing of cancer chemotherapeutic agents. *Journal of Urology* **95**: 51–7.

Chodak, G.W. and Summerhayes, I. (1984). Detection of angiogenesis activity in malignant bladder tissue cells. *Journal of Urology* **132**: 1032–5.

Chomette, G., Tranbaloc, P., De Frejacques, C. and Avriol, M. (1984). Non-transitional cell malignant tumors of the bladder: aratomo-pathological study. *Progress in Clinical and Biological Research* **162A**: 75–80.

Christensen, B., Kieler, J., Vilien, M., Don, P., Wang, C.Y. and Wolf, H. (1984). A classification of human urothelial cells propagated *in vitro*. *Anticancer Research* **4**: 319–37.

Clemmeson, J. and Nielsen, A. (1956). Cancer incidence in Denmark, 1943–1953. II: Tumours of the urinary system and prostate. *Danish Medical Bulletin* **3**: 36.

Cohen, S.M., Yang, J.P.S., Jacobs, J.B., Arai, M., Fukushima, S. and Friedell, G.H. (1981). Transplantation and cell culture of rat urinary bladder carcinoma. *Investigative Urology* **19**: 136–41.

Cole, P. (1971). Coffee drinking and cancer of the lower urinary tract. *Lancet* **1**: 1335–7.

Cooper, G.M. (1982). Cellular transforming genes. *Science* **218**: 801–6.

Cowell, J.K. (1979). Chromosome changes associated with epithelial cell transformation with special reference to *in vitro* systems. In *Neoplastic Transformation in Differentiated Epithelial Cell Systems* in vitro, p. 259. Edited by Franks, L.M. and Wigle, C.G. Academic Press, New York.

Croft, W.A., Nelson, C.E. and Nilsson, T. (1979). Scanning electron microscopy of exfoliated malignant and non-malignant human urothelial cells. *Scandinavian Journal of Urology and Nephrology* **13**: 49–57.

Czerniak, B., Darzynkiewicz, Z., Staiano-Coico, L., Herz, F. and Koss, L.G. (1984). Expression of Ca antigen in relation to cell cycle in cultured human tumor cells. *Cancer Research* **44**: 4342–6.

Daly, J.J. (1976). Carcinoma-in-situ of the urothelium. *Urologic Clinics of North America* **3**: 87–105.

Dan, K., Andreasen, A., Grondahl-Hansen, J., Kristensen, P., Nielsen, L.S. and Skriver, L. (1985). Plasminogen activators, tissue, degradation and cancer. In *Advances in Cancer Research*, vol. 44, pp. 139–266. Edited by Klein, G. and Weinhouse, S. Academic Press, New York.

Davies, J.M. (1982). Occupational and environmental factors in bladder cancer. In *Scientific Foundations of Urology*, 2nd edn., pp. 723–7. Edited by Chisholm, G.D. and Innes Williams, D. Heinemann, London.

Davis, B.H., Ludwig, M.E., Sole, S.R. and Pastuszak, W.T. (1983). Small cell neuroendocrine carcinoma of the urinary bladder: report of three cases with ultrastructural analysis. *Ultrastructural Pathology* **4**: 197–204.

Der, C., Krontiris, T., Cooper, G. (1982). Transforming genes of human bladder and lung carcinoma cell lines are homologons to the *ras* genes of Harvey and Kirsten sarcoma viruses. *Proceedings of the National Academy of Science* (USA) **79**: 3637–40.

Devonec, M., Fontaniere, B., Blanc-Brunat, N., Muchada, E. and Dubernard, J.M. (1985). Simultaneous staining of nuclear DNA and blood group cell surface antigens on cells from bladder irrigation fluid. *Analytical and Quantitative Cytology* **7**: 69–71.

Dimmette, R.M., Sproat, H.F. and Sayegh, E.S. (1956). The classification of carcinoma of the urinary bladder associated with schistosomiosis and metaplasia. *Journal of Urology* **75**: 680.

Doll, R., Muir, C. and Waterhouse, J. (1970). *Cancer Incidence in Five Continents*, vol. 2. Springer Verlag, New York.

Donagala, W., Kahan, A.V. and Koss, L.G. (1979). The ultrastructure of surfaces of positively identified cells in the human urinary sediment: a correlative light and scanning electron microscopic study. *Acta Cytologica* **23**: 147–55.

Droller, M.J. (1976). Differences in adenylate cyclase activities in murine normal cells and bladder tumor cells in tissue culture. *Investigative Urology* **14**: 249–52.

Droller, M.J., Perlmann, P. and Schneider, M.U. (1979). Enhancement of natural and antibody-dependent lymphocyte cytotoxicity by drugs which inhibit prostagland in production by tumor target cells. *Cellular Immunology* **39**: 154–64.

Druckrey, H., Preussman, R., Ivankovic, S. and Schmidt, C.H. (1964). Selektive Erzeugung von Blasenkrebs an ratten durch Dibutyl- und N-Butyl-N-butanol (4) nitrosamin. *A. Krebsforsch* **66**: 280–90.

Duong, H.N., Jackson, A.G., Kovi, J., Ransome, J.R. and Jones, G.W. (1981). Mixed mesodermal tumor of urinary bladder: a light and electron microscopic study. *Urology* **17**: 377–82.

Dus, D., Radzikowski, C., Debray, H. *et al.* (1985). Lectin binding to non-malignant and malignant human uro-epithelial cells *in vitro*. In *Lectins*, vol. IV, pp. 65–74. Edited by Bog-Hansen, T.C. de Gruyter, Berlin, New York.

Elliott, A.Y., Bronson, D.L., Cervenka, J., Stein, N. and Fraley, E.E. (1977). Properties of cell lines established from transitional cell cancers of the human urinary tract. *Cancer Research* **37**: 1279–89.

Elliott, A.Y., Bronson, D.L., Stein, N. *et al.* (1976). *In vitro* cultivation of epithelial cells derived from tumors of the human urinary tract. *Cancer Research* **36**: 365–9.

Elliott, A.Y., Stein, N. and Fraley, E.E. (1974). *In vitro* neoplastic transformation of bovine embryonic urothelium by Simian vacuolating virus 40 (SV$_{40}$). *Investigative Urology* **11**: 411.

Erturk, E., Cohen, S.M., Price, J.M. *et al.* (1969). Pathogenesis, histology and transplantability of urinary bladder carcinomas induced in albino rats by oral administration of N-[4-(5-nitro-2-furyl)-2-thiazolyl] formamide. *Cancer Research* **29**: 2219–28.

Erturk, E., Price, J.M., Morris, J.E. *et al.* (1967). The production of carcinomas of the urinary bladder in rats by feeding N-[4-(5-nitro-2-furyl)-2-thiazolyl] formamide. *Cancer Research* **27**: 1996–2002.

Falor, W.H. and Ward, R.M. (1976). Cytogenetic analysis: a potential index for recurrence of early carcinoma of the bladder. *Journal of Urology* **115**: 49–52.

Falor, W.H. and Ward, R.M. (1978). Prognosis in early carcinoma of the bladder based on chromosomal analysis. *Journal of Urology* **119**: 44–8.

Farsund, T., Hoestmark, J.G. and Laerum, O.D. (1984). Relation between flow cytometric DNA distribution and pathology in human bladder cancer: a report of 69 cases. *Cancer* **54**: 1771–7.

Farsund, T., Laerum, O.D. and Hoestmark, J.H. (1983). Ploidy disturbance of normal appearing bladder mucosa in patients with urothelial cancer: relationship to morphology. *Journal of Urology* **130**: 1076–82.

Fearon, E.R., Feinberg, A.P., Hamilton, S.H. and Vogelstein, B. (1985). Loss of genes on the short arm of chromosome 11 in bladder cancer. *Nature* **318**: 377–80.

Feitz, W., Beck, H., Smeets, A. *et al.* (1985). Tissue specific markers in flow cytometry of urological cancers: cytokeratins in bladder carcinoma. *International Journal of Cancer* **36**: 349–56.

Fogh, J. and Giovanella, B.C. (eds). (1978). *The Nude Mouse in Experimental and Clinical Research*. Academic Press, New York.

Fokkens, W. (1979). Phenacetin abuse related to bladder cancer. *Experimental Research* **20**: 192–8.

Fradet, Y., Cordon-Cardo, C., Thomson, T. *et al.* (1984). Cell surface antigens of human bladder cancer defined by tumour monoclonal antibodies. *Proceedings of the National Academy of Science* (USA) **81**: 224–8.

Franks, L. (1983). Tissue culture and transplantation of bladder. In *The Pathology of Bladder Cancer*, vol. II, pp. 184–212. Edited by Bryan, G. and Cohen, S. CRC Press, Boca Raton.

Frankfurt, O.S. and Huben, R.P. (1984). Clinical applications of DNA flow cytometry for bladder tumors. *Urology* **33** (suppl.): 29–34.

Friedman, L., Richardson, H.L., Richardson, M.E. *et al.* (1972). Toxic response of rats to cyclamate in chow and semi-synthetic dyes. *Journal of the National Cancer Institute* **49**: 751–64.

Fulker, M.J., Cooper, E.H. and Tanaka, T. (1971). Proliferation and ultrastructure of papillary transitional cell carcinoma of the human bladder. *Cancer* **27**: 71–82.

Fulker, M.J., Adamthwaite, S.J. and Anderson, C.K. (1976). Stereological measurements of bladder tumour morphology. *European Journal of Cancer* **12**: 575–9.

Gibas, Z. and Sandberg, A.A. (1984). Chromosomal rearrangements in bladder cancer. *Urology* **33** (suppl.): 3–9.

Gibas, Z., Prout, G.R., Connolly, J.G., Pontes J.E. and Sandberg, A.A. (1984). Nonrandom chromosomal changes in transitional cell carcinoma of the bladder. *Cancer Research* **44**: 1257–64.

Gibas, Z., Prout, G.R., Pontes, J.E., Connolly, T.J. and Sandberg, A.A. (1986). A possible specific chromosome change in transitional cell carcinoma of the bladder. *Cancer Genetics and Cytogenetics* **19**: 229–38.

Goldenberg, D.M. and Pavia, R.A. (1981). Malignant potential of murine stromal cells after transplantation of human tumors into nude mice. *Science* **212**: 65–7.

Graham, F.L. and van der Eb, A.J. (1973). A new technique for the assay of infectivity of human adenovirus 5 DNA. *Virology* **52**: 456–7.

Green, A.R. and Wyte, J.A. (1985). Anti-oncogenes: a subset of regulatory genes involved in carcinogenesis? *Lancet* **2**: 475–7.

Grossman, H.B. (1983). Hybridoma antibodies reactive with human bladder carcinoma cell surface antigens. *Journal of Urology* **130**: 610.

Grossman, H.B., Wedemeyer, G. and Ren. L. (1984). UM-UC-1 and UM-UC-2: characterization of two new human transitional cell carcinoma lines. *Journal of Urology* **132**: 834–7.

Guerrero, I., Villasante, A., Corces, V., Deamond, L., Altman, R. and Pellicer, A. (1985). Activation of c-*ras* oncogenes is associated with tumor induction in experimental animals. *Progressive Medical Virology* **32**: 72–85.

Gustafson, H., Tribukait, B. and Esposti, P.L. (1982a). The prognostic value of DNA analysis in primary carcinoma-in-situ of the urinary bladder. *Scandinavian Journal of Urology and Nephrology* **16**: 141–6.

Gustafson, H., Tribukait, B. and Esposti, P.L. (1982b). DNA profile and tumour progression in patients with superficial bladder tumours. *Urology Research* **10**: 13–18.

Hand, P.H., Thor, A., Wunderlich, D., Muraro, R., Caruso, A. and Schlom, J. (1984). Monoclonal antibodies of predefined specificity detect activated *ras* gene expression in human mammary and colon carcinomas. *Proceedings of the National Academy of Science* (USA) **81**: 5227–31.

Harn, G.L., Haynes, L. and Chlapowski, F.J. (1980). Variations of adenosine 3′,5′ cyclic monophosphate levels in four chemically transformed rat transitional epithelial cell lines. *Journal of the National Cancer Institute* **65**: 657–62.

Hashimoto, Y. Kitagawa, H.S. (1974). *In vitro* neoplastic transformation of epithelial cells of rat urinary bladder by nitrosamines. *Nature* **252**: 497.

Hastings, R.J. and Franks, L.M. (1981). Chromosome pattern, growth in agar and tumorigenicity in nude mice of four human bladder carcinoma cell lines. *British Journal of Cancer* **27**: 15–21.

Hastings, R.J. and Franks, L.M. (1983). Cellular heterogeneity in a tissue culture cell line derived from a human bladder carcinoma. *British Journal of Cancer* **47**: 233–44.

Heckl, W., Konyar, H. and Grumine, F. (1984). Presence of transforming growth factors in human bladder cancer. *Proceedings of the European Society of Urology, Oncology and Endocrinology* (4th Congress).

Hedley, D.W., Friedlander, M.L., Taylor, I.W., Rugg, C.A. and Musgrove, E.A. (1983). Method for analysis of cellular DNA content of paraffin embedded pathological material using flow cytometry. *Journal of Histochemistry and Cytochemistry* **31**: 1333–5.

Hepburn, P. and Masters, J. (1983). The biological characteristics of continuous cell lines derived from human bladder. In *The Pathology of Bladder Cancer*, vol. II, pp. 214–27. Edited by Bryan, G. and Cohen, S. CRC Press, Boca Raton.

Herz, F., Barlebo, H. and Koss, L.G. (1974). Modulation of alkaline phosphatase activity in cell cultures derived from human urinary bladder carcinoma. *Cancer Research* **34**: 1943–6.

Holsti, L.R. and Armala, R. (1955). Papillary carcinoma of the bladder in mice obtained after per oral administration of tobacco bar. *Cancer* **8**: 679–82.

Hueper, W.C., Wiley, F.H. and Wofe, H.D. (1938). Experimental production of bladder tumours in dogs by administration of beta-naphthylamine. *Journal of Industrial Hygene and Toxicology* **20**: 46.

Huland, H., Otto, U. and Paleske, A. (1985). Chemotherapy and human bladder carcinoma transplanted into NMRI nu/nu mice. *Journal of Urology* **134**: 601–6.

Ito, N., Hiasa, Y., Tamai, A., Okajima, E. and Kitamura, H. (1969). Histogenesis of urinary bladder tumors induced by N-butyl-N-(4-hydroxybutyl)nitrosamine in rats. *Gann* **60**: 401–10.

Jensen, O.M., Wahrendorf, J., Knudsen, J.B. and Sovenson, B.L. (1986). The Copenhagen case-control study of bladder cancer. II: Effect of coffee and other beverages. *International Journal of Cancer* **37**: 651–7.

Jacobs, J.B., Cohen, S.M., Farrow, G.M. and Friedell, G.H. (1981). Scanning electron microscopic features of human urinary bladder cancer. *Cancer* **48**: 1399–1409.

Jao, W., Soto, J.M. and Gould, V.E. (1975). Squamous carcinoma of bladder with pseudosarcomatous stroma. *Arch Pathology* **99**: 461–6.

Kakizoe, T., Kawachi, T. and Sugimura, T. (1979). Agglutination of bladder cells by concanavalin-A during the early phase of treatment of rats with N-Butyl-N-(4-hydroxybutyl) nitrosamine. *Cancer Research* **39**: 3353–6.

Kaufmann, J.J., Kaneshiro, W. and Roux, F. (1969). Further studies on human bladder and kidney tumors transplanted to the hamster cheek pouch. *Journal of Urology* **101**: 559–66.

King, H. and Bailar, J.C. (1966). Epidemiology of urinary bladder cancer. *Journal of Chronic Disease* **19**: 735–72.

Kinjo, M., Oka, K., Naito, S., Konga, S., Tanaka, K., Oboshi, S., Hayata, Y. and Yasumoto, K. (1979). Thromboplastic and fibrinolytic activities of cultured human cancer cell lines. *British Journal of Cancer* **39**: 15–23.

Kjaergaard, J., Storklint, H., Bierring, F. and Thybo, E. (1977). Surface topography of the healthy and diseased transitional cell epithelium of the human urinary bladder. *International Journal of Urology* **32**: 34–48.

Klein, G. and Klein, E. (1985). Evolution of tumours and the impact of molecular oncology. *Nature* **315**: 190–5.

Koss, L.G. (1975). Tumors of the urinary bladder. In *Atlas of Tumor Pathology* Second Series, fascicle 11.

Koss, L.G. (1977). Some ultrastructural aspects of experimental and human carcinoma of the bladder. *Cancer Research* **37**: 2824–35.

Kovnat, A., Buick, R.N., Connolly, J.G., Jewett, M.A., Keresteci, A.G. and Tannock, I.F. (1984). Comparison of growth of human bladder cancer in tissue culture or as xenografts with clinical and pathological characteristics. *Cancer Research* **44**: 2530–33.

Kovnat, A., Armitage, M. and Tannock, I. (1982). Xenografts of human bladder cancer in immune-deprived mice. *Cancer Research* **42**: 3696–3703.

Krontiris, T.G. and Cooper, G.M. (1981). Transforming activity of human tumor DNAs. *Proceedings of the National Academy of Science* (USA) **78**: 1181–4.

Kumar, S., Costello, C.B., Glashan, R.W. and Bjorklund, B. (1981). The clinical significance of tissue polypeptide antigen (TPA) in the urine of bladder cancer patients. *British Journal of Urology* **53**: 578–81.

Kyriazis, A.P., Yagoda, A., Keriakes, J.G., Kyriazis, A.A. and Whitmore, J.F. (1983). Experimental studies on the radiation-modifying effect of *cis*-diaminedichloroplatinum-II (DDP) in human bladder transitional cell carcinomas grown in nude mice. *Cancer* **52**: 452–7.

Land, H., Parada, L.F. and Weinberg, R.A. (1983). Cellular oncogenes and multistep carcinogenesis. *Science* **222**: 771–8.

Lee, U.K., Harriott, T.G., Kuchroo, V.K., Halliday, W.J., Hellstrom, I. and Hellstrom, K.E. (1985). Monoclonal anti-idiotypic antibodies related to a murine oncofetal bladder tumor antigen induce specific cell mediated tumor immunity. *Proceedings of the National Academy of Science* (USA) **18**: 6286–90.

Leighton, J. and Tchao, R. (1984). The propagation of cancer, a process of tissue remodelling: studies in histophysiologic gradient culture. *Cancer Metastasis Reviews* **3**: 81–97.

Lin, C.W., Lin, J.C. and Prout, G.R. (1985). Establishment and characterization of four human bladder tumor cell lines and sublines with different degrees of malignancy. *Cancer Research* **45**: 5070–79.

McCredie, M., Stewart, J.H., Ford, J.M. and MacLennon, R.A. (1983). Phenacetin-containing analgesics and cancer of the bladder or renal pelvis in women. *British Journal of Urology* **55**: 220–24.

McGrath, J.P., Capon, D.J., Goeddel, D.V. and Levinson, A.S. (1984). Comparative biochemical properties of normal and activated human *ras* p21 protein. *Nature* **310**: 644–9.

Marshall, C.J. (1984). Functions of *ras* oncogenes. *Nature* **310**: 448.

Masuko, T., Yagita, H. and Hashimoto, Y. (1984). Monoclonal antibodies against cell surface antigens present on human urinary bladder cancer cells. *Journal of National Cancer Institute* **72**: 523–30.

Masuko, T., Abe, J., Yagita, H. and Hashimoto, Y. (1985). Human bladder cancer cell surface antigens recognised by murine monoclonal antibodies raised against T24 bladder cancer cells. *Gann* **76**: 386–94.

Matthews, P.N., Grant, A.G. and Hermon-Taylor, J. (1982). The growth of human bladder and kidney cancers as xenografts in nude mice and rats. *Urological Research* **10**: 293–9.

Melamed, M.R. (1984). Flow cytometry of the urinary bladder. *Urologic Clinics of North America* **11**: 599–608.

Moore, G.E., Morgan, R.T., Quinn, L.A. and Woods, L.K. (1978). A transitional cell carcinoma cell line. *In vitro* **14**: 301–6.

Moriyama, N., Yokoyara, M. and Niijima, T. (1984). A morphometric study on the ultrastructure of well-differentiated tumours and inflammatory mucosa of the human urinary bladder. *Virchows Archives A: Pathological Anatomy and Histopathology* **405**: 25–39.

Morrison, A.S. and Cole, P. (1976). Epidemiology of bladder cancer. *Urologic Clinics of North America* **3**: 13–29.

Mostofi, F.K. and Sesterhenn, I.A. (1984). Pathology of epithelial tumors and carcinoma-in-situ of bladder. *Progress in Clinical and Biological Research* **162A**: 55–74.

Murphy, W.M. (1983). Current topics in the pathology of bladder cancer. *Pathology Annual*, pp. 1–25.

Murphy, W.M., Vandevoorde, J.P., Taoe, M.K. and Soloway, M.S. (1977). The clinical value of urinary CEA-like substances in urothelial cancer. *Journal of Urology* **118**: 806–8.

Naito, S., Isakawa, A., Tanaka, K. *et al.* (1980a). Heterotransplantation of human urinary bladder cancers in nude mice. *Investigative Urology* **18**: 285–8.

Naito, S., Tanaka, K., Kanamori, T. *et al.* (1980b). Heterotransplantation of human upper urinary tract tumors in nude mice. *Investigative Urology* **17**: 522–5.

Nadakavukaren, K.K., Summerhayes, I.C., Salcedo, B.F., Rheinwald, J.G. and Chen, L.B. (1984). A monoclonal antibody recognizing a keratin filament protein in a subset of transitional and glandular epithelium. *Differentiation* **27**: 209–20.

Nayak, S.K., O'Toole, C. and Price, Z.H. (1977). A cell line from an anaplastic transitional cell carcinoma of human urinary bladder. *British Journal of Cancer* **35**: 142–51.

Neal, D.E., Marsh, C., Bennett, M.K. *et al.* (1985). Epidermal growth factor receptors—human bladder cancer: comparison of invasive and superficial tumours. *Lancet* **1**: 366–8.

Nelson, C.-E., Croft, W.A. and Nilsson, T. (1979). Surface characteristics of malignant human urinary bladder epithelium studied with scanning electron microscopy. *Scandinavian Journal of Urology and Nephrology* **13**: 31–42.

Newbold, R. (1984). Mutant *ras* proteins and cell transformation. *Nature* **310**: 628–9.

Newman, J. and Hicks, R.M. (1977). Detection of neoplastic and preneoplastic urothelia by combined scanning and transmission electron microscopy of urinary surface of human and rat bladders. *Histopathology* **1**: 125–135.

Noda, M., Selinger, Z., Scolnick, E.M. and Bassin, R.H. (1983). Flat revertands isolated from kirsten sarcoma virus transformed cells are resistant to the actions of specific oncogenes. *Proceedings of the National Academy of Science* (USA) **80**: 5602–6.

Okajima, E., Hiramatsu, T., Motomiya, Y., Iriya, K., Ijuin, M. and Ito, N. (1971). Effect of DL-tryptophan on tumorigenesis in the bladder and liver of rats treated with N-nitrosodibutylamine. *Gann* **62**: 163–9.

Okajima, E., Hiramatsu, T., Hirao, K. *et al.* (1981). Urinary bladder tumors induced by N-butyl-N-(4-hydroxybutyl) nitrosamine in dogs. *Cancer Research* **41**: 1958–66.

O'Toole, C.M., Nayak, S., Price, Z., Gilbert, W.H. and Waisman, J. (1976). A cell line (SCaBER) derived from squamous cell carcinoma of the urinary bladder. *International Journal of Cancer* **17**: 707–14.

O'Toole, C.M., Povey, S., Hepburn, P. and Franks, C.M. (1983). Identity of some human bladder cancer cell lines. *Nature* **301**: 429–30.

Parada, L., Tabin, C., Shih, C. and Weinberg, R. (1982). Human EJ bladder carcinoma oncogene is homologue of Harvey sarcoma virus *ras* gene. *Nature* **297**: 474–8.

Paulie, S., Hansson, Y., Lundblad, M.-L. and Perlmann, P. (1983). Lectins as probes for identification of tumor-associated antigens on urothelial and colonic carcinoma cell lines. *International Journal of Cancer* **31**: 297–303.

Polvsen, C.O. (1978). Status of chemotherapy, radiotherapy, endocrine therapy and immunotherapy studies of human cancer in the nude mouse. In *The Nude Mouse in Experimental and Clinical Research*, pp. 427–56. Edited by Fogh, J. and Giovanella, B.C. Academic Press, New York.

Pontes, J.E., Morrison, K., Pierce, J.M., Gibas, Z. and Sandberg, A.A. (1984). Characterisation of a transitional cell carcinoma lines arising from a previously irradiated tumor. *Journal of Urology* **132**: 606–8.

Pugh, R.C.B. (1973). The pathology of cancer of the bladder: an editorial overview. *Cancer* **32**: 1267–74.

Pugh, R.C.B. (1982). Urothelium: histopathology. In *Scientific Foundations of Urology*, 2nd edn, pp. 701–11. Edited by Chisholm, G.D. and Innes-Williams, D. Heinemann, London.

Raber, M.N., Barlogie, B. and Luna, M. (1984). Flow cytometric analysis of DNA content in post-mortem tissue. *Cancer* **53**: 1705–7.

Raghavan, D. (1983). The study of oncodevelopmental markers in hetero-transplanted tumors. In *Oncodevelopmental Markers: Biologic, Diagnostic and Monitoring Aspects*, pp. 109–29. Edited by Fishman, W.H. Academic Press, New York.

Raghavan, D., Gibbs, J., Nogueira Costa, R. *et al.* (1980). The interpretation of marker protein assays: a critical appraisal in clinical studies and a xenograft model. *British Journal of Cancer* **41** (Suppl. IV): 191–4.

Ramaekers, F., Beck, H., Vooijs, G.P. and Herman, C.F. (1984). Flow cytometric analysis of mixed cell populations using intermediate filament antibodies. *Experimental Cell Research* **153**: 249–53.

Ramaekers, F., Juysmans, A., Moesker, O., Schaart, G., Herman, C. and Vooijs, P. (1985). Cytokeratin expression during neoplastic progression of human transitional cell carcinomas as detected by a monoclonal and a polyclonal antibody. *Laboratory Investigation* **52**: 31–8.

Reid, L.M., Lear, I., Kwan, P.W.L., Russell, P. and Merk, F.B. (1984). Characterization of a human sex steroid-responsive transitional cell carcinoma maintained as a tumor line (R198) in athymic nude mice. *Cancer Research* **44**: 4560–73.

Reyes, C.V. and Soneru, I. (1985). Small cell carcinoma of the urinary bladder with hypercalcemia. *Cancer* **56**: 2530–33.

Rigby, C.C. and Franks, L.M. (1970). A human tissue culture cell line from a transitional cell tumour of the urinary bladder: growth, chromosome pattern and ultrastructure. *British Journal of Cancer* **24**: 746–54.

Rosen, S.W., Weintraub, D. and Aaronson, S.A. (1980). Nonrandom ectopic protein production by malignant cells: direct evidence *in vitro*. *Journal of Clinical Endocrinology and Metabolism* **50**: 834–41.

Rubben, H. and Lutzeyer, W. (1984). Lectins in diagnostics and therapy of bladder carcinoma: *in vitro* studies. *Proceedings of the European Society of Urology, Oncology and Endocrinology* (4th Congress).

Russell, P., Raghavan, D., Gregory, P. *et al.* (1986). Bladder cancer xenografts: a model of tumor cell heterogeneity. *Cancer Research* **46**: 2035–40.

Russell, P.J., Wills, E.J., Philips, J., Jelbart, M., Gregory, P. and Raghavan, D. (submitted). Outgrowth of adenocarcinoma from a xenografted transitional cell carcinoma: evidence of a common histogenesis?

Russell, P.J., Jelbart, M., Wills, E., Wass, J., Wotherspoon, J. and Raghavan, D. Establishment and characterization of a new human bladder cancer cell line showing features of squamous and glandular differentiation. *International Journal of Cancer*, in press (1988).

Rygaard, J. and Povlsen, C.O. (1969). Heterotransplantation of human malignant tumour to 'nude' mice. *Acta Pathologica Microbiologica Scandinavica* **77**: 758–61.

Sanford, E.J., Geder, L., Dagen, J.E., Laychock, A.M., Ladda, R. and Rohner, T.J. (1978). Establishment and characterization of a new human urinary bladder carcinoma cell line (PS-1). *Investigative Urology* **16**: 246–52.

Santos, E., Martin-Zanca, D., Reddy, E.P., Pierotti, M.A., Della Porta, G. and Barbacid, M. (1984). Malignant activation of a K-*ras* oncogene in lung carcinoma but not in normal tissue of the same patient. *Science* **223**: 661–4.

Santos, E., Truick, S.R., Aaronson, S.A., Pulciani, S. and Barbacid, M. (1982). T24 human bladder carcinoma oncogene is an activated form of the normal human homologue of BALB- and Harvey-USV transforming genes. *Nature* **298**: 343–7.

Schneider, M.U., Troye, M., Paulie, S. and Perlmann, P. (1980a). Membrane associated antigens on tumor cells from transitional cell carcinoma of the human urinary bladder. I: Immunological characterization by xenogeneic antisera. *International Journal of Cancer* **26**: 185–92.

Schneider, M.U., Troye, M., Paulie, S. and Perlmann, P. (1980b). Membrane associated antigens on tumor cells from transitional cell carcinoma of the human urinary bladder. II: Identification at the molecular level of plasma membrane associated antigens. *International Journal of Cancer* **26**: 193–202.

Seeburg, P.H., Colby, W.W., Capon, D.J., Goedell, D.V. and Levinson, A.D. (1984). Biological properties of human c-Ha-*ras* genes mutated at codon 12. *Nature* **312**: 71–5.

Sharkey, F.E. and Fogh, J. (1979). Metastasis of human tumors in athymic nude mice. *International Journal of Cancer* **24**: 733–8.

Shih, C., Shilo, B.Z., Goldfarb, M.P., Dannenberg, A. and Weinberg, R.A. (1979). Passage of phenotypes of chemically transformed cells via transfection of DNA and chromatin. *Proceedings of the National Academy of Science* (USA) **76**: 5714–18.

Silverman, D.T., Hoover, R.N., Mason, T.J. and Swanson, G.M. (1986). Motor exhaust related occupations and bladder cancer. *Cancer Research* **46**: 2113–6.

Smith, A.F. (1981). An ultrastructural and morphometric study of bladder tumours (I). *Virchows Archives A: Pathological Anatomy and Histopathology* **390**: 11–21.

Smith, A.F. (1982). An ultrastructural and morphometric study of bladder tumours (II). *Virchows Archives A: Pathological Anatomy and Histopathology* **396**: 291–300.

Smith, A.F. (1985). An ultrastructural and morphometric study of bladder tumours (III). *Virchows Archives A: Pathological Anatomy and Histopathology* **406**: 7–16.

Soloway, M.S. and Murphy, W.M. (1979). Experimental chemotherapy of bladder cancer: systemic and intravesical. *Seminars in Oncology* **6**: 166–83.

Soloway, M.S., deKernion, J.B., Rose, D. *et al.* (1973). Effect of chemotherapeutic agents on bladder cancer: a new animal model. *Surgical Forum* **13**: 542–4.

Spitz, S., Maguigan, W.H. and Dobringer, K. (1950). The carcinogenic action of benzidine. *Cancer* **3**: 789–804.

Starling, J.J., Greig, S.M., Beckett, M.L. *et al.* (1982). Monoclonal antibodies to human prostate and bladder tumor-associated antigens. *Cancer Research* **42**: 3084–9.

Steel, G.G. and Peckham, M.J. (1980). Human tumour xenografts: a critical appraisal. *British Journal of Cancer* **41** (Suppl. IV): 133–41.

Steel, G.G., Courtenay, V.D. and Rostom, A.Y. (1978). Improved immune-suppression techniques for the xenografting of human tumours. *British Journal of Cancer* **37**: 224–32.

Sufrin, G., McGarry, M.P., Sandberg, A.A. and Murphy, G.P. (1979). Hetero-transplantation of human transitional cell carcinoma in athymic mice. *Journal of Urology* **121**: 159–61.

Tachibana, M. (1982). Studies on cellular adhesiveness in five different culture cell lines derived from carcinoma of the urinary bladder. *Keio Journal of Medicine* **31**: 127–48.

Takayama, H. (1984). Distribution of concanavalin-A binding sites on normal human urinary bladder mucosa and bladder tumors by transmission and scanning electron microscopy and x-ray microanalysis. *Urology Research* **12**: 135–41.

Taniguchi, K., Karre, K. and Klein, G. (1985). Lung colonization and metastasis by disseminated B16 melanoma cells: H-2 associated control at the level of the host and the tumor cell. *International Journal of Cancer* **36**: 503–70.

Tannenbaum, M. (1979a). Ultrastructural pathology of the human urinary bladder. In *Diagnostic Electron Microscopy*, vol. 2, pp. 221–67. Edited by Trump, B.F. and Jones, R.T. John Wiley, Chichester.

Tannenbaum, M. (1979b). Lowes urinary tract. In *Electron Microscopy in Human Medicine*, vol. 19, pp. 193–224. Edited by Johannesson, J.V. McGraw-Hill, New York.

Tannock, I.F., Choo, B. and Buick, R. (1984). The radiation response of human bladder cancer assessed *in vitro* or as xenografts in immune-deprived mice. *International Journal of Radiation Oncology, Biology and Physics* **10**: 1897–902.

Tiltman, A.J. and Friedell, G.H. (1971). The histogenesis of experimental bladder cancer. *Investigative Urology* **9**: 218–26.

Toyoshima, K., Valentich, S.D., Tchao, R. and Leighton, J. (1976). Conditions of cultivation required for the formation of hemicysts *in vitro* by rat bladder carcinoma R-4409. *Cancer Research* **36**: 2800–6.

Trejdosiewicz, L.K., Southgate, J., Donald, J.A., Masters, J.R., Hepburn, P.J. and Hodges, G.M. (1985). Monoclonal antibodies to human urothelial cell lines and hybrids: production and characterisation. *Journal of Urology* **133**: 533–8.

Trejdosiewicz, L.K., Southgate, J., Hodges, J.M. and Goodman, S.L. (1985). Microheterogeneous expression of peanut agglutinin-binding sites in the extracellular matrix of cultured cells. *Experimental Cell Research* **156**: 153–63.

Tribukait, B., Gustafson, H. and Esposti, P.L. (1982). The significance of ploidy and proliferation in the clinical and biological evaluation of bladder tumours: a study of 100 untreated cases. *British Journal of Urology* **54**: 130–35.

Vilien, M., Holf, H. and Rasmussen, F. (1981). Immunological characterization of cell lines establishing from malignant and normal human arothelium. *European Journal of Cancer* **17**: 321–7.

Wahren, B., Nilsson, B. and Zimmerman, R. (1982). Urinary CEA for prediction of survival time and recurrence in bladder cancer. *Cancer* **50**: 139–45.

Welte, K., Platzar, E., Lu, L., Gabriloua, J.L., Levi, E., Mertelsmann, R. and Moore, M.A. (1985). Purification and biochemical characterization of human pluripotent haematopoietic colony-stimulating factor. *Proceedings of the National Academy of Science* (USA) **82**: 1526–30.

Wijkstrom, H., Granberg-Ohman, I. and Tribukait, B. (1984a). Chromosomal and DNA patterns in transitional cell bladder carcinoma: a comparative cytogenic and flow cytometric DNA study. *Cancer* **53**: 1718–23.

Wijkstrom, H., Gustafson, H. and Tribukait, B. (1984b). Deoxyribonucleic acid analysis in the evaluation of transitional cell carcinoma before cystectomy. *Journal of Urology* **132**: 894–8.

Williams, R.D. (1980). Human urologic cell lines. *Investigative Urology* **17**: 359–63.

Wynder, E.L. and Goldsmith, R. (1977). The epidemiology of bladder cancer: a second look. *Cancer* **40**: 1246–68.

Zimmerman, R. (1979). *Carcinoembryonic Antigen in Urothelial Carcinoma*. PhD Thesis, National Bacteriological Laboratory, Stockholm. pp. 1–51.

Zinzor, S.N., Svet-Moldavsky, G.J., Fogh, J., Mann, P.E., Arlin, Z., Iliescu, K. and Holland, J.F. (1985). Elaboration of granulocyte–macrophage colony-stimulating factor by human tumor cell lines and normal urothelium. *Experimental Hematology* **13**: 574–80.

2

Developments in the pathology of bladder cancer

Catherine Limas and Paul H. Lange

Introduction

In the last decade, pathological analysis has become more important in the management of bladder cancer. This is because, in addition to determining the stage and grade of biopsy specimens, pathologists have been obliged to develop expertise in urinary cytology since this analysis has become increasingly important in management. Perhaps equally important, pathologists concerned with bladder cancer have increasingly focussed on subcellular elements of the tumour, particularly on analysis of chromosomes and the so-called tumour markers (see also Chapter 1).

Strictly speaking, a tumour marker is any molecule which is characteristic of the cancer. Initially it was hoped that tumour markers would prove to be produced only by the tumour and secreted into body fluids where they could be detected easily. As more was learned about suspected markers, it became apparent that most of them are also present in normal tissues, so that their utility depends on quantitative rather than qualitative differences.

Moreover, tumour markers are heterogeneous; they may originate in the tumour, in which case they may be either appropriate or inappropriate for the tissue, or they may be produced by normal tissue in response to the tumour's presence. They may be specific to a group of tumours or be associated non-specifically with any malignancy. They may be secreted by the cell or be a structural part of the cell (e.g. of the membrane) and may or may not be 'shed' into body fluids. However, most markers do share one characteristic: nearly all are proteins. Major exceptions are DNA and RNA, which are important in the study of oncogenes or in flow cytometry analysis. Therefore, because proteins are immunogenic in xenogeneic species, and because antibody-based detection methods are often more sensitive and specific than are classical biochemical methods, immunological assays have become the mainstay of tumour marker measurement, and tumour markers are often classified as 'antigens'.

Many substances have been explored as markers in transitional cell carcinoma (TCC) (see Table 2.1). However, few have retained the attention of investigators and even fewer have become established as clinically useful. The subject of tumour markers in TCC has been reviewed by Lange and Limas (1984).

In this chapter we discuss certain aspects of the histological and cytological analysis of tissue from bladder cancer as well as some of the more currently

Table 2.1 Molecular markers in transitional cell carcinoma. Reproduced with permission from Lange and Limas (1984).

Type	Examples
Acute-phase proteins	C-reactive protein, immunoglobulin, transferin, alpha-2-macroglobulin, haptoglobin
Oncodevelopmental proteins	CEA
Others	Fibrin degradation products, rheumatoid factor, tryptophan metabolites, polyamines, beta-amino-isobutyrate, beta-glucuronidase, glycosaminoglycans, tissue polypeptide antigen, endothelial cell migration factor
DNA/RNA associated factors	DNA/RNA content (flow cytometry), cellular oncogenes, and products
Blood-group antigens	ABH, T
Antigens defined by cellular immune responses	Lymphocyte mediated cytotoxicity, NK activity, lymphocyte subtypes
Antigens defined by antibody immune responses	Xenogeneic: polyclonal, monoclonal Allogeneic: polyclonal, monoclonal

important tumour markers. Aspects covered include automated cytometric analysis of DNA, the blood-group antigens, and several newer antigens as revealed by monoclonal antibodies.

Classical pathological analysis

Recent progress in the histological analysis of bladder cancer stems from the following concepts, which have been formulated and popularized in the past three decades:

1. Urothelial 'neoplasia' or 'carcinoma' encompasses a spectrum of clinicopathological entities, each of which can be identified by its distinct morphological characteristics and clinical course. A large body of literature has amply confirmed the validity of this concept and its applicability in the diagnosis and treatment of urothelial neoplasia.

2. Urothelial neoplasms are the end-product of a widespread biological abnormality which affects the mucosa of the urinary tract. In other words, they represent manifestations of a 'field' phenomenon rather than an isolated, localized process.

The spectrum of urothelial neoplasia

It is now well recognized that the terms 'neoplasia' and 'carcinoma' cover too broad a spectrum to be used without further qualifications when making a diagnosis and assigning prognosis to individual patients. The process should be defined at least for the two most important and generally accepted parameters: stage and grade. The biopsy material must be obtained with these requirements in mind so that it contains the necessary constituents in a well-preserved state. To evaluate the depth of invasion, and thus determine the stage, it is necessary that the biopsy include 'deep' tissues subjacent to the visible tumour. Interpretation of nuclear details sufficient to assign the correct grade is possible only in tissues free of artifacts, which can be induced by coagulation, delayed or poor fixation. Thus the demand for detailed classification of neoplasia in biopsies has generated an equal requirement for technical skill in obtaining and processing the diagnostic material. The fundamental importance of the quality of the submitted material for histological diagnosis has not been adequately emphasized in the urological literature.

Currently, both the grade and the stage form the basis for assessing the prognosis and formulating follow-up and therapy in each case (see Chapter 4). Urologists are very familiar with the significance of staging (Prout, 1980), but some controversies still exist concerning the grading of urothelial neoplasia.

Grading is known to be helpful in distinguishing neoplasms with different clinical evolution (Bergkvist et al., 1965; Schroeder et al., 1973; Friedell et al., 1976a; Cummings, 1980), but its practical value for an individual case is reduced by a number of unresolved problems. First, there is no single, unifying system of grading. Instead, numerous systems exist, and often more than one for each organ or tissue. This tends to confuse the general pathologist. Second, the criteria for grading urothelial neoplasms are semi-quantitative, which leaves a lot of room for subjective judgement (Mostofi et al., 1973; Koss, 1975; Friedell et al., 1976a). A brief account of the grading system which we use for papillary urothelial tumours is given in Table 2.2 and the major characteristics of each grade are illustrated in Figs. 2.1–2.4. This system can be learned and applied with good reproducibility after intensive training and frequent exposure to pertinent material. It is not unusual to encounter papillary transitional cell neoplasms which display a mixture of features of more than one grade. This suggests that a morphological as well as biological evolution may occur. Indeed, long-term follow-up shows that patients presenting with non-invasive grade-II lesions may later develop grade-III cellular changes and eventually progress to invasive stages (Limas and Lange, 1982a).

In biopsy specimens, in addition to the grade, the presence of invasion in the lamina propria (subepithelial connective tissue), muscularis, and vessels can also be evaluated provided an adequate amount of material has been submitted. In general, grade-I lesions are almost never invasive at the time of their discovery. Approximately 15 per cent of these lesions evolve into higher grades, and between 5 and 10 per cent of patients with grade-I lesions eventually develop invasive tumours. However, grade-I lesions may coexist with higher-grade neoplasias elsewhere in the urinary tract. Therefore, in order to assign the correct prognosis, all lesions must be discovered and biopsied whenever possible.

Some classifications of bladder neoplasms distinguish between 'papillomas' and grade-I transitional cell carcinoma, the former being regarded as benign and the latter as of low-grade malignancy (Pugh, 1973; Friedell et al., 1976a). The main distinguishing feature is the number of cellular strata, which in 'papillomas' are less than seven (Koss, 1975). The clinical implications of such classification will be that following excision of a 'papilloma' the patient is not at risk and need not be followed, as in the case of low-grade

Table 2.2 Grading of papillary transitional cell carcinomas

	Grade 1	Grade 2	Grade 3*	Grade 4†
Architectural design	Retained stratification	Mildly disturbed stratification˙	Disturbed with loss of orderly stratification	Absent: no consistent cell arrangement
Surface differentiation	Retained	Partly retained with areas of decreased cohesiveness	For the most part absent with loss of cohesiveness	Absent
Nuclear cytoplastic ratio	Normal or mildly increased	Mildly or moderately increased	Clearly increased	Very variable; very high in most cells
Chromatin density	Normal	Variable; usually mildly or moderately increased	Increased	Very high
Nuclear pleomorphism	None	Mild to moderate in some fields	Obvious throughout	Marked
Mitoses	Very rare	Rare to few	Several	Frequent
Necrosis	None	None or only individual cell degeneration	Variable‡	Patchy to extensive

*Such TCCs are often invasive (about 75 per cent).
†Such TCCs are almost invariably invasive.
‡More extensive in the invasive component.

carcinoma. We believe that the distinction is often more confusing than helpful for patient management and that the number of lesions which could be clearly classified as 'papillomas' is too few to be of consequence in the overall problem of urothelial neoplasia. It may be preferable to avoid the term 'carcinoma' by referring to these papillary growths as grade-I transitional cell 'neoplasms'.

The term 'inverted papilloma' has been applied to a smooth-surfaced tumour which consists of sheets and ribbons of transitional epithelium growing beneath the normal urothelial lining of the bladder (see Fig. 2.5) (DeMeester *et al.*, 1975). Although as originally described this tumour appeared to have very well-defined gross and microscopic characteristics and an invariably benign course, recent reports have cast some doubt on its identification and differential diagnosis from low-grade transitional cell neoplasms. Our experience indicates that, unless very strict criteria are applied, this entity may become a source of misinterpretation and clinical mismanagement. For example, low-grade, superficially invasive tumours misinterpreted as 'inverted papillomas' were later found to have progressed into deep-muscle invasion. In case of doubt, an expert on urothelial neoplasia should be consulted and, if possible, an evaluation of the tissue

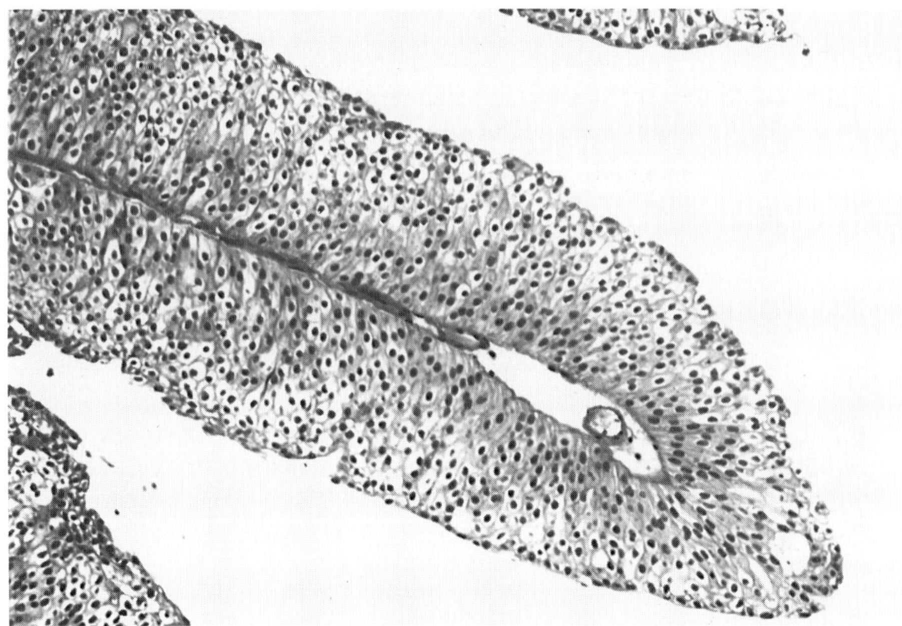

Fig. 2.1 Grade-I TCC, papillary non-invasive (Stage 0). The normal stratification, differentiation and cohesiveness of the transitional epithelium are preserved. The size and shape of the cells and the nuclei are uniform (×175)

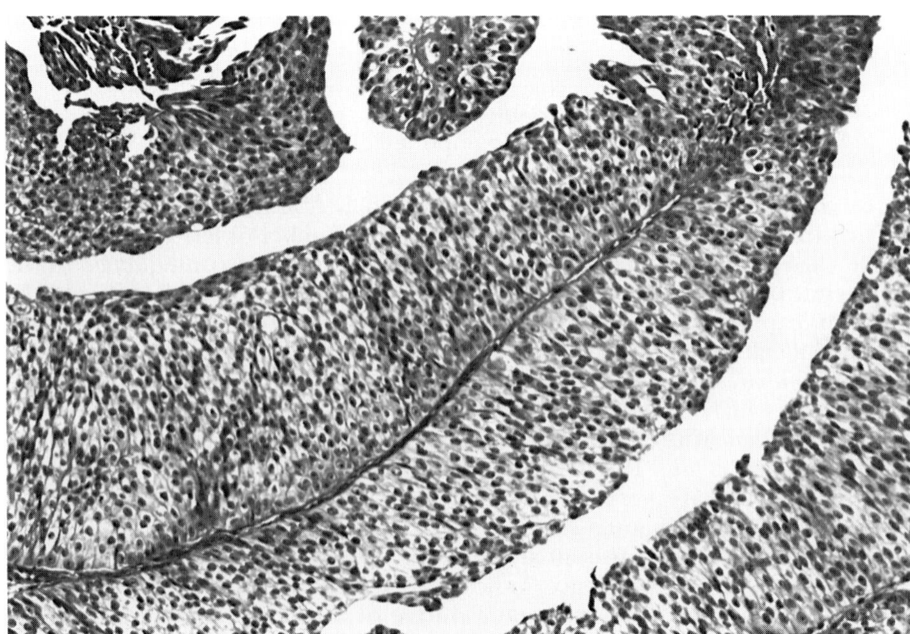

Fig. 2.2 Grade-II TCC, papillary non-invasive (Stage 0). Compared with Fig. 2.1, the orderly stratification of the cells appears disturbed with areas of crowding and irregular spacing of the nuclei. Also, compared with Fig. 2.1, many cells have an increased nuclear/cytoplasmic ratio (×175)

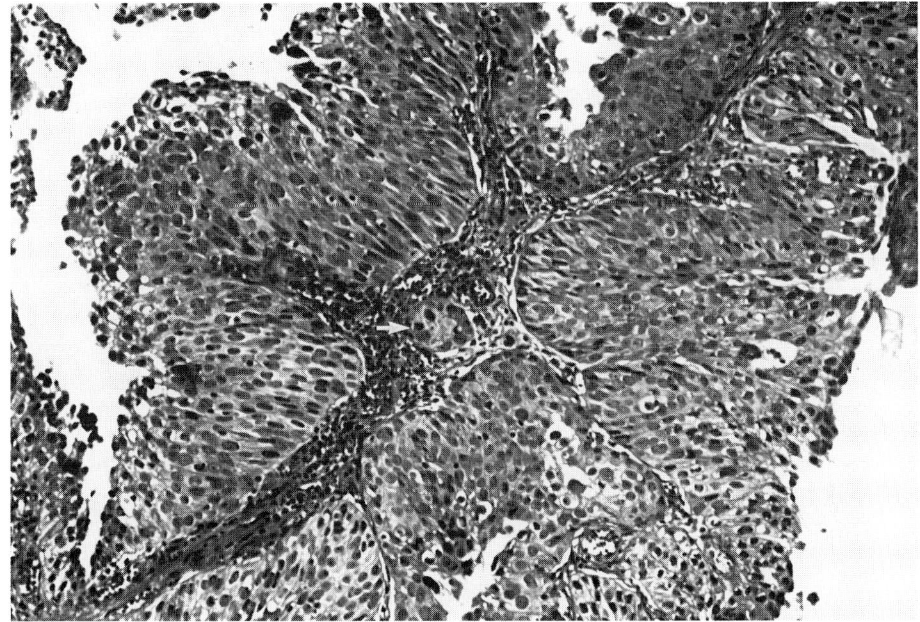

Fig. 2.3 Grade-III TCC, papillary with early invasion (Stage A). Compared with Figs. 2.1 and 2.2, there is a conspicuous absence of orderly stratification and poor differentiation of the surface epithelium, which also shows reduced cohesiveness. The nuclear/cytoplasmic ratio is markedly increased and the nuceli vary in size, shape and density (nuclear pleomorphism). The arrow points to a nest of malignant cells within the subepithelial tissue (×175)

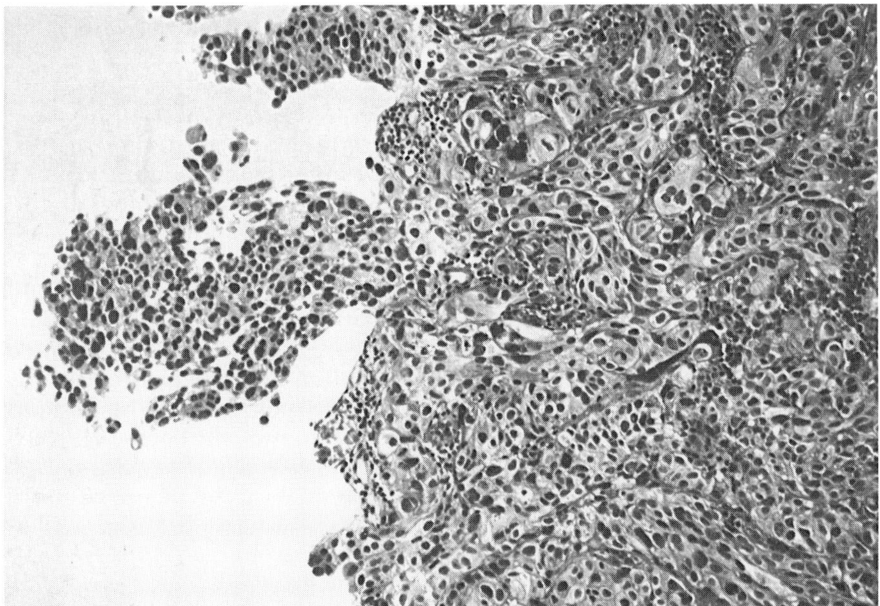

Fig. 2.4 Grade-III TCC, predominantly solid, invasive (Stage B). There is total absence of any orderly cell arrangement and of surface differentiation. The cellular cohesiveness is poor so that the cells of the superficial layers appear to fall apart. The nuclear pleomorphism is very obvious (×175)

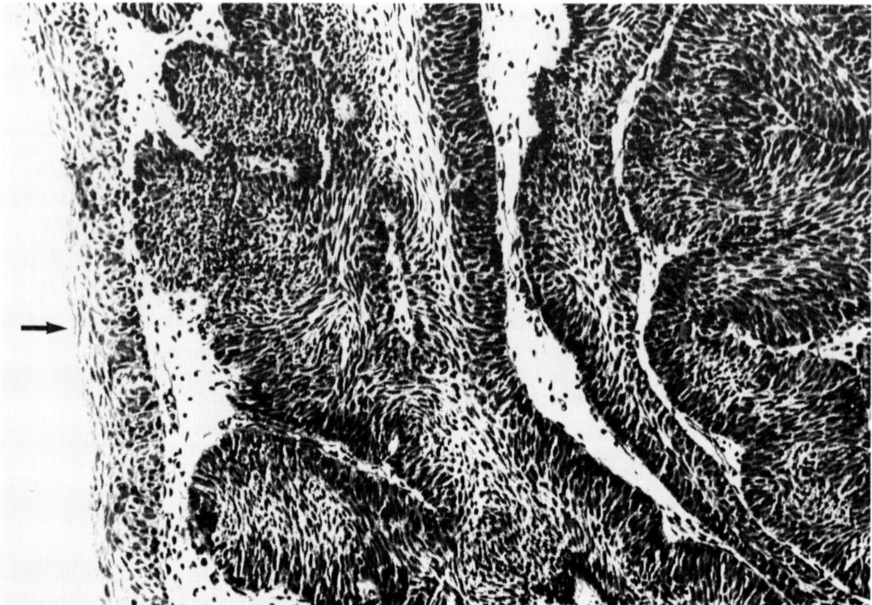

Fig. 2.5 Inverted papilloma of the bladder. This neoplasm consists of ribbon-like proliferations of the transitional epithelium beneath an intact normal surface epithelium (arrow). Note the characteristic nuclear 'palisading' at the periphery of the cellular sheets (×70)

blood-group antigen(s) may be helpful in this differential diagnosis (*vide infra*).

Approximately 80 per cent of grade-III tumours are associated with invasion at the time of diagnosis. Even if the presence of invasion has been excluded, these neoplasms have a poor prognosis and express their aggressive potential within 5 years (Bergkvist *et al.*, 1965; Koss, 1975; Friedell *et al.*, 1976a; Kern, 1984). Grade-IV neoplasms show no morphological differentiation and are almost invariably invasive, usually without associated papillary components.

Patients presenting with grade-II lesions have an unpredictable course. In about 50 per cent of the cases there will be progression to muscle invasion, but the time interval is extremely variable, as are the recurrences. As noted above, the progression to invasive stages is often accompanied or shortly preceded by an increase in grade. Roughly 50 per cent of the patients presently in non-invasive stages have grade-II tumours, the course of which is not predictable on the basis of morphological criteria. There are indications that grade-II lesions with aggressive potential can be identified using immunological tests (Limas *et al.*, 1979; Limas and Lange, 1982a) as well as chromosomal analysis (Summers *et al.*, 1983; Wijkstrom *et al.*, 1984; see also Chapter 1).

It is quite common to find areas of keratinization and/or gland formation in transitional cell neoplasms. This has been the cause of some confusion in the classification of bladder conditions with resultant significant variations in the reported incidence of squamous and adenocarcinomas of the urinary tract. Pure squamous carcinomas and adenocarcinomas account for a small fraction (1–7 per cent) of bladder tumours in Western countries (International Union Against Cancer, 1970; Thomas *et al.*, 1971; Pugh, 1973; Johnson *et al.*, 1976; Jacobo *et al.*, 1977; Alroy *et al.*, 1981).

Papillary neoplasms show all cytological gradations from nearly normal to overtly malignant. In contrast, solid transitional cell neoplasms are usually invasive and the overwhelming majority have overtly malignant cytology. The natural history of these solid tumours is still under study. At the present time, evidence suggests that some evolve from papillary lesions while others develop from flat carcinoma-in-situ without a preceding exophytic phase (Koss, 1979).

The concept of carcinoma-in-situ (CIS) of the urothelium was introduced three decades ago and is essentially the same as that known for other epithelia such as the uterine cervix, buccal mucosa and bronchus. The normal epithelium is replaced by epithelial cells which display malignant characteristics and which are distributed in a disorderly fashion from the deepest (basal) to the very top (superficial) layer. These cells do not penetrate beyond the basement membrane and, thus, have not expressed an ability to invade. Since invasion is the hallmark of malignancy in classical pathology, the use of the term 'carcinoma' to describe this process has been disputed, and the term 'intraepithelial neoplasia' has been proposed. Morphologically, the cells are recognized as malignant, and long-term observation as well as detailed studies of resected bladders strongly suggest that these cells may already have the potential for aggressive behaviour or are very prone to develop such potential. Because of their poor cohesiveness these cells shed easily, so that urine cytology is a reliable diagnostic tool for CIS (Melicow and Hollowell, 1952; Koss *et al.*, 1969; Barlebo *et al.*, 1972; Farrow *et al.*, 1977; Utz *et al.*, 1980; Murphy and Soloway, 1982a; Koss, 1982). CIS may be associated with synchronous invasive lesions. For this reason, once the diagnosis of CIS is made the patient must have his urinary tract re-evaluated and biopsies taken from suspicious lesions. About 50 per cent of patients presenting with CIS develop invasive neoplasms within a variable time interval, which ranges from months to more than 10 years (Koss *et al.*, 1969).

The concept of a 'field' phenomenon

Significant progress in our understanding and management of urothelial neoplasms was made with the recognition that, far from being the end-product of a localized process, carcinomas of the transitional epithelium may be the result of a widespread biological change which affects most if not the entire urothelium. Depending on still unknown factors, this widespread change may remain dormant or may be expressed as papillary tumours and/or flat CIS. It is possible for the various phases of the process to coexist. This was confirmed by the use of multiple biopsies from visible lesions as well as from apparently uninvolved bladder mucosa (Althausen *et al.*, 1976). Through the use of multiple random biopsies, a spectrum of mucosal changes classified as hyperplasias and atypias has come to our attention (Melicow, 1952; Cooper *et al.*, 1977; Soloway *et al.*, 1978). Hyperplasia is characterized by an increase in the number of cells which are often arranged in more than seven layers. Atypia is characterized by irregularities in the stratification as well as in the morphology of individual cells. The severity of atypia is graded into mild, moderate and severe.

Mild atypia can often be attributed to chemical, mechanical or inflammatory injury and is expected to regress following elimination of the irritating factors. Thus, in the presence of infection or calculi, the urothelium often shows mild atypia, which should be corrected with effective treatment. *Moderate* atypia may also be reactive but usually denotes a prolonged period of abnormal cellular environment and chronic injury interfering with normal growth. However, *severe* atypia exceeds the limits of a reactive process and should be viewed with suspicion unless an acceptable cause for its presence is found. Viral cytopathic effect, radiotherapy and some types of chemotherapy may cause severe urothelial atypias. If such an explanation cannot be found, the patient must be re-evaluated because of the frequent association of severe atypia with CIS or other neoplasias of the transitional epithelium. The presence of severe atypia in random biopsies from patients with non-invasive tumours increases the risk for recurrence and eventual invasion (Cooper *et al.*, 1973; Smith *et al.*, 1983).

Metaplasia, the phenomenon in which a fully differentiated but topographically inappropriate epithelium replaces the normal epithelium of an organ in part or in toto, has been involved in some misconceptions concerning bladder cancer. The cells lining the urinary tract normally differentiate into transitional epithelium but, depending on environmental conditions, these cells can differentiate into squamous or glandular, mucous-secreting (intestinal) epithelium. Both squamous or glandular metaplasia of the urothelium are benign processes which result as a reaction to an abnormal environment. This abnormal environment may also increase the risk for neoplasia and, therefore, carcinomas often coexist with metaplastic changes. However, metaplasia should not be regarded as 'premalignant', since there is no evidence that *per se* it predisposes to cancer. Ill-defined terminology such as 'premalignant', 'precancerous', and so forth, is best avoided altogether.

The clinical term 'leukoplakia' is also poorly defined with regard to its histological counterpart and its relationship to neoplasia. Squamous metaplasia with or without atypia or even superficial squamous cell carcinoma may clinically appear as 'leukoplakia'. For this reason, the clinical diagnosis of 'leukoplakia' is non-specific and of no prognostic significance unless further evaluated by histological examination (see Figs. 2.6 and 2.7) (Schabad, 1959; Widran *et al.*, 1974).

Urinary cytology

Although urinary cytology was first introduced in 1945 (Papanicolaou and Marshall, 1945), it did not achieve major clinical importance until the last decade, by which time the importance of CIS was generally appreciated. Another impediment to the clinical applicability of urinary cytology has been its relative lack of reliability. As is apparent from Table 2.2, urinary cytology would not be particularly helpful for the diagnosis of grade-I lesions, which have little tendency to shed cells or fragments of tissue that are distinguishable from normal or reactive epithelium. Grade-II lesions shed cellular

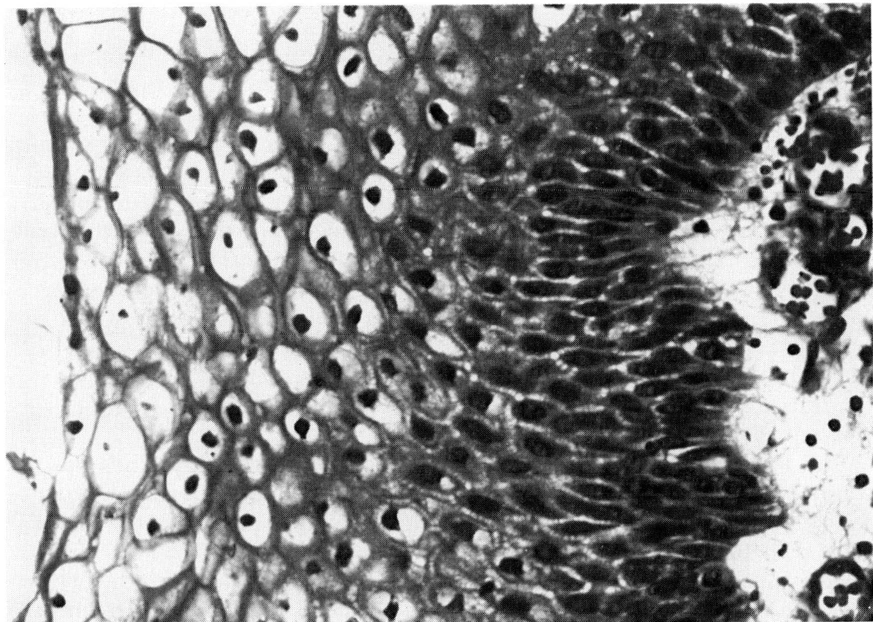

Fig. 2.6 Benign squamous metaplasia. Note the sharply demarcated cell borders, the very orderly cellular arrangement, maturation and low nuclear/cytoplasmic ratios of the squamous cells (×280). This is a reactive process which is expected to regress with appropriate treatment of the underlying disease

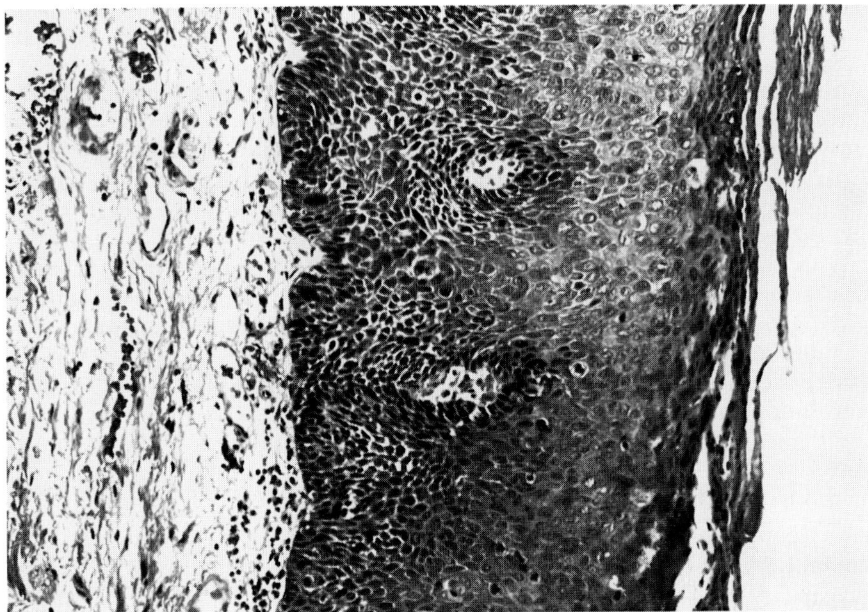

Fig. 2.7 Squamous metaplasia with severe atypia. There is obvious disturbance in the stratification and significant nuclear pleomorphism with frequent mitoses (×280). This lesion is often associated with squamous cell carcinoma of the bladder

clusters which are quite characteristic although they may lack the malignant features of individual cells. Grade-III and grade-IV neoplasms are characterized by poor cell-to-cell cohesiveness and, therefore, produce many dissociated individual cells as well as clusters with overtly malignant features. Thus the higher the grade, the greater the chances of producing positive cytologic findings in the urine. For example, low-grade tumours often have negative urinary cytology. In some series, only 3 per cent of low-grade papillary tumours showed cancer cells in the cytological smear, whereas more than 50 per cent of grade-II and a majority (80–90 per cent) of grade-III and grade-IV had positive findings (Esposti and Zajicek, 1972). The distinction between low-grade tumours and traumatic or inflammatory conditions may also lead to false-positive readings in as many as 15 per cent of samples (Geisse and Tweeddale, 1978).

The reliability of urinary cytology also depends on the methods used to obtain the specimen. The importance of good, standardized technique in the collection and preparation of the urine specimen cannot be overemphasized (Friedell *et al.*, 1976b; Loening *et al.*, 1978; Koss, 1975). For example, the second morning-voided specimen is superior to the first, which often contains cellular elements that have been shed during sleep and which have been exposed for a prolonged time period to the variable osmolarity and pH of the urine. Because some tumours shed more than others, the yield of positive cytologic specimens is enhanced when bladder washings, rather than voided specimens are obtained. With meticulous attention to detail, some centres have been able to increase the reliability of routine urinary cytology to a point where almost all grade-III and grade-IV tumours, and even 70 per cent of grade-II tumours, are detected (Murphy and Soloway, 1982b).

Also, any discrepancies between the cytology and the biopsy reports in the grading of urothelial tumours should be noted and the case re-evaluated. For example, if the biopsied lesion is grade-I or II but the cytology shows many overtly malignant cells, it is quite possible that the patient has both a low-grade tumour and diffuse carcinoma-in-situ (*vide infra*) or a high-grade process existent elsewhere in the urinary tract.

With the realization that most patients with potentially lethal bladder cancer have already progressed to the muscular invasive stage at the time of initial presentation (see Table 2.3), screening with urinary cytology has become an attractive idea for reducing bladder cancer mortality. To date, this approach does not seem practical because of the high cost and because conventional exfoliated urinary cytology, even with meticulous technique and expertise, will always suffer from a significant number of false negatives (Ellwein *et al.*, 1984). It is partially for this reason that computerized methods have been developed to assist in the diagnosis of malignant cells

Table 2.3 Onset of muscular invasive disease in relation to history

Series	Initially invasive	Prior bladder tumours
Kaye and Lange (1982)	139 (84%)	27 (16%)
Cutler *et al.* (1982)	84 (60%)	56 (40%)
Brawn (1982)	84 (81%)	20 (19%)
Hopkins *et al.* (1983)	82 (91%)	8 (9%)

from voided or aspirated urines. While such analysis has taken several different approaches, including computer-assisted recognition of cellular forms and patterns, the most popular method has been an analysis of cellular DNA content using automated flow cytometry.

Chromosomal analysis

Evidence that an analysis of chromosomes from transitional cell carcinoma can provide unique information has existed for a decade (Shigematsu, 1965), and to some extent this evidence has kept pace with advances in the technology of chromosomal analysis (see Chapter 1). Initially it was discovered that the modal chromosome number progressively increased with increasing stage. Thus, only 20 per cent of invasive tumours had a modal number, while more than 50 per cent of non-invasive tumours had a simple modal number (Falor, 1971). As banding techniques were developed, marker chromosomes in transitional cell carcinoma were observed and found to be an early indication of aggressive behaviour (Summers *et al.*, 1981). The combination of tetraploidy, markers, and invasion into the submucosa was a very strong indication that the patient would subsequently develop muscular invasive disease (Sandberg, 1984). Despite the prognostic power of chromosomal analysis, routine implementation is doubtful since this approach requires fresh tissue and special preparative techniques. Also, even in skilled hands, not all preparations can be properly analysed (Wijkstrom *et al.*, 1984).

Flow cytometry

In order to improve the results and efficiency of cytologic analysis, attempts have been made to analyse the individual cancer cell with sophisticated technology. While some investigators have used computerized image analysis to analyse anatomical patterns (Farsund *et al.*, 1983), the most popular technological application has been with automated flow cytometry (see Chapter 1). The simplest and most reliable of cellular alterations for analysis by flow cytometry is DNA content, because altered cancer cells have enlarged hyperchromatic nuclei from abnormally increased DNA content.

The usual method of flow cytometry DNA analysis involves specialized processing of bladder cell aspirates followed by cellular staining for DNA and RNA with the metachromatic fluorescent dye acridine orange. The properties of flow cytometry allow each cell to flow at high speeds through a blue laser light, which excites the acridine orange to fluorescent green when bound to DNA and red with RNA. Thus, RNA and DNA and nuclear size can be measured. Usually, 5000 cells per specimen are analysed, a process which takes less than one minute. Finally, using computer assistance the degree of aneuploidy (abnormal DNA content) can be measured and, using certain guidelines, the probability of the presence of cancer cells can be determined. Generally, RNA content is only useful for the diagnosis of papillomas, which are made up of cells with normal diploid DNA content and increased RNA (Melamed, 1984).

Many centres have now investigated the use of flow cytometry to analyse exfoliated cells from bladders. The exact statistics are still evolving and are outside the scope of this chapter. In general, DNA analysis by flow cytometry can detect 97 per cent of patients with CIS, 92 per cent with invasive disease, and 86 per cent with non-invasive papillary tumours. As with urinary cytology, low-grade papillary neoplasms are detected less well, with frequencies of approximately 30 per cent. False-positive results have averaged between 2 and 4 per cent. Several studies have shown flow cytometry to be (1) as good or better than urinary cytology in comparative studies, and (2) useful for follow-up studies in patients with CIS who are undergoing treatment with intravesical chemotherapeutic agents, including BCG (Melamed, 1984; deVere *et al.*, 1985). Because of the high cost of instrumentation and the fact that urinary aspirations are required, the superiority of flow cytometry to conventional urinary cytology and its generalized use in pathological laboratories or for screening studies needs to be determined. Nonetheless, because it is quantitative and because it requires no specialized pathological expertise, its future looks bright. For example, it now seems that paraffin-embedded material can be reliably analysed (Hedley *et al.*, 1983; Hofstadter *et al.*, 1986). Thus, more detailed applications of this technology to the nuances of bladder cancer behaviour will be possible. Perhaps the most important advantage of photocytometric applications, however, is that they can be used not only for DNA content but also for measuring changes in cell-surface antigens.

Blood-group antigen analysis

The development of morphological grading systems has improved our ability to differentiate between non-aggressive and aggressive urothelial neoplasia. There are, however, inherent weaknesses and limitations in these systems which are not likely to be overcome using conventional methods. A new approach which utilizes the antigenic abnormalities of neoplastic cells was suggested with the hope that such changes occur early in the process and are an indication of future cellular behaviour. In other words, instead of evaluating the shape or size of the nucleus, as is done in conventional grading, one tries to explore the antigenic make-up of the cells by testing for normally existing as well as aberrant antigenic determinants. For example, it was observed that the blood-group-associated antigens, A,B and H, which are normally detectable in the urothelium, were often undetectable in transitional cell neoplasms. Retrospective studies of patients who had been followed for 5 years or more showed that the detectability of the expected antigen in the initial diagnostic biopsy correlated with the clinical course (Decenzo *et al.*, 1975; Limas *et al.*, 1979; Richie *et al.*, 1980; Newman *et al.*, 1980). Transitional cell papillary tumours which preserve the expected antigen have a low probability (10–16 per cent) to evolve into high-stage lesions. When the expected antigen is reduced below a detectable level, the risk of an aggressive course is significantly increased, with between 62 and 66 per cent of the patients developing muscle invasion within the follow-up period. Testing the biopsy tissue for the blood-group-associated antigens may prove particularly helpful in patients who present with non-invasive grade-II neoplasms. These patients have very diverse outcomes despite the close morphological similarities of their tumours. By determining the A,B,H reactivity in the initial biopsy, it has been possible to identify those patients

with low-stage bladder tumours who subsequently develop invasive disease
(Limas *et al.*, 1979; Limas and Lange, 1982a; Lange and Limas, 1984).

In addition to the A,B,H antigens, the Lewis antigens have been detected
in normal and neoplastic urothelium (Limas and Lange, 1985). These
antigens are chemically and biosynthetically related to the A,B,H substances
and can be detected in tissues using a similar methodology. Most transitional
cell tumours in the non-invasive stages express the Lewis antigens even
when the expected A,B or H antigen is undetectable. Significant disturbance
in the expression of Lewis antigens was observed in grade-III transitional
cell carcinomas with poor prognosis.

While normally expressed antigens become undetectable, cryptic or
'masked' antigens may become spontaneously 'unmasked'. In particular, the
cryptic Thomsen–Friedenreich antigen, also referred to as T-antigen, has
been detected in bladder tumours. The spontaneous expression of the
T-antigen correlates with poor outcome and, together with the absence of
A,B,H antigen, can be used as a marker of existing or imminent invasion
(Coon *et al.*, 1982; Summers *et al.*, 1983; Lehman *et al.*, 1984). We found that
spontaneous unmasking of the T-antigen occurs in 60 per cent of invasive
tumours, in contrast to 10 per cent of non-invasive tumours (Limas and
Lange, 1986). It has been reported that the results of A,B,H and T-antigen
analysis may be refined still further by adding the results of karyotypic
analysis, specifically the finding of marker chromosomes or polyploidy. As in
previous studies, each test (ABH, T-antigen, chromosome) was more
accurate in predicting which patients would *not* have invasion than in
identifying those who would. The combination of T-antigen status and
modal chromosome number was accurate in 94 per cent of cases (Lange and
Limas, 1984).

The methodology for demonstrating A,B,H antigens in tissue sections
includes the red-cell adherence test (Figs. 2.8 and 2.9) and various immuno-
histochemical procedures. The antibodies used may be polyclonal or monoclonal and the tissues fresh-frozen or paraffin-processed. Each method has
advantages and disadvantages and there is also some variability in the results
(Limas and Lange, 1982b). We are currently analysing the results obtained
with monoclonal antibodies (Mabs) to the blood-group antigens, which
promise to increase the specificity of the reactions and permit accurate
localization of the reactive tissue components. We believe that currently the
methodology has not yet been standardized to the extent needed for its
routine introduction into the pathology laboratory.

Monoclonal antibodies

The development of hydridoma techniques has caused much excitement
because of the prospect of generating monoclonal antibodies not only to the
blood-group antigens, but also to other tumour-distinguishing antigens in a
variety of cancers (Moon *et al.*, 1985). Generally, the purposes of these
efforts are to reveal antigens which may be useful (1) for histochemical
analysis, cytologic analysis, or the development of serological markers; or (2)
for *in vivo* radio-immune detection; or (3) ultimately, for radio-immune or
chemo-immune therapy.

Efforts to produce Mabs preferential to transitional cell carcinoma are

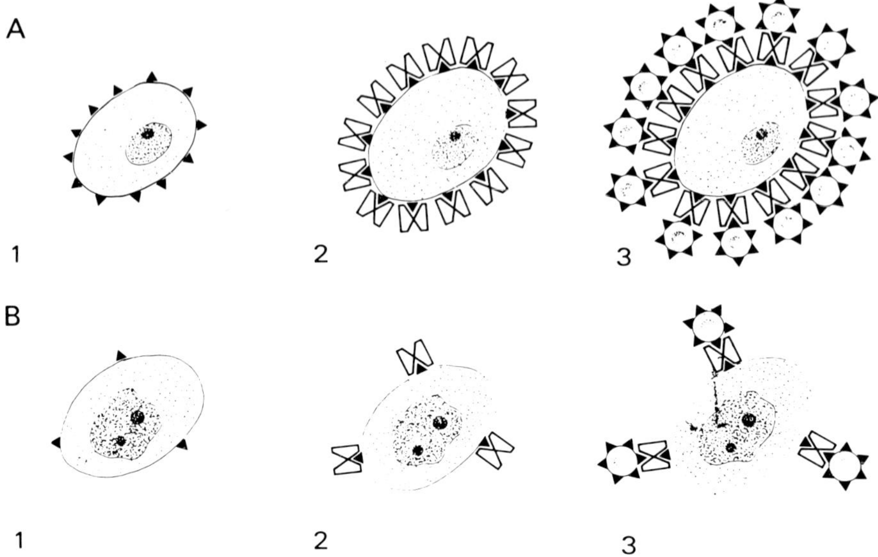

Fig. 2.8 Simplified representation of the red cell adherence test. (1) Cells in the tissue section or in suspension with (A) normal or (B) reduced surface sites for the expected blood-group antigen. (2) The sections are incubated with the antiserum and the specific antibody binds to the antigenic sites on the cell surface. (3) After washing away the unbound antibody the sections are incubated with a suspension of red blood cells of the corresponding blood group which carry the same antigenic sites as the tissue under testing. These red blood cells (RBCs) interact with the tissue-bound antibody and remain attached to the section against the force of gravity, thus acting as indicators of positive reactions

only beginning (see Chapter 1). One group of investigators immunized mice with bladder carcinoma cell lines or lysates of bladder papilloma and achieved a panel of Mabs which identified eleven distinct antigenic systems of assorted specificities. One of these, identified as OM5, is limited to a subset of bladder tumours (Fradet *et al.*, 1984). Masuko *et al.* (1984) also immunized mice with a transitional cell carcinoma cell line (K2-1) and generated several Mabs of interest. Chopin *et al.* (1985) developed Mabs to transitional cell carcinoma and compared Mab-based immunoperoxidase staining and conventional Papanicolaou staining of bladder washings from 75 patients with or without transitional cell carcinoma. They reported that the diagnostic value of Mab immunoperoxidase staining was similar to that of Papanicolaou staining in patients with high-grade transitional cell carcinoma, and that it provided some specific morphological criteria not possible by conventional cytology studies. It was recently reported that immunofluorescent staining of urine using transitional cell carcinoma-preferential Mabs is highly specific in identifying tumour cells in bladder washings and may improve tumour detection (Young *et al.*, 1985). Obviously, the ultimate diagnostic value of Mabs in transitional cell carcinoma will require further experience.

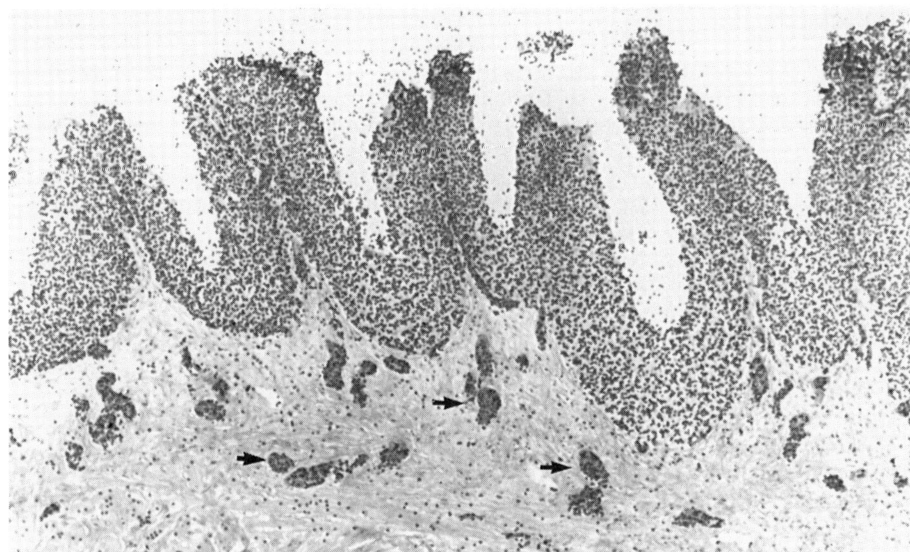

Fig. 2.9 Red-cell adherence test showing positive tissue reactivity for the blood-group antigen A in a case of benign papillomatosis of the bladder. The indicator RBCs are seen adhering to the transitional epithelium and to the blood vessels (arrows) (×70)

Conclusions

Over the last decade, the significant advances made in the pathological analysis of bladder cancer have substantially widened the scope of inquiry. In some respects, the knowledge already exists to predict successfully the outcome of and manage appropriately the patient with initially superficial transitional cell carcinoma. The next major challenge in this field today is to develop less expensive and more reliable methods for screening.

References

Alroy, J., Roganovic, D., Banner, B.F., Jacobs, J.B., Merk, F.B., Ucci, A.A., Kwan, P.W., Coon, J.S. and Miller, A.W. (1981). Primary adenocarcinomas of the human urinary bladder: histochemical, immunological and ultrastructural studies. *Virchows Archives A: Pathological Anatomy and Histopathology* **393**: 165–81.

Althausen, A.F., Prout, G.R. and Daly, J.J. (1976). Non-invasive papillary carcinoma of the bladder associated with carcinoma-in-situ. *Journal of Urology* **116**: 575–80.

Barlebo, H., Sorensen, B.L. and Ohlsen, A.S. (1972). Carcinoma-in-situ of the urinary bladder. *Scandinavian Journal of Urology and Nephrology* **6**: 213–18.

Bergkvist, A., Ljungqvist, A. and Moberger, G. (1965). Classification of bladder tumours based on the cellular pattern: preliminary report of a clinical–pathological study of 300 cases with a minimum follow-up of eight years. *Acta Chirurgica Scandinavica* **130**: 371–8.

Brawn, P.N. (1982). The origin of invasive carcinoma of the bladder. *Cancer* **50**: 515–19.

Chopin, D.K., deKernion, J.B., Rosenthal, D.L. and Fahey, J.L. (1985). Monoclonal antibodies against transitional cell carcinoma for detection of malignant urothelial cells in bladder washing. *Journal of Urology* **134**: 260–65.

Coon, J.S., Weinstein, R.S. and Summers, J.L. (1982). Blood group precursor T-antigen expression in human urinary bladder carcinoma. *American Journal of Clinical Pathology* **77**: 692–9.

Cooper, P.H., Waisman, J., Johnston, W.H. and Skinner, D.G. (1973). Severe atypia of transitional epithelium and carcinoma of the urinary bladder. *Cancer* **31**: 1055–60.

Cooper, T.P., Wheelis, R.F., Correa, R.J., Gibbons, R.P., Mason, J.R. and Cummings, K.B. (1977). Random mucosal biopsies in the evaluation of patients with carcinoma of the bladder. *Journal of Urology* **117**: 46–8.

Cummings, K.B. (1980). Carcinoma of the bladder: predictors. *Cancer* **45**: 1849–55.

Cutler, S.J., Heney, N.M. and Friedell, G.H. (1982). Longitudinal study of patients with bladder cancer: factors associated with disease recurrence and progression. In *Bladder Cancer*, vol. 1, pp. 35–46. Edited by Bonney, W.W. and Prout, G.R. (American Urological Association Monographs). Williams and Wilkins, Baltimore.

Decenzo, J.M., Howard, P. and Irish, C.E. (1975). Antigenic deletion and prognosis of patients with stage-A transitional cell bladder carcinoma. *Journal of Urology* **114**: 874–8.

DeMeester, L.J., Farrow, G.M. and Utz, D.C. (1975). Inverted papillomas of the urinary bladder. *Cancer* **36**: 505–13.

deVere White, R.W. and Cockburn, A.G. (1985). Predicting the invasive potential of bladder carcinoma. *World Journal of Urology* **3**: 73–5.

Ellwein, L.B., Farrow, G.M., Friedell, G.H. and Greenfield, R.E. (1984). An assessment of the impact of urine cytology screening using a computer-based model of bladder cancer. *Urologic Clinics of North America* **11**: 585–98.

Esposti, P.L. and Zajicek, J. (1972). Grading of transitional cell neoplasms of the urinary bladder from smears of bladder washings: a critical review of 326 tumours. *Acta Cytologica* **16**: 529–37.

Falor, W.H. (1971). Chromosomes in non-invasive papillary carcinoma of the bladder. *Journal of the American Medical Association* **216**: 791–4.

Farrow, G.M., Utz, D.C., Rife, C.C. and Green, L.F. (1977). Clinical observations on sixty-nine cases of *in situ* carcinoma of the urinary bladder. *Cancer Research* **37**: 2794–8.

Farsund, T., Laerum, O.D. and Hostmark, J. (1983). Polyploidy disturbance of normal-appearing bladder mucosa in patients with urothelial cancer: relationship to morphology. *Journal of Urology* **130**: 1076–82.

Fradet, Y., Cordon-Cardo, C., Thompson, T., Daly, M.E., Whitmore, W.F., Lloyd, K.O., Melamed, M.R. and Old, L.J. (1984). Cell surface antigens of human bladder cancer defined by mouse monoclonal antibodies. *Proceedings of the National Academy of Science* (USA) **81**: 224–8.

Friedell, G.H., Bell, J.R., Burney, S.W., Soto, E.A. and Tiltman, A.J. (1976a). Histopathology and classification of urinary bladder carcinoma. *Urologic Clinics of North America* **3**: 53–70.

Friedell, G.H., Soto, E.A. and Nagy, G.K. (1976b). Cytologic and histopathologic study of bladder cancer patients. *Urologic Clinics of North America* **3**: 71–8.

Geisse, L.J. and Tweeddale, D.N. (1978). Pre-clinical cytological diagnosis of bladder cancer. *Journal of Urology* **102**: 51–6.

Hedley, D.W., Friedlander, M.L., Taylor, I.W., Rugg, C.A. and Musgrove, E.A. (1983). Method for analysis of cellular DNA content of paraffin-embedded pathological material using flow cytometry. *J. Histochemistry and Cytochemistry* **31**: 1333–5.

Hofstadter, F., Delgado, R., Jakse, G. and Judmaier, W. (1986). Urothelial dysplasia and carcinoma-in-situ of the bladder. *Cancer* **57**: 356–61.

Hopkins, S.C., Ford, K.S. and Soloway, M.S. (1983). Invasive bladder cancer: support for screening. *Journal of Urology* **130**: 61–4.

International Union Against Cancer (1970). *Cancer Incidence in Five Continents: a Technical Report*, vol. 2. Edited by Doll, R., Payne, P. and Waterhouse, J. Springer-Verlag, Berlin.

Jacobo, E., Loening, S., Schmidt, J.D. and Culp, D.A. (1977). Primary adenocarcinoma of the bladder: a retrospective study of 20 patients. *Journal of Urology* **117**: 54–6.

Johnson, D.E., Schoenwald, M.B., Ayala, A.G. and Miller, L.S. (1976). Squamous cell carcinoma of the bladder. *Journal of Urology* **115**: 542–4.

Kaye, K.W. and Lange, P.H. (1982). Mode of presentation of invasive bladder cancer: reassessment of the problem. *Journal of Urology* **128**: 31–3.

Kern, W.H. (1984). The grade and pathologic stage of bladder cancer. *Cancer* **53**: 1185–9.

Koss, L.G., Melamed, M.R. and Kelly, E. (1969). Futher cytologic and histologic studies of bladder lesions in workers exposed to paraaminodiphenyl: progress report. *Journal of the National Cancer Institute* **43**: 233–43.

Koss, L.G. (1975). Tumors of the urinary bladder. In *Atlas of Tumor Pathology*, series 2, fasc. 11, pp. 13–46. Armed Forces Institute of Pathology, Washington, DC.

Koss, L.G. (1979). Mapping of the urinary bladder: its impact on the concepts of bladder cancer. *Human Pathology* **10**: 533–48.

Koss, L.G. (1982). Evaluation of patients with carcinoma-in-situ of the bladder. *Pathology Annual* **17**: 353–9.

Lange, P.H. and Limas, C. (1984). Molecular markers in the diagnosis and prognosis of bladder cancer. *Urology* **23** (Suppl.): 46–54.

Lehman, T.P., Cooper, H.S. and Mulholland, S.G. (1984). Peanut lectin binding sites in transitional cell carcinoma of the urinary bladder. *Cancer* **53**: 272–7.

Limas, C., Lange, P.H., Fraley, E.E. and Vessella, R.L. (1979). A,B,H antigens in transitional cell tumors of the urinary bladder: correlation with the clinical course. *Cancer* **44**: 2099–107.

Limas, C. and Lange, P.H. (1980). Altered reactivity for A,B,H antigens in transitional cell carcinomas of the urinary bladder: a study of the mechanisms involved. *Cancer* **46**: 1366–73.

Limas, C. and Lange, P.H. (1982a). Tissue blood-group-associated antigens in urothelial neoplasia: theory and clinical application. *World Urology Update Series*, vol. 1, lesson 10.

Limas, C. and Lange, P.H. (1982b). A,B,H, antigen detectability in normal and neoplastic urothelium: influence of methodologic factors. *Cancer* **49**: 2476–84.

Limas, C. and Lange, P.H. (1985). Lewis antigens in normal and neoplastic urothelium. *American Journal of Pathology* **121**: 176–83.

Limas, C. and Lange, P.H. (1986). T-antigen in normal and neoplastic urothelium. *Cancer* **58**: 1236–45.

Loening, S., Narayana, A., Yoder, L., Slymen, D., Weinstein, S., Penick, G. and Culp, D. (1978). Longitudinal study of bladder cancer with cytology and biopsy. *British Journal of Urology* **50**: 496–501.

Masuko, T., Yagita, H. and Hashimoto, Y. (1984). Monoclonal antibodies against cell surface antigens present on human urinary bladder cancer cells. *Journal of the National Cancer Institute* **72**: 523–30.

Melamed, M.R. (1984). Flow cytometry of the urinary bladder. *Urologic Clinics of North America* **11**: 599–608.

Melicow, M.M. (1952). Histological study of vesical urothelium intervening between gross neoplasms in total cystectomy. *Journal of Urology* **68**: 261–79.

Melicow, M.M. and Hollowell, J.W. (1952). Intra-urothelial cancer: carcinoma-in-situ, Bowen's disease of the urinary system: discussion of thirty cases. *Journal of Urology* **68**: 763–72.

Moon, T.D., Vessella, R.L. and Lange, P.H. (1983). Monoclonal antibodies in urology. *Journal of Urology* **130**: 584–92.

Mostofi, F.K., Sobin, L.H. and Torloni, H. (1973). Histological typing of urinary bladder tumours. In *WHO International Histological Classification of Tumours*, no. 10, pp. 9–35.

Murphy, W.M. and Soloway, M.S. (1982a). Developing carcinoma (dysplasia) of the urinary bladder. *Pathology Annual* **17**: 197–217.

Murphy, W.M. and Soloway, M.S. (1982b). Urothelial dysplasia. *Journal of Urology* **127**: 849–54.

Newman, A.J., Carlton, C.E. and Johnson, S. (1980). Cell surface A,B or O(H) blood group antigens as an indicator of malignant potential in stage A bladder carcinoma. *Journal of Urology* **124**: 27–9.

Papanicolaou, G.N. and Marshall, V.F. (1945). Urine sediment smears as a diagnostic procedure in cancers of the urinary tract. *Science* **101**: 519–21.

Prout, G.R. (1980). Classification and staging of bladder carcinomas. *Cancer* **45**: 1832–41.

Pugh, R.C.B. (1973). The pathology of cancer of the bladder. *Cancer* **32**: 1267–74.

Richie, J.P., Blute, R.D. and Waisman, J. (1980). Immunologic indicators of prognosis in bladder cancer: the importance of cell surface antigens. *Journal of Urology* **123**: 22–4.

Sandberg, A.A. (1984). Karyotypic findings in bladder carcinoma. In *Bladder Cancer*, pp. 45–59. Edited by Smith, P.H. and Prout, G.R. Butterworth International Medical Reviews, London.

Schabad, A.L. (1959). Is bladder leukoplakia to be regarded as precarcinomatous? *Zeitschrift fur Urologie* **52**: 520–25.

Schroeder, E., Christensen, T.B., Jacobsen, F. and Sjolin, K.E. (1973). Carcinoma of the urinary bladder. *Acta Chirurgica Scandinavica* **43** (Suppl.): 126–31.

Shigematsu, S. (1965). Significance of the chromosome in vesical cancer. In *XIII Congres de la Societe Internationale d'Urologie*, vol. 2, pp. 111–21. E. & S. Livingstone Ltd, Edinburgh.

Smith, G., Elton, R.A., Beynon, L.L., Newsam, J.E., Chisholm, G.D. and Hargreave, T.B. (1983). Prognostic significance of biopsy results of normal-looking mucosa in cases of superficial bladder cancer. *British Journal of Urology* **55**: 665–9.

Soloway, M.S., Murphy, W., Rao, M.K. and Cox, C. (1978). Serial multiple-site biopsies in patients with bladder cancer. *Journal of Urology* **120**: 56–9.

Summers, J.L., Falor, W.H. and Ward, R. (1981). A 10-year analysis of chromosomes in non-invasive papillary carcinoma of the bladder. *Journal of Urology* **125**: 177–8.

Summers, J.L., Coon, J.S., Ward, R.M., Falor, W.H., Miller, A.W. and Weinstein, R.S. (1983). Prognosis in carcinoma of the urinary bladder based upon tissue blood group ABH and Thomsen–Friedenreich antigen status and karyotype of the initial tumor. *Cancer Research* **43**: 934–9.

Thomas, D.G., Ward, A.M. and Williams, J.L. (1971). A study of 52 cases of adenocarcinoma of the bladder. *British Journal of Urology* **43**: 4–15.

Utz, D.C., Farrow, G.M., Rife, C.C., Segura, J.W. and Zincke, H. (1980). Carcinoma-in-situ of the bladder. *Cancer* **45**: 1842–8.

Widran, J., Sanchez, R. and Gruhn, J. (1974). Squamous metaplasia of the bladder: a study of 450 patients. *Journal of Urology* **112**: 479–82.

Wijkstrom, H., Granberg-Ohman, I. and Tribukait, B. (1984). Chromosomal and DNA patterns in transitional cell bladder carcinoma: a comparative cytogenetic and flow-cytofluorometric DNA study. *Cancer* **53**: 1718–23.

Young, D.A., Lin, C.W. and Prout, G.R. (1985). Detection of tumor cells in bladder washings by monoclonal antibody. *Journal of Urology* **133** (no. 4, part 2), p. 126A, abstract #50.

3

Laboratory assessment of new approaches to treatment: the human tumour cloning system*

Carlos L. Arteaga, Gary M. Clark and Daniel D. Von Hoff

Introduction

For many years, investigators have tried to develop an *in vitro* system that could accurately predict the cnemosensitivity of malignant tumours. Hamburger and Salmon (1977a,b) described a two-layer agar tissue culture system which supported the growth of a variety of tumours. A number of retrospective reports indicate that this human tumour cloning system (HTCS) can predict *in vivo* chemosensitivity with a 50–70 per cent accuracy (Salmon *et al.*, 1978; Von Hoff *et al.*, 1981; Bertelsen *et al.*, 1984). In this chapter we describe our experience using a human tumour cloning system for growth and chemosensitivity testing of transitional cell carcinoma of the bladder.

Growth of bladder cancer in soft agar

During the last six years, we have received a total of 185 specimens from patients with transitional cell carcinoma (TCC) of the bladder for culture in soft agar. The methodology for culturing these specimens has been extensively reviewed (Hamburger and Salmon, 1977; Von Hoff *et al.*, 1983). One hundred and seventy-five specimens were plated. Ten specimens were not plated owing to contamination or lack of an adequate number of cells. Of the 175 remaining specimens, 126 were primary lesions, 41 were from metastatic sites, and 8 were from unknown sites. Evaluable growth, defined by at least 30 colonies (aggregates of 50 or more cells) per 500 000 cells plated in each petri dish, was obtained in 59 tumours (34 per cent). Table 3.1 details the overall growth and its distribution according to the primary or metastatic origin of the tumour specimen. By chi-squared analysis, there are no statistically significant differences in the evaluable growth rate from primary tumours versus metastases ($p = 0.07$).

Table 3.1 also summarizes the specimens with evaluable growth according to site. The numbers are too small to establish any meaningful conclu-

* The work reported in this chapter was supported by the US Department of Health and Human Sciences, National Institute of Health (grant numbers CA 09434 and CA 27733), the American Cancer Society (grant number CH-162-D) and the American Cancer Society, Texas Division Fellowship Program.

Table 3.1 Evaluable growth statistics (at least 30 colonies per plate)

	Evaluable growth/attempted (numbers)	Evaluable growth (%)
By source		
All	59/175	34
Primary	47/126	37
Metastatic	9/41	22
Unknown	3/8	37
By site		
Bladder	45/119	38
Washings	1/7	17
Urine	0/7	0
Lymph nodes	3/11	27
Soft tissues	2/7	29
Liver	0/1	0
Ileum	0/1	0
Bone	1/3	33
Ascites	1/3	33
Pleural fluid	2/7	29
Previous exposure		
Prior therapy	14/30	47
No prior therapy	21/66	32

sion, but we should point out that none of seven urine samples with cytology positive for malignancy formed colonies in the soft agar assay.

Table 3.1 finally details the specimens with evaluable growth according to previous exposure to chemotherapeutic agents. There was no statistically significant difference between the growth achieved with specimens previously exposed versus those not exposed to chemotherapy ($p = 0.16$ by chi-squared analysis).

Drug sensitivity testing

Cell suspensions from the human tumours that formed at least 30 colonies per 500 000 cells plated in each petri dish were exposed either for one hour or continuously to different conventional and investigational agents at a clinically achievable concentration (one-tenth of peak plasma level in man). The use of this one-hour exposure is based on the finding that it appears to be more predictive of chemotherapeutic sensitivity in a murine bladder tumour model while continuous drug exposure overestimates drug sensitivity (Niell *et al.*, 1985). Overall, 59 of 175 specimens (34 per cent) were considered to have adequate growth for drug sensitivity testing. *In vitro* drug sensitivity was defined as not more than 50 per cent survival in tumour colony-forming units. This last criterion has been shown to have a 60 per cent true-positive and an 85 per cent true-negative rate for predicting for response or lack of response of an individual patient's tumour to a single agent tested in the HTCS (Von Hoff *et al.*, 1983).

Table 3.2 *In vitro* sensitivity of transitional cell carcinoma of the bladder to standard agents

Drug	Exposure (h)	Concen- tration (µg/ml	Number evaluable	Number with ≤50% colony survival
5-fluorouracil	1	6.0	7	0 (0%)
Adriamycin	1	0.04	29	6 (20%)
m-AMSA	1	10.0	1	0 (0%)
Carmustine	1	0.1	5	2 (40%)
Bleomycin	1	0.2	1	0 (0%)
Chlorambucil	1	0.2	2	0 (0%)
Cyclophosphamide	1	3.0	2	0 (0%)
Melphalan	1	0.1	2	0 (0%)
Mitomycin C	1	0.1	9	0 (0%)
Methotrexate	1	0.3	6	1 (16%)
Cisplatin	1	0.2	24	4 (16%)
Cisplatin	1	1.0	14	5 (35%)
Vinblastine	1	0.05	11	0 (0%)
Vinblastine	Continuous	0.05	4	2 (50%)
Etoposide	1	3.0	2	0 (0%)

Table 3.2 details the *in vitro* activity of standard agents against TCC of the bladder. We were not able to document any activity against TCC for mitomycin C (0/9) which is commonly used intravesically for locally recurrent disease or carcinoma-in-situ. Our results are in contrast to the work of others (Hashimura *et al.*, 1984; Zabbo *et al.*, 1984) who found *in vitro* activity for mitomycin C. However, they used continuous exposure and higher concentrations of mitomycin C. We have found *in vitro* activity against TCC of the bladder when testing vinblastine (continuous exposure) (50 per cent) and carmustine (40 per cent). Vinblastine has been used in patients in a single dose as part of the M-VAC regimen (methotrexate, vinblastine, doxorubicin, cisplatin) which, in a recent pilot study (Sternberg *et al.*, 1984), achieved a 72 per cent response rate in patients with advanced TCC of the bladder. Our *in vitro* experience, as well as the favourable results with continuous infusion of vinblastine, in other malignancies, when compared with bolus injection (Yap *et al.*, 1980), may provide some basis for further phase-II trials with vinblastine either as a continuous exposure or intravesically for patients with TCC of the bladder. We are not aware of any clinical trials with carmustine, but our results would suggest that a phase-II trial with this drug in transitional cell carcinoma of the bladder is indicated. The only agent in which there appeared to be a dose-response *in vitro* effect was cisplatin. This would suggest that higher doses of this agent could possibly achieve better therapeutic results.

There are few reports of large numbers of *in vitro* drug sensitivity tests in TCC of the bladder. Hashimura *et al.* (1982) found *in vitro* activity from cisplatin (15 per cent) and vincristine (17 per cent) using a continuous type of exposure and a drug concentration ten times higher than ours. Another report (Zabbo *et al.*, 1984) describes *in vitro* chemosensitivity of TCC of the

Table 3.3 *In vitro* and *in vivo* response (single-agent trials) of TCC of the bladder to chemotherapeutic agents

Drug	Concentration (µg/ml)	Response in vivo (%)	Response in vitro (%)
Cisplatin	0.2	30	16
Adriamycin	0.04	18	20
Vinblastine	0.05 (1 h)	13	0
Bisantrene	0.5	0	28
Mitoxantrone	0.05	0	0
Mitomycin C	0.1	19	0
Cyclophosphamide	3.0	7	0
5-fluorouracil	6.0	7	0
Methotrexate	0.3	29	16
Bleomycin	0.2	8	0

bladder to thiotepa (35 per cent) and doxorubicin (25 per cent), but the type of exposure and *in vitro* drug concentrations are not mentioned. Finally, Stanisic *et al.* (1981), using *in vitro* drug concentrations similar to ours, for one hour, describes chromosensitivity to cisplatin (17 per cent), doxorubicin (33 per cent), and mitomycin (17 per cent). Although the *in vitro* experience is somewhat small, it appears that the agents with *in vitro* activity against TCC of the bladder are the ones that have been effective in the *in vivo* trials. Table 3.3 correlates our *in vitro* experience with the *in vivo* data from single-agent trials in TCC of the bladder (Yagoda, 1983; Yagoda *et al.*, 1977; Blumenreich *et al.*, 1982; Panduro *et al.*, 1981; Early *et al.*, 1973; Ducheck *et al.*, 1980; Turner *et al.*, 1979; Van Oosterom *et al.*, 1984).

A number of investigational agents have also been tested *in vitro* (one-hour exposure time at one -tenth the clinically achievable peak plasma concentration) and the results are summarized in Table 3.4. Of these agents, Bisantrene, BW301 (a new antifole), methylglyoxal-bis guanylhydrazone (MGBG), and carbetimer, a new polymer in clinical trials, showed *in vitro* activity against TCC of the bladder. It appears reasonable that they should be examined in prospective clinical trials in patients with advanced disease who fail first-line chemotherapy.

In vitro/in vivo correlations

There are not enough data in the literature to support the use of this human tumour cloning assay to predict the response or resistance to chemotherapeutic agents in patients with TCC of the bladder. Stanisic *et al.* (1983) reported five positive *in vitro/in vivo* drug sensitivity correlations in patients with carcinoma-in-situ of the bladder and suggested that this assay may have potential usefulness in selecting agents for intravesical chemotherapy. In our experience, out of nine patients with metastatic bladder cancer, only two were treated with drugs tested in the assay. Neither patient responded (one patient was treated with Bisantrene and the second one with methotrexate) to the drugs to which their tumours showed *in vitro* resistance.

The principal limitation of the human tumour cloning system is limited

Table 3.4 *In vitro* sensitivity of TCC of the bladder to investigational agents

Drug	Concen-tration (µg/ml)	Number evaluable	Number with ⩽50% colony survival
MGBG	10.0	24	5 (20%)
Bisantrene	0.5	7	2 (28%)
Mitoxantrone	0.05	3	0 (0%)
Carbetimer	100.0	2	2 (100%)
Fludarabine	1.0	2	0 (0%)
BW301	0.5	1	1 (100%)
Trimetrexate	0.1	1	0 (0%)
Echinomycin	0.001	1	0 (0%)

growth *in vitro*. There is a need to improve the growth of these specimens. A number of new approaches are being tried. Our group has developed a cloning system (Von Hoff, 1984) in which tumour cells are suspended in soft agar in square 100 µl capillary tubes. The tubes are sealed with clay at each end and colonies are counted under an inverted microscope on day 14. Drug sensitivity testing can easily be accomplished using this system, the number of tumour cells needed per drug test being one-tenth of that needed with the conventional petri dish technique. We hope that this system will avoid the need for a large tumour cell sample and in this way extend its applicability in the treatment of recurrent TCC of bladder or carcinoma-in-situ. This test could be extensively useful in selecting intravesical chemotherapy. We also hope that it will improve the number of tumours that form colonies. Once this is accomplished, a prospective clinical trial using the capillary cloning system in TCC of the bladder would allow us to define its role in the selection of chemotherapy for patients with this disease.

Prediction of prognosis

The human tumour cloning system has provided some important prognostic information. Colony growth has been noticed in urine samples from patients with dysplasia of the urothelium or in patients with a history of TCC of the bladder who are presumably at risk for recurrence (Niell *et al.*, 1983; Stanisic *et al.*, 1981). In a recently published study, bladder washings from patients with recurrent TCC of the bladder showed a higher growth rate in a modified double-layer soft agar system when compared with washings from patients who remained tumour-free (Noronha *et al.*, 1985). All these data would suggest a possible predictive value of the human tumour cloning assay in identifying patients with a higher risk of recurrence.

Summary

Overall, in our experience, 34 per cent of transitional cell carcinoma of the bladder specimens will achieve evaluable growth using the conventional soft agar cloning assay. Clearly, efforts are required to improve the *in vitro* growth of bladder cancer. Based on *in vitro* drug sensitivity tests, there are several agents that probably merit a phase-II trial in patients with metastatic

TCC of the bladder that fail first-line chemotherapy. Those agents are vinblastine (continuous infusion), carmustine, and methyl-glyoxal-bis guanylhydrazone.

Until the growth rate of this tumour in the soft agar cloning assay is significantly improved, we cannot recommend it as part of the routine clinical care of patients with TCC of the bladder. However, this system can be used to follow the malignant potential of the urothelium in patients at risk of recurrence, as well as to screen new anti-neoplastic agents for activity against TCC of the bladder.

References

Bertelsen, C.A., Sondak, V.K., Mann, B.D. *et al.* (1984). Chemosensitivity testing of human solid tumors: a review of 1582 assays with 258 clinical correlations. *Cancer* **53**: 1240–5.

Blumenreich, M.S., Yagoda, A., Natale, R.B. *et al.* (1982). Phase II trial of vinblastine sulfate for metastatic urothelial tract tumors. *Cancer* **50**:435–8.

Ducheck, M., Edsmyr, F. and Naeslund, I. (1980). 5-Fluorouracil in the treatment of recurrent cancer of the urinary bladder. In *Bladder Tumors and Other Topics in Urology Oncology*, pp. 381–5. Edited by Pavone-Macaluso, M., Smith, P. and Edsmyr, F. Plenum Press, New York.

Early, K., Elias, E.G., Mittleman, A. *et al.* (1973). Mitomycin C in the treatment of metastatic transitional cell carcinoma of the bladder. *Cancer* **31**: 1150–3.

Hamburger, A.W. and Salmon, S.E. (1977a). Primary bioassay of human myeloma stem cells. *Journal of Clinical Investigation* **60**: 846–54.

Hamburger, A.W. and Salmon, S.E. (1977b). Primary bioassay of human tumor stem cells. *Science* **197**: 461–5.

Hashimura, T., Tanigawa, J., Okada, K. *et al.* (1984). Clonogenic assay for Urologic malignancies. *Gann* **75**: 724–8.

Niell, H.B. and Soloway, M.S. (1983). Use of the tumor colony assay in the evaluation of patients with bladder cancer. *British Journal of Urology* **55**: 271–4.

Niell, H.B., Soloway, M.S. and Wood, C.A. (1985). Effect of concentration and time of drug exposure on clonal growth of murine bladder cancer. *Urology* **25**: 267–72.

Noronha, R.F.X., Goodall, C.M., Beagley, K.W. *et al.* (1985). Correlation of human bladder tumor recurrence with changes in clonogenicity of urothelial cells. *Cancer* **56**: 1574–7.

Panduro, J., Hansen, M. and Hansen, H.H. (1981). Oral VP-16-213 in transitional cell carcinoma of the bladder: a phase II study. *Cancer Treatment Reports* **65**: 703–4.

Salmon, S.E., Hamburger, A.W., Soehnlen, B. *et al.* (1978). Quantitation of differential sensitivity of human tumor stem cells to anticancer drugs. *New England Journal of Medicine* **298**: 1321–7.

Stanisic, T.H., Buick, R.N., Trent, J.M. *et al.* (1981). An *in vitro* clonal assay for the bladder cancer: studies of the biologic potential of the urothelium and determination of *in vitro* sensitivity to cytotoxic agents. *Journal of Surgical Oncology* **18**: 67–72.

Stanisic, T.H., Owens, R. and Graham, A.R. (1983). Use of clonal assay in determination of urothelial drug sensitivity in carcinoma *in situ* of the bladder: clinical correlations in 5 patients. *Journal of Urology* **129**: 949–52.

Sternberg, C., Yagoda, A., Scher, H. *et al.* (1984). Methotrexate, vinblastine, adriamycin, and cisplatin for transitional cell carcinoma (TCC) of the urothelium. *Proceedings of the American Society of Clinical Oncology* **3**: 156.

Turner, A.G., Durrant, K.R. and Malpas, J.S. (1979). A trial of bleomycin vs. adriamycin in advanced carcinoma of the bladder. *British Journal of Urology* **51**: 121–4.

Von Hoff, D.D., Casper, J., Bradley, E. *et al.* (1981). Association between human tumor colony-forming assay results and response of an individual patient's tumor to chemotherapy. *American Journal of Medicine* **70**: 1027–32.

Von Hoff, D.D., Clark, G.M., Stogdill, B.J. *et al.* (1983). Prospective clinical trial of a human tumor cloning system. *Cancer Research* **43**: 1926–31.

Von Hoff, D.D. (1984). Plating efficiencies of human tumors in capillaries versus petri dishes. In *Human Tumor Cloning*, pp. 153–62. Edited by Salmon, S.E. and Trent, J.M. Grune and Stratton, New York.

Van Oosterom, A.T., Fossa, S.D., Bergerat, J.R. *et al.* (1984). Phase II studies with mitoxantrone in renal cell and bladder cancer. *Investigational New Drugs* **2**: 108.

Yagoda, A., Watson, R.C., Grabstald, H. *et al.* (1977). Adriamycin and cyclophosphamide in advanced bladder cancer. *Cancer Treatment Reports* **61**: 97–9.

Yagoda, A. (1983). Chemotherapy for advanced urothelial cancer. *Seminars in Urology* **1**: 60–74.

Yap, H.Y., Blumenschein, G.R., Keating, M.J. *et al.* (1980). Vinblastine given a continuous five-day infusion in the treatment of refractory advanced breast cancer. *Cancer Treatment Reports* **64**: 279–83.

Zabbo, A., Monte, J.E., Budd, G.T. *et al.* (1984). Initial observations and problems with *in vitro* predictive assay in genitourinary malignancies. *Urology* **23**: 370–3.

4

Diagnosis and management of primary bladder cancer: a British perspective

W.F. Hendry

Introduction

The recognition that bladder tumours often occur as part of a widespread neoplastic change in the urothelium as a whole (Melicow, 1945) coincided with increasing interest in the possible existence of chemical carcinogens in the urine. Careful epidemiological and biochemical studies led to the definition of significant industrial hazards which had been suspected as a cause of bladder cancer for over half a century, and as a result the most potent carcinogens were identified and banned (Case *et al.*, 1954). At the same time the urologist began to think of bladder cancer as part of a generalized urothelial disease, and this led to a policy of long-term surveillance of the whole urinary tract in all patients who developed a transitional cell tumour irrespective of the exact primary site.

Most superficial urothelial tumours can be eliminated by local therapy, and yet many recur a year or two later; more deeply invasive tumours require radiotherapy and/or radical surgery, and in these cases the long-term results of treatment are often disappointing. The successful control or eradication of this disease is entirely dependent on the correct assessment of its extent and malignant potential when the patient first presents. Failure to define the nature of the tumour and to predict its probable future behaviour at an early stage may allow the opportunity of curing the disease to be missed. In other cases failure to adhere to a strict follow-up regimen may give recurrent disease time to spread so extensively that local therapy can no longer control it. Knowledge of the natural history of urothelial cancers, including the sites, patterns of growth and methods of spread will enable the clinician to determine the most appropriate treatment regime for a particular patient (see Chapters 1 and 2).

Distribution of the disease

Tumours of the renal pelvis

One case of carcinoma of the renal pelvis can be expected for every 64 cases of carcinoma of the bladder (Williams and Mitchell, 1973a). Coexisting tumours may be present in the ipsilateral ureter in as many as 15 per cent of cases (Newman *et al.*, 1967); this incidence rises to 33 per cent in a small ureteric stump after incomplete nephroureterectomy and 56 per cent in a longer segment left after simple nephrectomy (Kinder and Wallace, 1962). About 10 per cent of cases have coexisting bladder tumours and up to 50 per cent can be expected to develop bladder tumours later after an average interval of 15 months. Bladder recurrence is about twice as common if the nephroureterectomy is incomplete (Williams and Mitchell, 1973a). By contrast tumours of the opposite renal pelvis and ureter are relatively uncommon (Talavera *et al.*, 1970). Multiple tumours occur most commonly, though not exclusively, when the lesion in the renal pelvis is of the papillary type.

Tumours of the renal pelvis are discussed further in Chapter 16.

Ureteric tumours

One ureteric tumour can be expected for every 51 cases of bladder cancer. These may present *de novo* as carcinomas of ureter, or they may occur in patients with pre-existing bladder tumours (Williams and Mitchell, 1973b). Scott and McDonald (1970) reviewed the literature on ureteric tumours and found that bladder tumours were associated previously in 13.7 per cent, simultaneously in 11 per cent, and subsequently in 14 per cent of reported cases. The lower third of the ureter was the most common site, with the middle third and upper third affected much less often. In a few cases the tumours were multiple within the ureter and bilateral tumours were rare. Babaian and Johnson (1980) reviewed 44 patients with ureteric tumours treated between 1951 and 1977. The distal ureter was affected in 73 per cent and one-fifth had multiple lesions. Seven had a history of, and four had concomitant, bladder tumours. Two developed asynchronous contralateral urothelial tumours. Thirteen subsequently developed bladder tumours, after a median time of 10 months.

Bladder tumours

About 80 per cent of bladder tumours are papillary, and after adequate treatment about half of the affected patients never develop a recurrence; the other half continue to form more tumours either singly or in progressively increasing numbers. The recurrences 'breed true' usually for a substantial time with the same histological features as the original tumour, although eventually a new tumour of greater malignancy may develop (Melicow, 1974). Most invasive tumours present as solid infiltrating growths, and only 10–15 per cent have a previous history of papillary superficial tumours (Hopkins *et al.*, 1983; Kaye and Lange, 1982).

Bladder tumours most commonly occur on the posterior and lateral walls, especially near the ureteric orifices, and are much less common on the bladder neck, dome and anterior walls on first presentation (Melicow, 1974). However, papillary non-invasive tumours commonly recur in these areas, especially near the air bubble, suggesting possible implantation after initial treatment (Page *et al.*, 1978).

Urethral tumours

These occur in association with about 4 per cent of bladder tumours (Ashworth, 1956), although a much higher microscopical incidence (18 per cent) of multifocal *in situ* carcinomatous change has been observed in patients dying of bladder cancer (Gowing, 1960).

Patterns of local tumour growth

There are four main factors which affect the rate and pattern of tumour growth: cell type, grade of malignancy, growth pattern and depth of infiltration. All of these factors are interrelated to some extent, and all have an influence on the patients' prognosis (see Chapters 1 and 2).

The cell type which normally forms the urothelium is transitional, but these cells are capable of undergoing metaplasia into squamous or glandular epithelium. The vast majority of tumours are transitional cell in origin (Miller *et al.*, 1969).

The grade of malignancy is based on the degree of anaplasia of the tumour (WHO, 1973). The term 'papilloma' is strictly reserved for the rare benign papillary tumour which has epithelium indistinguishable from normal. Three grades of malignancy are recognized: Grade I applies to tumours that have the least degree of cellular anaplasia compatible with a diagnosis of malignancy, and this corresponds to 'well-differentiated' or 'low-grade' tumours. Grade III applies to tumours with the most severe degree of cellular anaplasia, which may no longer be clearly recognizable as of transitional cell origin: this corresponds to 'poorly differentiated' or 'high-grade' tumours. Grade II lies in between and corresponds to 'moderately well-differentiated' tumours.

The growth pattern may be papillary, infiltrating, papillary and infiltrating, or non-papillary and non-infiltrating (carcinoma-in-situ) (WHO, 1973). There is a correlation between the grade of malignancy and the pattern of growth: most differentiated tumours are papillary, non-infiltrating, and have a relatively good prognosis, whereas most anaplastic tumours are infiltrating and have a poorer prognosis. An intermediate group of 'papillary and infiltrating' tumours exists in which the prognosis abruptly worsens in comparison with the non-infiltrating tumours. Carcinoma-in-situ is the term employed for lesions in which there is definite anaplasia of surface epithelium without formation of papillary structures and without infiltration: this lesion constitutes about 3 per cent of cases of bladder tumours.

Depth of infiltration can be determined pathologically from a deep biopsy specimen taken with a resectoscope and correctly orientated and cut by the pathologist. This information is of fundamental importance to the urologist in assessment of infiltration in early cases of bladder tumours; in more advanced cases, it can only indicate a minimum depth of invasion if bladder perforation during resection is to be avoided.

Distant spread of tumours

In 50 per cent of cases in which the tumour has infiltrated superficial muscle, and in all cases with infiltration of deep muscle, malignant cells may be found within lymphatics in the wall of the bladder at a considerable distance from the primary tumour (Baker, 1968). Local lymph nodes are involved in 40 per cent of patients once bladder muscle is invaded (Kerr and Colby, 1951); and once the tumour has reached the perivesical fat, the disease can be expected to have spread to the lymph nodes or beyond in 84 per cent of cases (Jewett and Strong, 1946).

Blood spread of urothelial cancer is usually a late event, and while it is generally associated with invasive anaplastic lesions, it may also occur in some patients with well-differentiated tumours. The most common sites affected are lungs, liver, vertebrae and pelvic bones (Melicow, 1974). Blood-borne dissemination is not uncommonly seen with infiltrating tumours of the anterior urethra in males, where only a delicate basement membrane separates the tumour from the vascular spaces of the corpus spongiosum.

Cell-surface antigens and immunological factors

The growth and spread of any cancer is dependent not only on the aggressiveness of the tumour, but also on the innate resistance of the host. Recently there has been increasing interest in the prognostic significance of the antigens on the surface of the tumour cells, and in the immunological defence mechanisms of patients with urothelial tumours (as discussed in Chapter 2). Many studies have demonstrated that the absence of blood-group iso-antigens on the surface of the tumour cells correlates well with their potential for invasiveness and hence with prognosis, both for tumours in the bladder (Lange *et al.*, 1978; Chapter 2) and in the renal pelvis and ureter (Lippert *et al.*, 1983). This test may well become useful in identifying patients with potentially invasive tumours *before* such invasion has taken place. However, variability in the sensitivity of the assay has led to the recommendation that it should be used only as a research tool at present (Wolk and Bishop, 1983).

Another marker of the likelihood of a tumour pursuing an aggressive course is the presence of certain chromosomal abnormalities in the tumour cells (Falor and Ward, 1978; see also Chapter 1).

Turning to the defence mechanisms of the host, it is known that most patients with early tumours show *in vitro* cell-mediated and humoral reactions against bladder tumour cells, but this reaction appears to be blocked in patients with more extensive or less well-differentiated disease (Catalona and Chretien, 1973).

Presentation and investigation

Haematuria is the presenting symptom of urothelial malignancy in 85–90 per cent of cases, but 15 per cent of patients have some dysuria or frequency as well, and 10 per cent never have haematuria at all. Wallace and Harris (1965) pointed out that most bladder tumours are probably curable when the first symptoms appear, and showed that the 3-year survival rate for infiltrating tumour falls from 60 to 25 per cent when treatment is delayed for more than one month after the onset of bleeding. Analysis of the delay showed that three-quarters of patients went to their doctors within a month of developing haematuria, and that most general practitioners referred these patients quickly for specialist investigation (although it was estimated that only one case of bladder tumour occurs for every 30 cases with haematuria). By far the most important source of delay was in the hospitals, where patients had to wait for admission and then frequently had to wait for referral for specialist treatment. Wallace pointed out that it is much better for the patient to wait three hours as an urgent addition to an outpatient list than to wait three weeks for a specified appointment.

The effectiveness of a haematuria diagnostic service has been studied both at the Royal Marsden Hospital (Turner *et al.*, 1977a) and at St Bartholomew's Hospital (Hendry *et al.*, 1980). Both studies confirmed that most patients presented to their doctors quickly after developing haematuria: 85 and 57 per cent of patients respectively had had their symptoms for less than one month; in a similar study in the USA, 46 per cent had had symptoms for less than one month on presentation (Hopkins *et al.*, 1983). Comparison of 108 bladder cancer patients diagnosed before the introduction of the haematuria diagnostic service with 65 patients detected afterwards showed that the proportion of early, potentially curable (T2) tumours was increased, and the proportion of probably incurable (T3) tumours decreased in the population with the infiltrating tumours (Hendry *et al.*, 1980; Table 4.1). Ta and T1 tumours are mostly non-invasive and the proportion of these is likely to remain the same, irrespective of the degree of delay in diagnosis. However, infiltrating carcinoma invades the wall of the bladder progressively and the depth of invasion increases with time. It is for these patients (who comprise about one-third of all patients with bladder cancer) that early diagnosis is essential if conservative methods of treatment, sparing the bladder, are to have a reasonable chance of success and if radical surgery is to have a maximum chance of cure in more advanced cases.

Table 4.1 Distribution of bladder tumours at diagnosis by T-category before and after the introduction of a haematuria service (Hendry *et al.*, 1980)

Classification	*Routine service, 1973–76* (*N*=108)	*Haematuria service, 1977–79* (*N*=65)
Ta and T1	69 (63.9%)	43 (66.2%)
T2	10 (9.2%)	10 (15.4%)
T3	21 (19.4%)	9 (13.8%)
T4a	2 (1.9%)	1 (1.5%)
T4b	3 (2.8%)	0 (0%)
TX	3 (2.8%)	2 (3.1%)

Urinary cytology shows a positive correlation with the presence of urothelial neoplasia in about 62 per cent of cases (Sarnacki *et al.*, 1971). However, a false-negative rate of 38 per cent indicates the need for full investigation of all cases of haematuria (Curling *et al.*, 1986). This investigation is of particular value in screening large numbers of 'at risk' workers (Parkes, 1975).

Bladder washings, obtained by irrigation with normal saline, produce better cellular detail and a slightly higher malignancy pick-up rate than examination of exfoliated cells in voided urine (Murphy *et al.*, 1981).

Malignant cells may be detected in bladder washings even though cytoscopy is apparently clear (Flanagan and Miller, 1978), and this technique appears to be particularly useful for confirmation of the nature of upper tract lesions (Leistenschneider and Nagel, 1980). Flow cytometry can bring automated technology and possible improved sensitivity to the cytological diagnosis of urothelial malignancy (Devonec *et al.*, 1981).

The intravenous urogram should be of good quality in the investigation of haematuria, and if there is any doubt about the upper tracts it should be repeated with a high dose of contrast medium and tomography. This investigation should always precede cystoscopy, as some renal pelvic tumours and most ureteric tumours show no dye excretion from the affected kidney. An ascending ureterogram will usually outline these tumours; but if this is technically difficult—perhaps due to an enlarged prostate—antegrade pyelography should be done. If cystoscopy shows a bladder tumour overlying the ureteric orifice, it may be assumed that this is the cause of the obstruction if it is deeply infiltrating and poorly differentiated. On the other hand, if the tumour is papillary and appears to be causing undue obstruction, a coexisting ureteric tumour should be suspected and this can also be demonstrated most easily by antegrade pyelography. Ureteroscopy may also be helpful in assessing ureteric tumours.

Cystourethroscopy should be done under general anaesthesia if tumour is suspected. Only then can an adequate biopsy be taken, the tumour resected if suitable, and most important of all, bimanual examination made with the patient's abdominal muscles fully relaxed. Too many patients have been frightened away by cystoscopy under local anaesthesia, only to return once all hope of cure has gone. The demand for immediate cystoscopy while the patient is bleeding has little relevance today with the accuracy of modern investigations, except for the occasional patient with unexplained haematuria even after full assessment. The use of immediate cystoscopy in outpatients to reduce the load on the x-ray department is mentioned only to be condemned, revealing as it does complete lack of understanding of the many possible sites and combinations that may be affected by urothelial neoplasia.

The tumour itself is always biopsied or resected, and tissue submitted for histological study. Additionally, mucosa adjacent to and remote from the tumour should be biopsied to find out whether there is a 'field change' in the apparently normal mucosa of the bladder (Wallace *et al.*, 1979; Smith *et al.*, 1983).

Lymphography is unnecessary for superficial tumours, but this investigation can be used in the assessment of infiltrating tumours. Although the nodes in the immediate vicinity of the bladder may not be filled by bilateral pedal lymphography, these nodes are easily included within the fields of radical surgical excision or radiotherapy. The importance of lymphography lies in demonstrating involvement of nodes beyond the immediate regional nodes, so that inadequate radical surgery can be avoided, and the volume to be irradiated appropriately extended.

Chest x-ray should, of course, be done as a routine, and *bone scan* should be included in the work-up prior to radical treatment for infiltrating tumours. *CT* and *NMR scanning* will often show the tumour clearly and indicate the depth of invasion and any possible involvement of adjacent organs. This is particularly of value in determining the extent of the disease and in staging (see Chapter 5).

Management

The successful treatment of bladder cancer starts with the correct assessment of the size, site, multiplicity, grade and depth of invasion of the tumour, which can only be done adequately under general anaesthesia. As discussed in Chapter 16, the treatment plan of primary bladder cancer must be designed in the context that urothelial malignancy is often multifocal, and that tumours may also be present in the upper tracts. Most tumours are still curable if appropriate treatment is undertaken soon after the onset of symptoms. The temptation to pursue a 'wait and see' policy following immediate transurethral diathermy of an incompletely assessed bladder tumour is often great, but by the time the tumour has recurred, revealing its true malignant potential, the opportunity to eradicate the disease may have gone forever.

The serious prognosis with invasive bladder cancer has been amply demonstrated in many careful clinicopathological studies. When the surgeon is faced with a new bladder tumour he must make a firm decision: either the tumour is obviously papillary, superficial and suitable for immediate and complete removal, in which case this should be done straight away; or the tumour appears to be too large, too extensive, or too infiltrating for immediate eradication. In this situation the surgeon should take a representative biopsy, carefully palpate the tumour bimanually to assess its depth of invasion, and then await the histology and the results of other relevant staging investigations. Once this information is available the tumour can be accurately classified, and the most effective treatment can be chosen after due consideration of all aspects of the case.

The TNM system (IUCC, 1978; Fig. 4.1) was revised to allow bladder tumours to be classified whether the surgeon decides upon immediate resection, or simply on biopsy and bimanual examination prior to definitive treatment. The classification applies only to epithelial tumours. Papilloma is excluded, but such cases should be listed under the category 'GO'. Papillary non-invasive carcinoma should be listed under the category Ta. There should be histological or cytological verification of the disease. Any unconfirmed cases must be reported separately.

The following are the *minimal requirements* for assessment of the T, N and M categories. If these cannot be met the symbols TX, NX or MX should be used:

T categories: Clinical examination, urography, cystoscopy, bimanual examination under anaesthesia and biopsy *or* transurethral resection of the tumour (if indicated) prior to definitive treatment.

N categories: Clinical examination and radiography, including lymphography and urography.

M categories: Clinical examination and radiography. In the more advanced primary tumours or when clinical suspicion warrants it, radiographic or isotope studies are recommended.

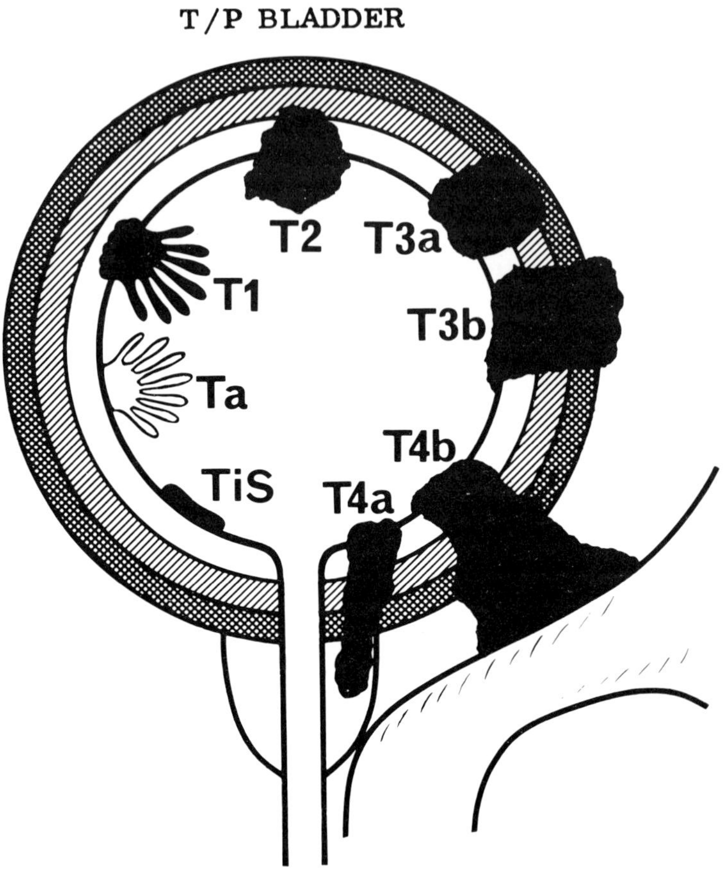

Fig. 4.1 TNM classification for bladder tumours (UICC, 1978)

The *regional lymph nodes* are the pelvic nodes below the bifurcation of the common iliac arteries. The *juxta-regional lymph nodes* are the inguinal nodes, the common iliac nodes and the para-aortic nodes.

TNM pretreatment clinical classification

T—Primary tumour

TIS   Preinvasive carcinoma (carcinoma-in-situ): 'flat tumour'

Ta   Papillary non-invasive carcinoma

T0   No evidence of primary tumour

T1   On bimanual examination a soft freely mobile mass may be felt: this should not be felt after complete transurethral resection of the lesion *and/or* microscopically the tumour does not invade beyond the lamina propria

T2   On bimanual examination there is induration of the bladder wall which is mobile. There is no residual induration after complete transurethral resection of the lesion *and/or* there is microscopic invasion of superficial muscle

T3   On bimanual examination induration *or* a nodular mobile mass is palpable in the bladder wall which persists after transurethral resection of the exophytic portion of the lesion *and/or* there is microscopic invasion of deep muscle, or of extension through the bladder wall
    T3a: Invasion of deep muscle
    T3b: Invasion through the bladder wall

T4   Tumour fixed or extending to neighbouring structures *and/or* there is microscopic evidence of such involvement
    T4a: Tumour infiltrating the prostate, uterus or vagina
    T4b: Tumour fixed to the pelvic wall *and/or* abdominal wall

TX   The minimum requirements to assess the primary tumour cannot be met.
    NOTE: The suffix (m) may be added to the appropriate T category to indicate multiple tumours, e.g. T2(m)

N—Regional and juxta-regional lymph nodes

N0   No evidence of regional lymph node involvement

N1   Evidence of involvement of a single homolateral regional lymph node

N2   Evidence of involvement of contralateral *or* bilateral *or* multiple regional lymph nodes

N3   Evidence of involvement of fixed regional lymph nodes (there is a fixed mass on the pelvic wall with a free space between this and the tumour)

NX   The minimum requirements to assess the regional *and/or* juxta-regional lymph nodes cannot be met

M—Distant metastases

N0   No evidence of distant metastases

M1   Evidence of distant metastases

MX   The minimum requirements to assess the presence of distant metastases cannot be met.

Treatment by stage (UICC)

TIS N0 M0—Carcinoma-in-situ (see also Chapter 6)

This description applies solely to flat, non-invasive carcinoma-in-situ which often presents with symptoms resembling interstitial cystitis in men of middle age. Sterile pyuria and atypical cells may be present in the urine and on cystoscopy areas of reddened 'unstable mucosa' are usually seen. Multiple small mucosal biopsies show a progression of changes from hyperplasia, through cellular atypia, to frank carcinoma-in-situ which is usually rather poorly differentiated (Pugh, 1973, 1981).

About two-thirds of these patients can be expected to develop progressive disease, with widespread instability of the bladder mucosa and a high incidence of infiltration of the bladder wall (Utz *et al.*, 1970). Most of these patients have severe symptoms and radical treatment is clearly necessary. In approximately one-third of cases, however, the finding of carcinoma-in-situ appears to be incidental, symptoms are few and the disease process is indolent. It may be very difficult to know which course the disease is likely to run when the patient first presents. Initially, a policy of close surveillance would seem reasonable with repeated cystoscopies and biopsy of unstable, red areas. If symptoms get worse, or if there is clear evidence of disease progression, treatment should be started without delay.

Intravesical chemotherapy may be tried first, and doxorubicin (Adriamycin) appears to be an effective agent. Glashan (1983) used 50 mg Adriamycin dissolved in 50 ml sterile saline, instilled into the bladder for 2 hours and repeated at weekly intervals for 6 weeks. Overall, 82 per cent of 17 patients with primary carcinoma-in-situ, and 67 per cent of 22 patients with carcinoma-in-situ following previous bladder tumours, responded as judged by cystoscopy with biopsies and by cytological examination of the urine; most patients remained clear with follow-up extending to 2.5 years. Alternatively, systemic cyclophosphamide can be used, and complete regression of TIS has been reported in 12 of 15 patients lasting for up to 15 months (England *et al.*, 1981).

The experience of Riddle *et al.* (1976) indicates that radiotherapy probably has little to offer in the management of widespread superficial carcinoma-in-situ. There seems to be little doubt that if there is clear evidence of disease progression, especially if symptoms are severe, that does not clear quickly with chemotherapy, then the bladder should be removed since the disease is often more extensive than cystoscopy reveals, and the prognosis becomes much worse once infiltration has occurred (see Chapter 6).

Ta and T1 N0 M0 tumours

These categories make up 70–80 per cent of all bladder tumours, including all papillary tumours, both non-infiltrating (Ta) and infiltrating submucosa (T1), in which biopsy shows no evidence of invasion of muscle, and in which there is no palpable tumour or thickening of the bladder wall once transurethral treatment has been completed. Most of these tumours are suitable for endoscopic treatment by cystodiathermy or transurethral resection. About 50 per cent of these patients will develop recurrences. Eighty per cent of patients with differentiated (grade I) tumours, and only 40 per cent of those with undifferentiated (grades II and III) tumours, will be alive at 5 years (Miller *et al.*, 1969). Progression, indicated by development of muscle invasion or metastases, has been observed in only 2 per cent of patients with grade I tumours, in 11 per cent of grade II and in no less than 45 per cent of patients with grade III growths (Heney *et al.*, 1983). Only 4 per cent of patients with Ta tumours had progression, compared with 30 per cent of those with T1 growths (see Table 4.2). The majority of those whose disease progressed did so within two years of diagnosis. Other factors associated with a high likelihood of progression were (a) size greater than 5 cm (35 per cent progressed), and (b) moderate to severe dysplasia in mucosa taken from non-tumour-bearing areas of the bladder (33 per cent progressed). Positive urine cytology showed a striking correlation with tumour grade (Table 4.3). These observations indicate clearly that between a quarter and a third of papillary bladder tumours might be termed 'wolves in

Table 4.2 Incidence of progression to muscle invasion or metastases in patients with superficial tumours related to grade and stage (Heney *et al.*, 1983)

Stage	Grade I	Grade II	Grade III
Ta	2/85 (2%)	3/50 (6%)	1/4 (25%)
T1	0/7	6/29 (21%)	13/27 (48%)

Table 4.3 Association between urinary cytology and grade of bladder tumour (Heney *et al.*, 1983)

		Cytological findings	
Grade	Number of patients	Negative	Positive
0	4	4	0
I	68	62	6 (9%)
II	60	41	19 (32%)
III	20	6	14 (70%)

sheep's clothing'—they look to the urologist like fairly innocent growths which should respond to cystoscopic treatment and regular surveillance, whereas in fact they are destined for a progressively invasive, probably metastatic and ultimately fatal course.

With modern equipment, most papillary bladder tumours can be removed endoscopically when the patient first presents. However, if the tumour is too large for immediate transurethral treatment, the bladder may be opened and the tumour removed transvesically with no deterioration in 5-year survival rate compared with endoscopic treatment, although about 3 per cent of patients will develop scar recurrence (Miller *et al.*, 1969). An alternative approach to the treatment of large superficial tumours was introduced by Helmstein (1972). Under epidural anaesthesia a specially constructed balloon catheter is introduced into the bladder and inflated to 25 cm of water above diastolic blood pressure for 6 hours. This causes ischaemic necrosis of the bulk of tumour, which is subsequently passed per urethram: at review cystoscopy 4–6 weeks later any small residual tumour can usually be dealt with endoscopically. England *et al.* (1973) confirmed the efficacy of this treatment, and showed that the best results are obtained with large long-fronded well-differentiated papillary tumours.

All patients with Ta and T1 tumours should be followed with regular check cystoscopies until the bladder has been clear for at least five years: thereafter patients may be transferred to annual cytological follow-up as outpatients. Ideally all check cystoscopies should be performed under general anaesthesia, if men with recurrent tumours are not to be frightened away. Recurrences are to be expected in about 50 per cent of patients and these can usually be controlled cystoscopically. The administration of compounds like retinoids and perhaps also pyridoxine (vitamin B_6)—the former to inhibit and perhaps reverse premalignant epithelium changes and the latter to reduce urinary tryptophan metabolites, which may act as urothelial carcinogens—may come to play an important role in preventing the formation of new bladder tumours, especially in patients with flat carcinoma-in-situ or with multiple recurring papillary tumours (Alfthan *et al.*, 1983; Studer *et al.*, 1984).

Intravesical chemotherapy, as outlined in Chapter 6, can be used to clear a bladder of multiple superficial tumours if they are too numerous for endoscopic treatment, or the drug can be instilled into the bladder following cystoscopic removal of the tumour with the intention of reducing the incidence and the number of recurrences. Two recent reviews (Soloway, 1980; Prout, 1984) confirmed that such treatment can be effective for both purposes. Approximately one-third of superficial non-invasive (Ta) tumours can be cleared by intravesical chemotherapy, one-third will temporarily improve but later recur, and one-third will not respond; lack of response is usually seen with less-well-differentiated tumours often with a degree of basement membrane breakthrough (i.e. T1 tumours). Following endoscopic treatment, a statistically significant reduction in recurrence rate of tumours can be achieved.

There seems little to choose between the following regimens:

Epodyl: 100 ml of 1% solution retained in the bladder for 1 hour, once a week for 3 months, then monthly so long as control persists (Riddle and Wallace, 1971)

Thiotepa: 30 mg in 50 ml normal saline instilled via a catheter for 2 hours on postoperative days 1, 3 and 5 following endoscopic removal of as much tumour as possible. (Dose reduced to 15 mg if blood counts show evidence of marrow depression.) Review cystoscopy at 3 months, and repeat treatment as necessary (England *et al.*, 1981)

Adriamycin: 80 mg in 100 ml normal saline given intravesically for 60 minutes once a month for 3 months, then 3-monthly (Edsmyr, 1981)

Mitomycin C: 30–40 mg in 40 ml sterile water, in the bladder for 2 hours weekly for 8 weeks, then monthly for 1 year (Soloway and Ford, 1983)

Side effects are few so long as the patient is not allergic to the drug. Thiotepa may be absorbed systemically and so white blood cell and platelet counts should precede each treatment. Systemic myelotoxicity does not occur with Epodyl, Adriamycin and mitomycin C which are not absorbed from the bladder. An alternative approach has been used by Morales and colleagues (1981) using bacillus Calmette–Guerin: 120 mg of BCG in 50 ml normal saline are instilled into the bladder for at least 2 hours, together with an intradermal dose of 5 mg; both treatments are repeated weekly for 6 weeks. Ten of 17 patients with incompletely resected superficial tumours (Ta or T1) experienced complete ablation of residual disease with a mean follow-up of 19 months. Six of the 7 unresponsive patients had less differentiated tumours. Untoward reactions were generally brief and mild.

If a patient has multiple superficial tumours which fail to respond to intravesical chemotherapy or immunotherapy, it is very likely that the growths will continue to recur and are likely to metastasize. Fitzpatrick *et al.* (1979) have shown that patients whose tumours do not respond to such therapy have a poor prognosis, and suggested that failure of response is an indication for early cystourethrectomy.

Once it becomes clear that cystoscopic treatment is failing to control the tumours, especially if intravesical chemotherapy has been tried and failed, the bladder should be removed without further delay. Radiotherapy is ineffective in controlling superficial tumours, and, indeed, may make matters worse by inducing telangiectasia and encouraging bleeding. Bracken *et al.* (1981) have described their experiences with preoperative radiotherapy in 109 patients with stage 0 and A (Ta and T1) bladder tumours unmanageable transurethrally who underwent radical cystectomy and ileal loop diversion. The operative mortality was 2.75 per cent and the overall 5-year survival rate was 76 per cent. Those who were *not* given preoperative ratiotherapy (53 patients) showed slightly better survival than those (56 patients) who received 5000 cGy (rads) in 5 weeks prior to surgery. Use of preoperative radiotherapy was not randomized, but neither was it related to tumour grade or the patients' general health. There seems little point in using such therapy for these early-stage cases.

Two groups of patients with papillary bladder tumours deserve special mention. First, if the tumour is situated in or close to a diverticulum, it should be excised completely with the diverticulum, since the results of endoscopic treatment under those circumstances are poor (Bracken *et al.*, 1981). Second, the coexistence of ureteric obstruction with a papillary tumour demands particularly careful evaluation. If the bladder tumour is non-invasive, there is almost certainly coexisting papillary tumour in the ureter. This can usually be demonstrated by antegrade pyelogram if the presence of tumour overlying the ureteric orifice makes an ascending ureterogram impossible. Depending on the extent of the tumour, nephro-uretero-cysto-urethrectomy may be required for panurothelial disease.

T2 N0/N1 M0 tumours

In this group there is invasion into the superficial muscle, and this is possibly the most difficult group to assess. Cystoscopically one may suspect infiltration such as in a solid, broad-based tumour. On bimanual examination there may be a little thickening of the bladder wall but there should be no residual induration after complete transurethral resection of the lesion. In practice, this classification is usually based on a deep resectoscopic biopsy which shows invasion of the superficial muscle layers, when bimanual examination reveals no induration of the bladder wall.

Once the tumour has invaded the superficial muscle of the bladder wall, it becomes a life-threatening disease which is unlikely to be satisfactorily controlled endoscopically, although it may be possible to treat it effectively by other means while still conserving the bladder. With invasion into deep muscle (T3) the prognosis becomes very poor, and local treatment is much less likely to eradicate the disease. It is therefore most important to distinguish accurately between these two categories (T2 and T3). Fortunately, the combination of deep biopsy and careful bimanual examination under general anaesthetic has been shown to be over 90 per cent accurate in differentiating superficial from deep infiltration (Jewett, 1973), although Magri (1962) showed that there is a greater tendency to understage (27 per cent) than overstage (12 per cent). The advent of CT and NMR scanning has helped to define the depth of invasion with greater accuracy.

In a few carefully selected cases with lesions situated towards the bladder vault, partial cystectomy may be feasible, and approximately 50 per cent of patients treated by this method will be alive 5 years later (Magri, 1962); follow-up treatment with radiotherapy or chemotherapy is probably advisable.

If the tumour is situated at the bladder base or too extensive for local excision, the choice lies between external-beam irradiation, total cystectomy, or preoperative irradiation and cystectomy. Analysis of reported results of these treatments is difficult because in many series T2 tumours have not been separated from mucosal or deep-muscle tumours.

On present evidence it appears that radical external-beam radiotherapy (Caldwell *et al.*, 1967) followed if necessary by 'salvage' cystectomy (Crawford and Skinner, 1980; Swanson *et al.*, 1981) should be recommended for cases in which these relatively early but serious tumours are not suitable for local excision (see also Chapters 8 and 17). Open excision and interstitial irradiation is seldom done today, although this treatment gave quite good results in the past.

Improvements in anaesthetic and operative techniques, together with better postoperative care, have produced such marked improvement in the morbidity and mortality associated with cystectomy that some surgeons have suggested that radical cystectomy with clearance of pelvic lymph nodes may give results which are comparable to those obtained by radical radiotherapy (Chapter 7). The need for even preoperative radiotherapy is now being questioned in relatively early (T2) cases (Radwin, 1980). Skinner *et al.* (1982) have reported an operative mortality of less than 1 per cent in 131 single-stage radical cystectomies with node dissection and urinary diversion, preceded by high-dose, short-course (16 cGy in 4 days) radiation therapy. Some investigators (Montie *et al.*, 1984) have now dispensed with the radiotherapy and the results of prospective trials of radical surgery alone versus radiotherapy (with or without surgery) are awaited with interest.

T3 N0/N1 M0 tumours
There should be little difficulty in recognizing a tumour in this category: either the biopsy shows evidence of invasion of deep muscle, or a hard mobile lump is felt on bimanual examination which is still palpable even if the surgeon decides to resect the part of the tumour projecting into the bladder. In fewer than 10 per cent of cases is the surgeon likely to miss the palpable lump if he examines the patient bimanually under general anaesthesia, either because of thick or unrelaxed abdominal wall, or because of inaccessible location—for example, adherent to the back of the symphysis pubis (Jewett, 1973).

Once the diagnosis of a deeply infiltrating poorly differentiated tumour has been made, the prognosis is extremely grave. A few tumours may be small enough to permit partial cystectomy, in which case postoperative external-beam radiotherapy can substantially increase the chance of survival (Magri, 1962). The very criteria that make these cases suitable for local treatment ensure that they have a less serious prognosis. The larger T3 tumours have given equally poor 5-year survival rates (generally less than 30 per cent) following either external irradiation (Edsmyr, 1975) or radical cystectomy (Whitmore and Marshall, 1962). Since radiotherapy spares the patient a major mutilating operation, this method of treatment has been favoured in Britain for the past 15 to 20 years (Blandy *et al.*, 1980). The use of hyperbaric oxygenation to try to increase the radiosensitivity of bladder cancer has not produced any improvement in results (Dische, 1973).

In about 75 per cent of cases, the tumour can be expected not to disappear completely or to recur within 5 years of radical radiotherapy. In some cases 'salvage' cystectomy may be possible, but under these circumstances the operation is likely to be difficult and a higher complication rate is to be expected compared with patients who received planned preoperative therapy or no radiotherapy (Droller and Walsh, 1983). Nevertheless, operative mortality rates of 5 per cent or less have been recorded for salvage cystectomy in large series of patients following radical radiotherapy (for a review see Hendry (1986)).

The high incidence of therapeutic failure with deeply invasive bladder cancer led Whitmore (1969) to try the combination of a sub-radical dose of planned preoperative irradiation followed by cystectomy. Whitmore's patients received doses of 4000 cGy given to the whole pelvis in 4 weeks, followed by cystectomy 4–12 weeks later. Subsequently, a regime of 2000 cGy in 1 week with immediate cystectomy was used. Analysis showed that 32–41 per cent of patients with high-stage tumours survived for 5 years after the latter combined treatment.

Werf-Messing (1973) has shown a significant improvement in survival of T3 cases when there was reduction in the depth of invasion in the cystectomy specimen after preoperative irradiation. Five-year actuarial survival was 80 per cent for 35 patients with so-called 'downstaging' (i.e. reduction in stage in the surgical specimen following irradiation). On the other hand, of 19 patients without such 'downstaging' none survived 5 years. The overall survival rate was 45 per cent in this series of 54 cases, irrespective of any change in the stage in the cystectomy specimen.

A trial of radical radiotherapy (6000 cGy in 6 weeks) versus preoperative radiotherapy (4000 cGy in 4 weeks) was done in London under the sponsorship of the Institute of Urology (Wallace and Bloom, 1976; Bloom et al., 1982). The corrected 5-year actuarial survival rate for all 98 patients, without exclusions, randomized to receive preoperative irradiation followed by radical cystectomy, was 38 per cent compared with 29 per cent for 91 patients in the radical radiotherapy group (Fig. 4.2). Of the 85 patients in the radical radiotherapy group, 18 ultimately came to salvage cystectomy with 60 per cent surviving for 5 years (Fig. 4.3).

Patients whose tumours responded to preoperative irradiation had a greater survival than did those showing no such response. Thus, the survival rate in patients with downstaged tumours was more than twice as great as that for those patients showing no tumour reduction: at 5 years, 64 per cent of the patients with pT0-pT2 tumours were alive, compared with only 27 per cent for those with persistent pT3 or pT4 lesions (Fig. 4.4).

The 5-year survival rate for patients less than 60 years old, receiving the combined treatment, was 49 per cent compared with 25 per cent for radical radiotherapy. The same trend in results was seen in patients aged 60–64 years with 41 and 28 per cent alive, respectively. On the other hand, for patients aged 65–70 years the trend was reversed, with a possible slight advantage for radical irradiation, the 5-year survival rates being 35 and 43 per cent respectively.

Results from two controlled trials in which the data available permit comparison are shown in Table 4.4. Evidence is mounting that, for deeply infiltrating bladder cancer, a combination of preoperative irradiation and

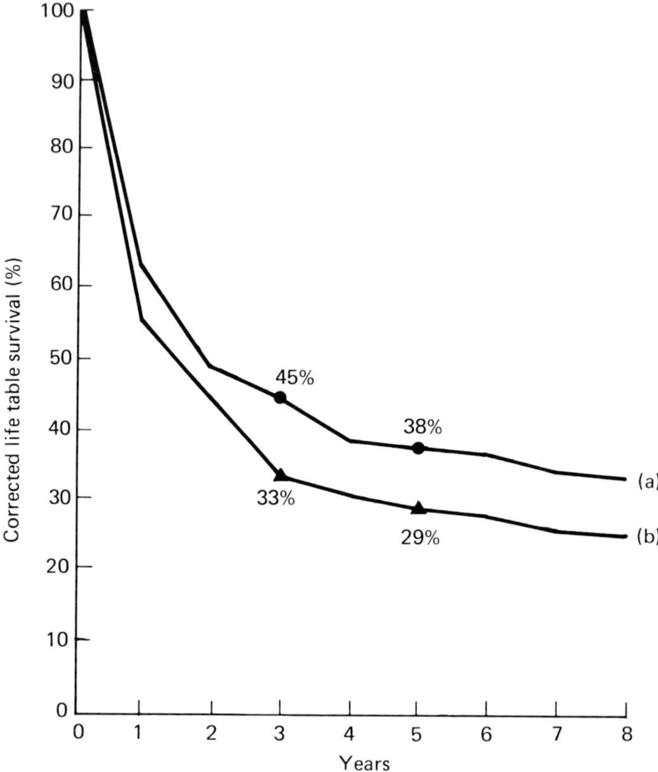

Fig. 4.2 Institute of Urology T3 bladder carcinoma trial results: survival by protocol treatment allocated. (a) 4000 cGy + cystectomy (98 cases); (b) 6000 cGy (91 cases). $p=0.2$ (Bloom *et al.*, 1982)

Table 4.4 Results from allocated randomized treatment in two controlled studies: crude 5-year survival rates for radical radiotherapy and for preoperative radiotherapy and elective cystectomy

Treatment	Reference	Number of patients*	Crude 5-year survival (%)
Preoperative radiotherapy (5000 cGy/5 weeks and simple cystectomy)	Miller (1977)	35	46
Radical radiotherapy (7000 cGy/7 weeks)	Miller (1977)	34	22
Preoperative radiotherapy (4000 cGy/4 weeks and radical cystectomy)	Wallace and Bloom (1976)	98	34
Radical radiotherapy (6000 cGy/6 weeks)	Wallace and Bloom (1976)	91	25

*All randomized patients included.

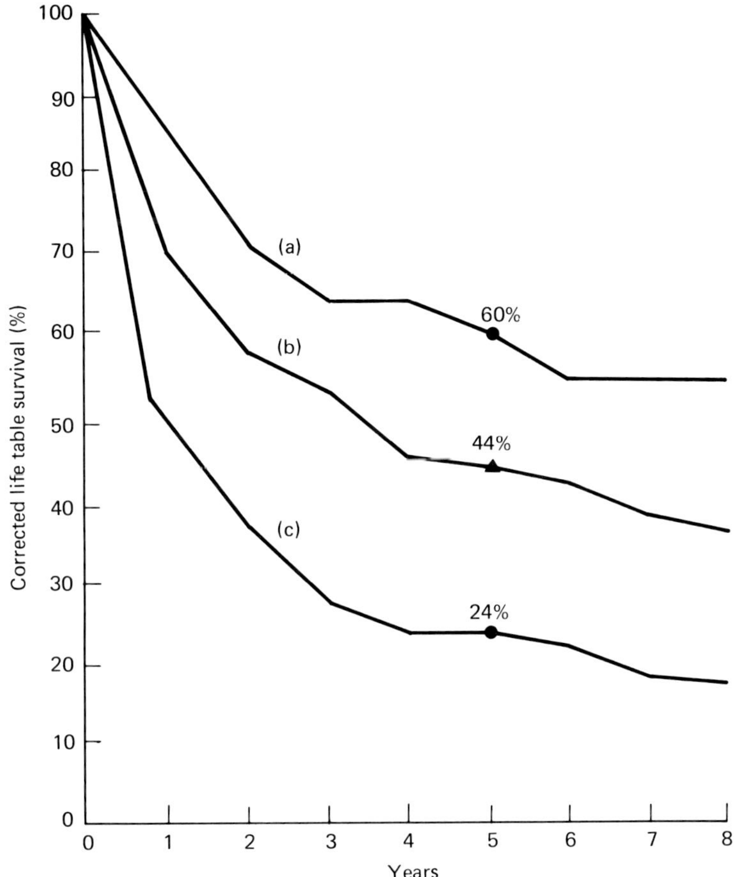

Fig. 4.3 Institute of Urology T3 bladder carcinoma trial results: survival by treatment received. (a) 6000 cGy + salvage cystectomy (18 cases); (b) 4000 cGy + cystectomy (77 cases); (c) 6000 cGy only (67 cases) (Bloom *et al.*, 1982)

cystectomy produces greater control of the primary tumour and regional nodes and higher survival rates than either modality alone, especially among those patients showing a good response to the preliminary irradiation. The benefit of the combined treatment, however, seems to be restricted to patients under 65 years of age.

In the Institute of Urology study, the operative mortality within 2 months of radical cystectomy following preoperative radiotherapy was 7.8 per cent but ranged from 5.5 per cent for patients under 60 years of age to 11 per cent for those aged between 65 and 70 years. The successful use of preoperative irradiation and radical cystectomy in the treatment of this disease is dependent on patients surviving the cystectomy. Mortality rates of between 10 and 15 per cent have commonly been reported in the past, mainly owing to complications arising with anastomosis of irradiated ureters, especially to the colon. The use of high ureteroileal anastomosis (above the field of irradiation) as described by Wallace (1970) and improvements in anaesthesia and postoperative management have reduced the mortality to

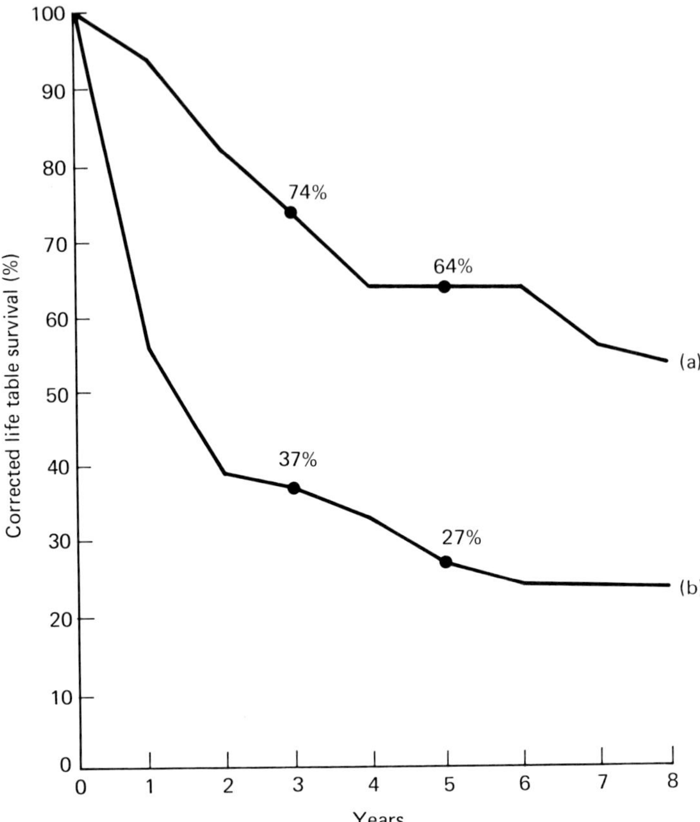

Fig. 4.4 Institute of Urology T3 bladder carcinoma trial results: survival according to whether or not there was reduction of pathological tumour stage in the radical cystectomy specimen following 4000 cGy. (a) pT0–pT2 (36 cases); (b) pT3–pT4 (38 cases). $p<0.01$ (Bloom *et al.*, 1982)

less than 5 per cent (Hendry, 1986). Ureterocolic diversion is not recommended: it has a high incidence of postoperative complications and subsequent renal dysfunction especially after radiotherapy, and in cases with recurrent disease terminal nursing care is often malodorous and unpleasant.

N1: local lymph node involvement

Until quite recently, the presence of node involvement in patients with bladder cancer was considered to indicate a hopeless prognosis, and this is supported by the high mortality in patients at the Royal Marsden Hospital with positive lymphograms (Turner *et al.*, 1976; Fig. 4.5). However, this radiological investigation demonstrates only nodes with gross disease, and radiotherapy may be of value in patients with nodal micrometastases. There is, in fact, evidence that strictly limited node involvement is compatible with survival for 5 years or more following radical surgery (Dretler *et al.*, 1973).

The 5-year survival rate for node-negative cases treated by preoperative

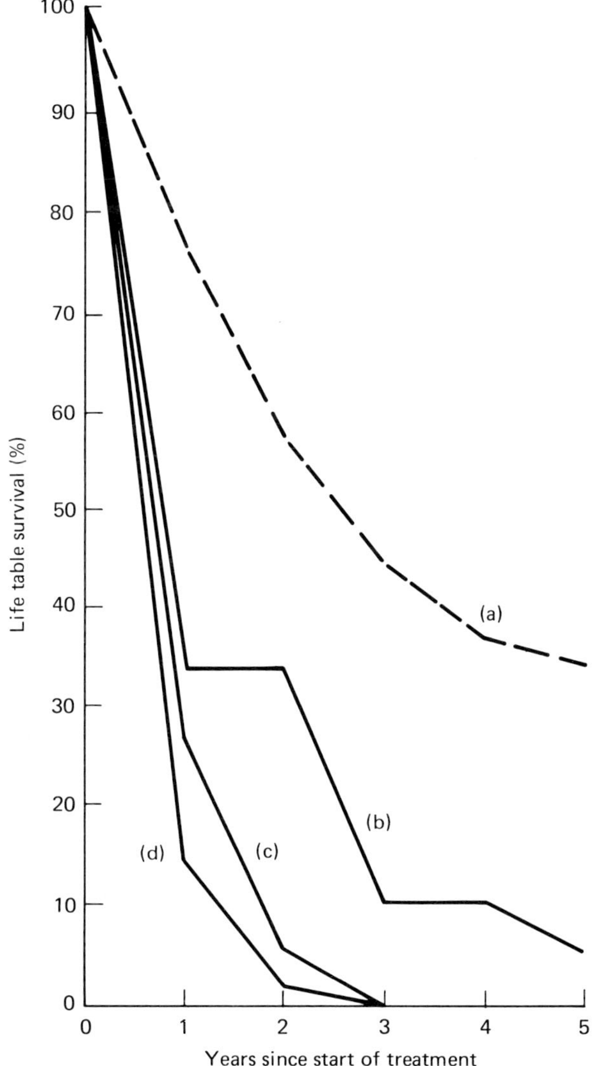

Fig. 4.5 Survival of patients with bladder cancer related to findings on lymphography. (a) negative (131 cases); (b) unilateral positive (30 cases); (c) bilateral positive (22 cases); (d) para-aortic positive (39 cases) (Turner *et al.*, 1976)

irradiation and cystectomy in the Institute of Urology trial was 53 per cent compared with 16 per cent for those with persistent node involvement (Fig. 4.6).

T4 tumours

Tumours may become T4 by virtue of invasion of adjacent organs (T4a) or by local fixation (T4b). Some tumours, especially the multifocal type, tend to involve the prostate by *in situ* change in the prostatic ducts and acini. These

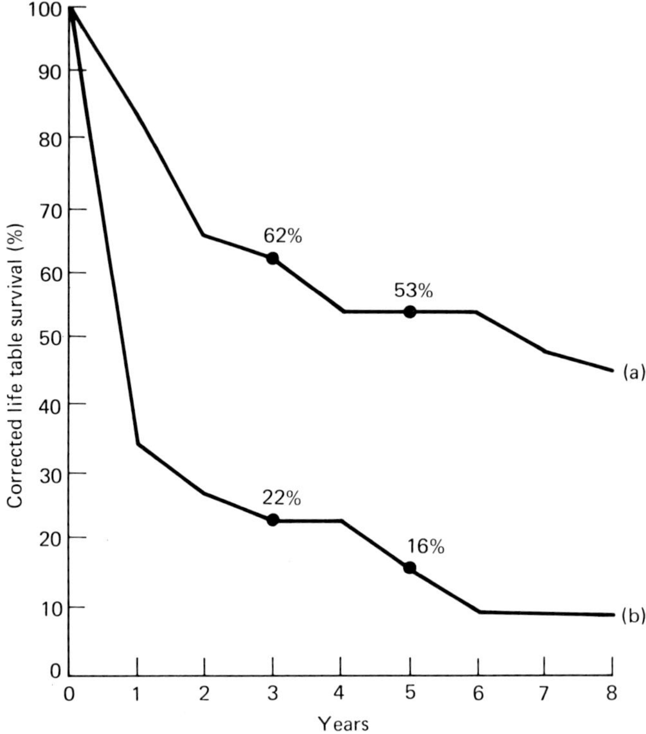

Fig. 4.6 Institute of Urology T3 bladder carcinoma trial results: survival following preoperative radiotherapy and radical cystectomy according to the presence or absence of pelvic node metastases in the surgical specimen. (a) node negative (60 cases); (b) node positive (15 cases). $p<0.05$ (Bloom *et al.*, 1982)

tumours are essentially non-invasive and should be classified and treated according to the category of the bladder tumour. Much more ominous is true invasion of the prostate, which should be treated in the same way as T3 tumours (Chibber *et al.*, 1981; Kirk *et al.*, 1981).

Once the tumour has become fixed the prognosis is very poor. Green and George (1974) found that average survival for 74 patients in this category was only 10 months, although most derived considerable benefit from palliative radiotherapy.

M1: metastatic disease

Subjective and objective evidence of tumour response has been reported with a number of chemotherapeutic agents in patients with advanced bladder cancer. Although the response has often been short-lived in patients with disseminated disease, it seems likely that in future these agents may be used singly or in combination as adjuvants for patients in whom there is a clearly defined high risk of developing distant metastases, since it is well established that chemotherapy is more effective with micrometastases. Only carefully controlled clinical trials will establish whether such adjuvant chemotherapy provides any benefit in patients with tumours of established poor prognosis (see Chapters 15 and 17).

Urethral tumours

Tumours in the prostatic urethra may be infiltrating or non-infiltrating, and should be treated according to their extent in a similar manner to bladder tumours. Infiltrating tumours have a poor prognosis and require radical treatment.

Tumours of the anterior urethra present a more difficult problem, since only a delicate basement membrane separates them from the large vascular spaces of the corpus spongiosum. Many reports have shown that these tumours are associated with a poor prognosis and should be considered a serious complication of bladder cancer (Hendry *et al.*, 1974). Accordingly, when cystectomy is performed for multiple papillary bladder tumours, the urethra should always be removed simultaneously as a one-stage cystourethrectomy. When the bladder is removed for single anaplastic tumours, urethral cytology (Trott, 1971) may be helpful in selecting cases for cystourethrectomy. Urethral recurrence after previous cystectomy is a serious and life-threatening complication, which should be treated by early secondary urethrectomy. If pathological examination shows invasive cancer in the anterior urethra, it may be advisable to give postoperative chemotherapy for up to six months.

In women, care should be taken to remove the whole urethra with the bladder, since this adds little to the extent of the operation, and prevents stump recurrence after cystectomy which can carry a grave prognosis.

Acknowledgements

I wish to thank the *British Journal of Urology* for permission to reproduce Figs. 4.2–4.6.

References

Alfthan, O., Tarkkanen, J., Grohn, P., Heinonen, E., Pyrhonen, S. and Saila, K. (1983). Tigason (eretinate) in prevention of recurrence of superficial bladder tumours: a double blind clinical trial. *European Urology* **9**: 6–9.

Ashworth, A. (1956). Papillomatosis of the urethra. *British Journal of Urology* **28**: 3–11.

Babaian, R.J. and Johnson, D.E. (1980). Primary carcinoma of the ureter. *Journal of Urology* **123**: 357–9.

Baker, R. (1968). The accuracy of clinical versus surgical staging. *Journal of the American Medical Association* **206**: 1770–3.

Blandy, J.P., England, H.R., Evans, S.J.W., Hopestone, H.F., Mair, G.M.M., Mantell, B.S., Oliver, R.T.D., Paris, A.M.I. and Risdon, R.A. (1980). T3 bladder cancer—the case for salvage cystectomy. *British Journal of Urology* **52**: 506–10.

Bloom, H.J.G., Hendry, W.F., Wallace, D.M. and Skeet, R.G. (1982). Treatment of T3 bladder cancer: controlled trial of pre-operative radiotherapy and radical cystectomy versus radical radiotherapy (second report and review). *British Journal of Urology* **54**: 136–51.

Bracken, R.B., McDonald, M.W. and Johnson, D.E. (1981). Cystectomy for superficial bladder cancer. *Urology* **18**: 459–63.

Caldwell, W.L., Bagshaw, M.A. and Kaplan, H.S. (1967). Efficacy of linear accelerator X-ray therapy in the cancer of the bladder. *Journal of Urology* **97**: 294–303.

Case, R.A.M., Hosker, M.E., McDonald, D.B. and Pearson, J.T. (1954). Tumours of the urinary bladder in workmen engaged in the manufacture and use of certain dyestuff intermediates in the British Chemical Industry. *British Journal of Industrial Medicine* **11**: 75–104.

Catalona, W.J. and Chretien, P.B. (1973). Correlation among host immunocompetence and tumour stage, tumour grade and vascular permeation in transitional carcinoma. *Journal of Urology* **110**: 526–8.

Chibber, P.J., McIntyre, M.A., Hindmarsh, J.R., Hargreave, T.B., Newsam, J.E. and Chisholm, G.D. (1981). Transitional cell carcinoma involving the prostate. *British Journal of Urology* **53**: 605–9.

Crawford, E.D. and Skinner, D.G. (1980). Salvage cystectomy after irradiation failure. *Journal of Urology* **123**: 32–4.

Curling, M., Broome, G. and Hendry, W.F. (1986). How accurate is urine cytology? *Journal of the Royal Society of Medicine* (in press).

Devonec, M., Darzynkiewicz, Z., Whitmore, W.F. and Melamed, M.R. (1981). Flow cytometry for follow-up examinations of conservatively treated low stage bladder tumours. *Journal of Urology* **126**: 166–70.

Dische, S. (1973). The hyberbaric oxygen chamber in the radiotherapy of carcinoma of the bladder. *British Journal of Radiology* **46**: 13–17.

Dretler, S.P., Ragsdale, B.D. and Leadbetter, W.F. (1973). The value of pelvic lymphadenectomy in the surgical treatment of bladder cancer. *Journal of Urology* **109**: 414–16.

Droller, M.J. and Walsh, P.C. (1983). Therapeutic efficacy of salvage cystectomy. *Urology* **22**: 118–22.

Edsmyr, F. (1975). Radiotherapy in the management of bladder cancer. In *The Biology and Clinical Management of Bladder Cancer*, pp. 229–54. Edited by Gooper, E.H. and Williams, L.E. Blackwell Scientific Publications, Oxford.

Edsmyr, F. (1981). Intravesical therapy with adriamycin in patients with superficial bladder tumours. In *Bladder Cancer: Progress in Combination Therapy*. Edited by Oliver, R.T.D., Hendry, W.F. and Bloom, H.J.G. Butterworth, London.

England, H.R., Molland, E.A., Oliver, R.T.D. and Blandy, J.P. (1981). Systemic cyclophosphamide in flat carcinoma-in-situ of the bladder. In *Bladder Cancer: Principles of Combination Therapy*, pp. 97–105. Edited by Oliver, R.T.D., Hendry, W.F. and Bloom, H.J.G. Butterworth, London.

England, H.R., Paris, A.M.I. and Blandy, J.P. (1981). Intravesical thiotepa as adjuvant to cystodiathermy in multiple recurrent superficial bladder tumours. In *Bladder Cancer: Progress in Combination Therapy*. Edited by Oliver, R.T.D., Hendry, W.F. and Bloom, H.J.G. Butterworth, London.

England, H.R., Rigby, C., Shepheard, B.G.F., Tresidder, G.C. and Blandy, J.P. (1973). Evaluation of Helmstein's distension method for carcinoma of the bladder. *British Journal of Urology* **45**: 593–9.

Falor, W.H. and Ward, R.M. (1978). Prognosis in early carcinoma of the bladder based on chromosomal analysis. *Journal of Urology* **199**: 545–8.

Fitzpatrick, J.M., Khan, O., Oliver, R.T.D. and Riddle, P.R. (1979). Longterm follow-up in patients with superficial bladder tumours treated with intravesical epodyl. *British Journal of Urology* **51**: 545–8.

Flanagan, M.J. and Miller, A. (1978). Evaluation of bladder washing cytology for bladder cancer surveillance. *Journal of Urology* **119**: 42–3.

Ghazizadeh, M., Takigawa, H., Fujimura, N. and Kurokawa, K. (1983). Direct immunofluorescence for ABH blood group 180 antigens: use of FITC-confugated lectius. *Urology* **22**: 381–4.

Glashan, R.W. (1983). Treatment of carcinoma-in-situ of the bladder with doxorubicin (adriamycin). *Cancer Chemotherapy and Pharmacology* **11** (Suppl.): 535–7.

Gowing, N.F.C. (1960). Urethral carcinoma associated with cancer of the bladder. *British Journal of Urology* **32**: 428–38.

Green, N. and George, F.W. (1974). Radiotherapy of advanced localised bladder cancer. *Journal of Urology* **111**: 611–12.

Hawtrey, C.E. (1971). Fifty-two cases of primary urethral carcinoma: a clinical–pathological study. *Journal of Urology* **105**: 188–93.

Helmstein, K. (1972). Treatment of bladder carcinoma by a hydrostatic pressure technique. *British Journal of Urology* **44**: 434–50.

Hendry, W.F. (1986). The morbidity and mortality of radical cystectomy (1971–1981 and 1978–1985). *Journal of the Royal Society of Medicine.*

Hendry, W.F., Gowing, N.F.C. and Wallace, D.M. (1974). Surgical treatment of urethral tumours associated with bladder cancer. *Proceedings of the Royal Society of Medicine* **67**: 304–7.

Hendry, W.F., Manning, N., Perry, N.M., Whitfield, H.N. and Wickham, J.E.A. (1981). The effects of a haematuria service on the early diagnosis of bladder cancer. In *Bladder Cancer: Progress in Combination Therapy.* Edited by Oliver, R.T.D., Hendry, W.F. and Bloom, H.J.G. Butterworth, London.

Heney, N.M., Ahmed, S., Flanagan, M.J., Frable, W., Corder, M.P., Hafermann, M.D. and Hawkins, I.R., for National Bladder Cancer Collaborative Group A (1983). Superficial bladder cancer: progression and recurrence. *Journal of Urology* **130**: 1083–6.

Heney, N.M., Nocks, B.N., Daly, J.J., Blitzer, P.H. and Parkhurst, E.C. (1981). Prognostic factors in carcinoma of the ureter. *Journal of Urology* **125**: 632–6.

Hopkins, S.C., Ford, K.S. and Soloway, M.S. (1983). Invasive bladder cancer: support for screening. *Journal of Urology* **130**: 61–3.

Jewett, H.J. (1973). Cancer of the bladder: diagnosis and staging. *Cancer* **32**: 1072–7.

Jewett, H.J. and Strong, G.H. (1946). Infiltrating carcinoma of bladder: relation of depth and penetration of the bladder wall to incidence of local extension and metastases. *Journal of Urology* **55**: 366.

Kaye, K.W. and Lange, P.H. (1982). Mode of presentation of invasive bladder cancer: reassessment of the problem. *Journal of Urology* **128**: 31–3.

Kerr, W.S. and Colby, F.H. (1951). Carcinoma of bladder: a correlation of pathology with treatment and prognosis. *Journal of Urology* **65**: 841–844.

Kim, K.H., Leiter, E. and Brendler, H. (1972). Primary tumours of the ureter. *Journal of Urology* **107**: 955–8.

Kinder, C.H. and Wallace, D.M. (1962). Recurrent carcinoma in the ureteric stump. *British Journal of Surgery* **50**: 202–5.

Kirk, D., Savage, A., Makepeace, A.R. and Gostelow, B.W. (1981). Transitional cell carcinoma involving the prostate—an unfavourable sign in the management of bladder cancer. *British Journal of Urology* **53**: 610–612.

Lange, P.H., Limas, C. and Fraley, E.E. (1978). Tissue blood-group antigens and prognosis in low stage transitional cell carcinoma of the bladder. *Journal of Urology* **199**: 52–5.

Leistenschneider, W. and Nagel, R. (1980). Lavage cytology of renal pelvis and ureter with special reference to tumours. *Journal of Urology* **124**: 597–600.

Lippert, M., Bergman, S., Walker, P., Berger, C. and Javadpour, N. (1983). Detection of cell surface antigen in cancer of renal pelvis and ureter. *Urology* **22**: 366–8.

Magri, J. (1962). Partial cystectomy: a review of 104 cases. *British Journal of Urology* **34**: 74–87.

McDonald, J.R. and Priestley, J.T. (1944). Carcinoma of renal pelvis: histologic study of 75 cases with special reference to prognosis. *Journal of Urology* **51**: 245–58.

Melicow, M.M. (1945). Tumours of the urinary drainage tract: urothelial tumours. *Journal of Urology* **54**: 186–93.

Melicow, M.M. (1974). Tumours of the bladder: a multifaceted problem. *Journal of Urology* **112**: 467–78.

Miller, A., Mitchell, J.P. and Brown, N.J. (1969). The Bristol Bladder Tumour Registry. *British Journal of Urology* **41** (Suppl.): 17–43.

Miller, L.S. (1977). Bladder cancer: superiority of pre-operative irradiation and cystectomy in clinical stages B2 and C. *Cancer* **39**: 973–80.

Montie, J.E., Straffon, R.A. and Stewart, B.H. (1984). Radical cystectomy without radiation therapy for carcinoma of the bladder. *Journal of Urology* **131**: 477–81.

Morales, A., Ottenhoff, P. and Emerson, L. (1981). Treatment of residual, non-infiltrating bladder cancer with bacillus Calmette–Guerin. *Journal of Urology* **125**: 649–51.

Murphy, W.N., Crabtree, W.N., Jukkola, A.F. and Soloway, M.S. (1981). The diagnostic value of urine versus bladder washing in patients with bladder cancer. *Journal of Urology* **126**: 320–22.

Narayana, A.S., Loening, S.A., Slymen, D.J. and Culp, D.A. (1983). Bladder cancer: factors affecting survival. *Journal of Urology* **130**: 56–60.

Newman, D.M., Allen, L.E., Wishard, W.N., Nourse, M.H. and Mertz, J.H.O. (1967). Transitional cell carcinoma of the upper urinary tract. *Journal of Urology* **98**: 322–7.

Page, B.H., Levison, V.B. and Curwen, M.P. (1978). Site of recurrence of non-infiltrating bladder tumours. *British Journal of Urology* **50**: 237–42.

Parkes, H.G. (1975). Occupational bladder cancer. *Practitioner* **214**: 80–86.

Prout, G.R. (1984). Superficial bladder cancer. In *Bladder Cancer*, pp. 151–71. Edited by Smith, P.H. and Prout, G.R. Butterworth, London.

Pugh, R.C.B. (1973). The pathology of cancer of the bladder. *Cancer* **32**: 1267–74.

Pugh, R.C.B (1981). The diagnosis of carcinoma-in-situ of the urinary bladder. In *Recent Advances in Urology/Andrology*, vol. III, pp. 271–7. Edited by Hendry, W.F. Churchill Livingstone, Edinbugh.

Radwin, H.M. (1980). Radiotherapy and bladder cancer: critical review. *Journal of Urology* **124**: 43–6.

Riddle, P.R., Chisholm, G.D., Trott, P.A. and Pugh, R.C.B. (1976). Flat carcinoma-in-situ of bladder. *British Journal of Urology* **47**: 829–33.

Riddle, P.R. and Wallace, D.M. (1971). Inactivity chemotherapy for multiple non-invasive bladder tumours. *British Journal of Urology* **43**: 181–4.

Sarnacki, C.T., McCormack, L.J., Kiser, W.S., Hazard, J.B., McLaughlin, T.C. and Belovich, D.M. (1971). Urinary cytology and the clinical diagnosis of urinary tract malignancy: a clinico-pathologic study of 1400 patients. *Journal of Urology* **106**: 761–4.

Skinner, D.G., Tift, J.P. and Kaufman, J.J. (1982). High dose, short course pre-operative radiation therapy and immediate single stage radical cystectomy with pelvic node dissection in the management of bladder cancer. *Journal of Urology* **127**: 671–4.

Smith, G., Elton, R.A., Beynon, L.L., Newsam, J.E., Chisholm, G.D. and Hargreave, T.B. (1983). Prognostic significance of biopsy results of normal-looking mucosa in cases of superficial bladder cancer. *British Journal of Urology* **55**: 665–9.

Soloway, M.S. (1980). The management of superficial bladder cancer. *Cancer* **45**: 1856–65.

Soloway, M.S. and Ford, K.S. (1983). Subsequent tumour analysis of 36 patients who have received intravesical mitomycin C for superficial bladder cancer. *Journal of Urology* **130**: 74–7.

Studer, V.E., Biedermann, C., Chollet, D., Karrer, P., Kraft, R., Toggenberg, H. and Vonbank, F. (1984). Prevention of recurrent superficial bladder tumours by oral etretinate: preliminary results of a randomised, double blind multicenter trial in Switzerland. *Journal of Urology* **131**: 47–9.

Swanson, D.A., von Eschenbach, A.C., Bracken, R.B. and Johnson, D.E. (1981). Salvage cystectomy for bladder carcinoma. *Cancer* **46**: 2275–9.

Talavera, J.M., Carney, J.A. and Kelasis, P.P. (1970). Bilateral, synchronous, primary transitional cell carcinoma of the ureter: report of 2 cases and review of the literature. *Journal of Urology* **104**: 679–83.

Trott, P.A. (1971). Detection of urethral carcinoma using a soluble swab. *British Journal of Surgery* **58**: 66–9.

Trott, P.A. and Edwards, L. (1973). Comparison of bladder washings and urine cytology in the diagnosis of bladder cancer. *Journal of Urology* **110**: 664.

Turner, G.A., Hendry, W.F., MacDonald, J.S. and Wallace, D.M. (1976). The value of lymphography in the management of bladder cancer. *British Journal of Urology* **48**: 579–86.

Turner, A.G., Hendry, W.F., Williams, G.B. and Wallace, D.M. (1977a). A haematuria diagnostic service. *British Medical Journal* **2**: 29–31.

Turner, A.G., Hendry, W.F., Williams, G.B. and Bloom, H.J.G. (1977b). The treatment of advanced bladder cancer with methotrexate. *British Journal of Urology* **49**: 673–8.

Union Internationale Contre Cancer (1978). TNM classification of malignant tumours. Geneva, UICC.

Utz, D.C., Hanash, K.A. and Farrow, G.M. (1970). The plight of the patient with carcinoma-in-situ of the bladder. *Journal of Urology* **103**: 160–64.

Wallace, D.M. (1970). Uretero-ileostomy. *British Journal of Urology* **42**: 529–34.

Wallace, D.M. and Bloom, H.J.G. (1976). The management of deeply infiltrating (T3) bladder carcinoma: controlled trial of radical radiotherapy versus pre-operative radiotherapy and radical cystectomy (first report). *British Journal of Urology* **48**: 587–94.

Wallace, D.M. and Harris, D.L. (1965). Delay in treating bladder tumours. *Lancet* **2**: 332–4.

Wallace, D.M.A., Hindmarsh, J.R., Webb, J.N., Busuttil, A., Hargreave, T.B., Newsam, J.E. and Chisholm, G.D. (1979). The role of multiple mucosal biopsies in the management of patients with bladder cancer. *British Journal of Urology* **51**: 535–40.

Werf-Messing, B. van der (1973). Carcinoma of the bladder treated by pre-operative irradiation followed by cystectomy. *Cancer* **32**: 1084–8.

Whitmore, W.F. (1969). Combined radiotherapy and surgical treatment. *Journal of the American Medical Association* **207**: 349–50.

Whitmore, W.F. and Marshall, V.F. (1962). Radical total cystectomy for cancer of bladder: 230 consecutive cases five years later. *Journal of Urology* **87**: 853–68.

WHO (1973). Histological typing of urinary bladder tumours. World Health Organisation, Geneva.

Williams, C.B. and Mitchell, J.P. (1973a). Carcinoma of the renal pelvis: a review of 43 cases. *British Journal of Urology* **45**: 370–76.

Williams, C.B. and Mitchell, J.P. (1973b). Carcinoma of the ureter: a review of 54 cases. *British Journal of Urology* **45**: 377–87.

Wolk, F.N. and Bishop, M.C. (1983). The specific red cell adherence test in transitional cell carcinoma of the bladder before and after radiotherapy in patients with blood group A. *Journal of Urology* **130**: 71–3.

5

Non-invasive investigation of the patient with bladder cancer

Janet E. Husband

Introduction

Non-invasive imaging, which includes radionucleide scanning, ultrasound, computed tomography (CT) and now magnetic resonance imaging (MRI), has been one of the most exciting fields of development in the management of patients with cancer during recent years. With respect to bladder cancer both ultrasound and CT may be employed to assess the primary tumour as well as the presence of metastatic disease, whereas radionucleide scanning is restricted to the detection of metastases in the liver, bone and brain. Thus, all these techniques can provide overlapping information and the clinician may be faced with the dilemma of whether to refer a patient for radionucleide scanning, for ultrasound or CT, or whether to perform all the tests with the hope that one will provide additional information with respect to the others. The decision to employ ultrasound or CT in a given clinical situation will also depend on the availability of equipment as well as on the expertise and experience of personnel in the imaging department.

The value of MRI with regard to body imaging has not been firmly established. However, the technique may provide new information in some aspects of pelvic pathology; for example, by providing images of tumours in the coronal and sagittal planes for radiotherapy planning, and by detecting the presence of persistent or recurrent tumour in patients who have developed postirradiation pelvic fibrosis (Hricak *et al.*, 1983; Fisher *et al.*, 1985).

Staging

Optimum treatment of bladder cancer is a major challenge to the clinician as survival rates have not improved significantly over the last few decades (Schmidt and Weinstein, 1976; Oliver *et al.*, 1981; Narayana *et al.*, 1983). Apart from tumour grading, a critical factor determining survival is the depth of tumour infiltration, and accurate staging is therefore of paramount importance for appropriate management (Jewett and Strong, 1946). Traditional methods of staging bladder cancer have been disappointing, with failure to demonstrate the extent of local tumour spread in up to 30–35 per cent of patients (Richie *et al.*, 1975; Schmidt and Weinstein, 1976; Prout 1977). These conventional methods of staging include cytoscopy with biopsy, transurethral resection and bimanual examination under general anaesthesia. Arteriography with intravesical and perivesical air insufflation has also been used in some centres but this has not gained widespread acceptance; it is now rarely employed because it is invasive and carries a certain risk. Other investigations used include intravenous urography, chest radiography, lymphangiography, bone and liver radionucleide scanning and ultrasound scanning of the liver. Although ultrasound is now being used in several centres to assess the primary tumour, CT is more widely used and is currently employed as an additional staging procedure on a routine basis in many departments. For this reason emphasis will be placed on the findings of CT in bladder cancer but the relationship of ultrasound and CT will also be discussed. The findings will be described according to the TNM classification (UICC, 1978; see Chapter 4).

Primary tumours

Computed tomography

As with all pelvic CT examinations, meticulous attention to technique is essential if optimum results are to be obtained. All patients are scanned with a full bladder and dilute oral contrast medium is given at least one hour before the scan to opacify the small bowel. Rectal contrast medium is also helpful, particularly in patients with posterior bladder tumours. In female patients a tampon is placed in the vagina to delineate the vaginal vault. A computed radiograph is taken routinely for preliminary localization. This view is also used after the examination to relate the position of the CT slices demonstrating the tumour and bladder to anatomical bony landmarks for radiotherapy planning. (Fig. 5.1).

Intravenous contrast medium is used routinely in many centres for evaluating bladder tumours because it delineates the bladder lumen with positive contrast and shows the position of the ureters. However, it is our practice to take an initial series of scans without contrast medium because the difference in density between the urine and bladder wall is usually sufficient to identify the tumour, and the use of intraluminal contrast medium does not influence the ability to detect extravesical extension. Intravenous contrast medium should be given to solve specific problems encountered on the first series of scans. For example, bladder opacification is helpful for evaluating tumours at the bladder base or dome which may otherwise be difficult to identify because the tumour has a similar density to the bladder wall. (Fig. 5.2).

Several authors have recommended special techniques for investigating bladder cancer with the intention of improving the contrast between the bladder lumen and the tumour. Seidelman *et al.* (1978) reported a series of patients in whom the bladder was filled with carbon dioxide prior to the CT examination, and others have used fat emulsion and peanut oil (Hidell *et al.*, 1981; Sager *et al.*, 1983). Double-contrast techniques using either carbon dioxide or air with dilute contrast medium introduced by a Foley catheter have also been employed (Hamlin *et al.*, 1981; Morgan *et al.*, 1981). Those who advocate these techniques state that the advantage of the double-contrast method is that polypoid soft-tissue masses can be clearly delineated

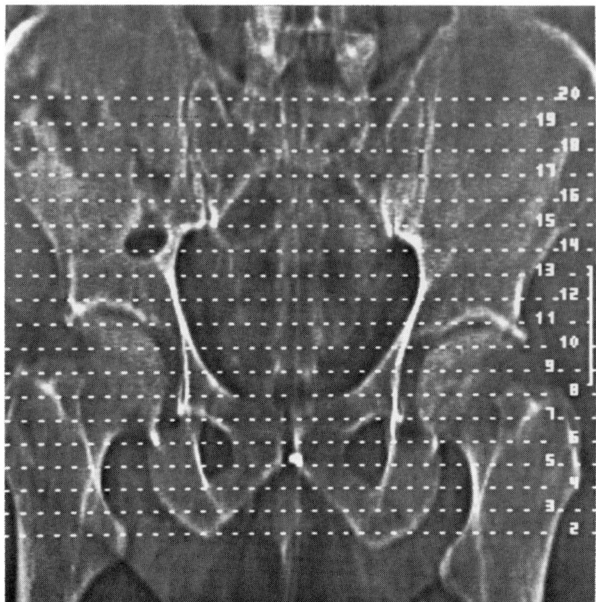

Fig. 5.1 Computed radiograph showing the position and number of CT slices taken for assessment of a patient with bladder cancer

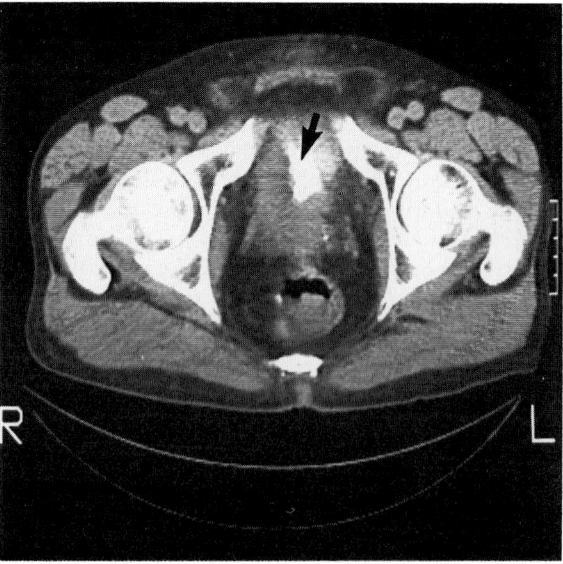

Fig. 5.2 A patient with a large tumour involving the bladder base. The bladder lumen (arrowed) has been opacified with contrast medium to delineate tumour extent

from the bladder lumen because contrast medium coats the inner surface of the bladder wall. However, the major role of CT is the detection of extravesical tumour spread since intraluminal tumour is still best evaluated at cystoscopy. The possible small advantage offered by these specialized techniques must be weighed against the major drawback that catheterization is required (which is unpleasant for the patient, increases the risk of urinary tract infection and prolongs the examination time).

For staging bladder cancer, high-dose scanning techniques should be employed to provide the highest quality images. A small field of view further improves spatial resolution. If scanning is employed for radiotherapy planning, the field of view must contain the whole body contour. Contiguous slices of 8–10 mm thickness are taken through the pelvis to the middle of the 5th lumbar vertebra. If a small tumour is identified, thin slices of 4–6 mm collimation may be repeated through the region of interest. An advantage of using contiguous thin slices is that good-quality reconstructed images in the longitudinal and oblique planes can be obtained from the cross-sectional scans (Fig. 5.3). Occasionally altering the patient's position may be helpful, particularly for evaluation of tumours at the bladder base if prostatic or rectal invasion is suspected. In many centres the CT examination is extended to include the abdomen. CT slices at 1.5 or 1.6 cm intervals are usually sufficient for identification of retroperitoneal lymphadenopathy or hydronephrosis. If liver metastases are suspected the liver should be examined using 8 or 10 mm contiguous slices.

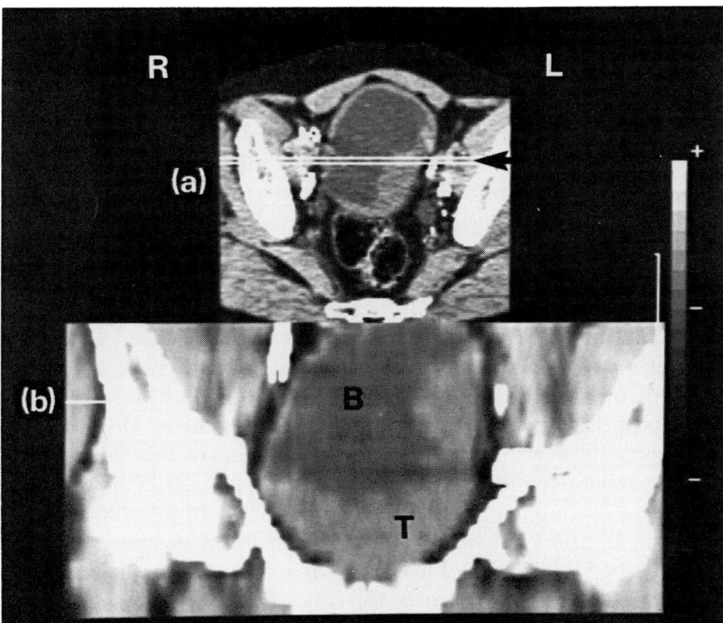

Fig. 5.3 (a) is a CT scan showing tumour occupying the left lateral and posterior bladder walls. Multiple CT sections through the bladder can be reconstructed in the coronal plane (black arrow). (b) shows the final reconstruction in the coronal plane. Bladder (B), tumour (T)

CT findings

The intraluminal component of bladder tumour is shown on CT as a soft tissue mass projecting into the bladder lumen. Occasionally, the surface of the tumour is encrusted with calcium or with blood clot (Fig. 5.4). The configuration of the tumour may be sessile, peduncular or may appear simply as a localized area of bladder wall thickening (Fig. 5.5).

With CT, tumours involving the lamina propria cannot be distinguished from those involving superficial muscle and the technique is also unreliable for distinguishing superficial from deep-muscle invasion. Thus, the technique is impractical for staging tumours less than T3A (Hodson *et al.*, 1979; Jeffrey *et al.*, 1981; Morgan *et al.*, 1981) and its major advantage lies in the ability to distinguish extravesical spread from those tumours confined to the bladder wall. Extravesical tumour spread is identified in early cases by an increase in density of the perivesical fat in the region of the tumour and because the tumour itself has an irregular ill-defined outer aspect (see Fig. 5.4(b)). Thin slices are helpful if there is doubt regarding the presence of extravesical extension, and careful comparison of the abnormal area with normal portions of the bladder wall is also useful. In more advanced cases of extravesical tumour spread there is little difficulty in making the diagnosis (Fig. 5.6) as soft-tissue tumour is seen as a mass extending beyond the pelvic fat. Spread to the pelvic side wall (T4B) is diagnosed if the tumour extends through the pelvic fat and is continuous with the pelvic side wall muscles; for example, the obturator internus muscle (Fig. 5.7). Since there is no clear fat plane between the bladder wall and such organs as the uterus, prostate, rectum and vagina, invasion of adjacent organs (T4A) can be difficult to identify. Caution should therefore be exercised in diagnosing invasion of organs unless the structure is partially or completely surrounded by tumour (Fig. 5.8). Invasion of the seminal vesicles is easier to identify because there is a fat angle between the posterior bladder wall and the anterior surface of the seminal vesicles; this has been termed the seminal vesicle fat angle (Seidelman *et al.*, 1978). Tumours extending into the seminal vesicle obliterate this fat angle by contiguous tumour spread (Fig. 5.9).

The major drawbacks of CT for staging bladder cancer are the difficulties of identifying minimal extravesical tumour spread and spread of tumour into adjacent organs. However, other limitations of the technique may be encountered in patients who have previously been investigated by cystoscopy or treated with radiotherapy. If endoscopy has been carried out within a few days prior to the CT examination, oedema and inflammation of the bladder wall may be misinterpreted as tumour. Furthermore, blood clot in the bladder may simulate an intraluminal tumour mass (Hodson *et al.*, 1979). Patients who have previously been treated with radiotherapy present a particular problem because irradiation decreases bladder capacity and produces thickening of the bladder wall and generalized increase in perivascular tissue density (Fig. 5.10). These features make the diagnosis of persistent or recurrent tumour within the bladder wall frequently impossible.

Rarely bladder cancer may develop in a diverticulum or in a persistent urachus and these anomalies may also lead to difficulty in interpretation of the CT appearances (Figs. 5.5 and 5.11).

Although hydronephrosis and ureteric dilatation can be demonstrated

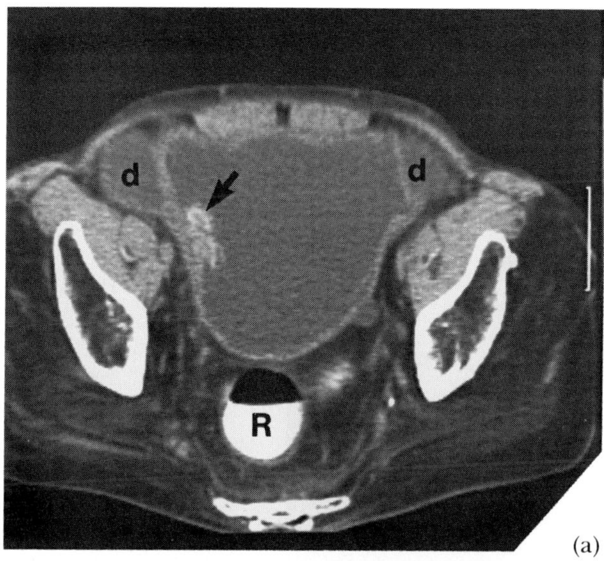

(a)

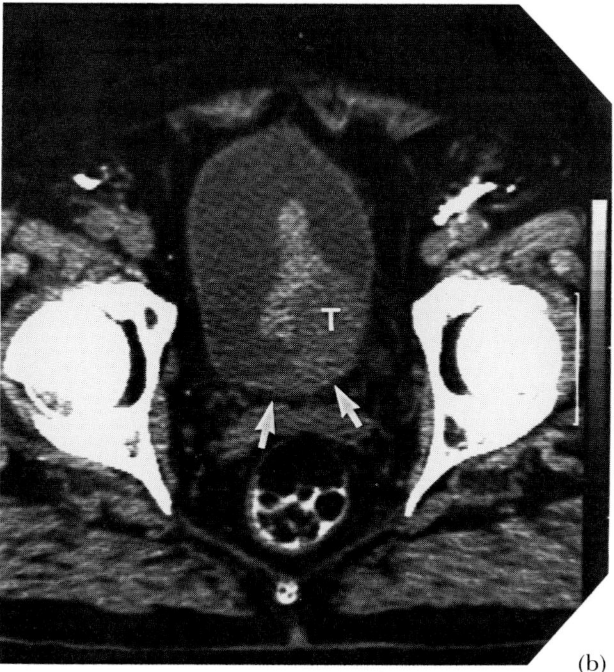

(b)

Fig. 5.4 (a) Small tumour on the right bladder wall. Note high-density calcification encrusted on the inner surface (arrowed). The bladder shows bilateral diverticula (d), contrast in rectum (R). (b) Intraluminal bladder tumour (T) has a soft-tissue density. The higher-density material on the surface of the tumour represents blood clot. Note the irregular outer aspect of the tumour, indicating early extravesical extension (arrowed)

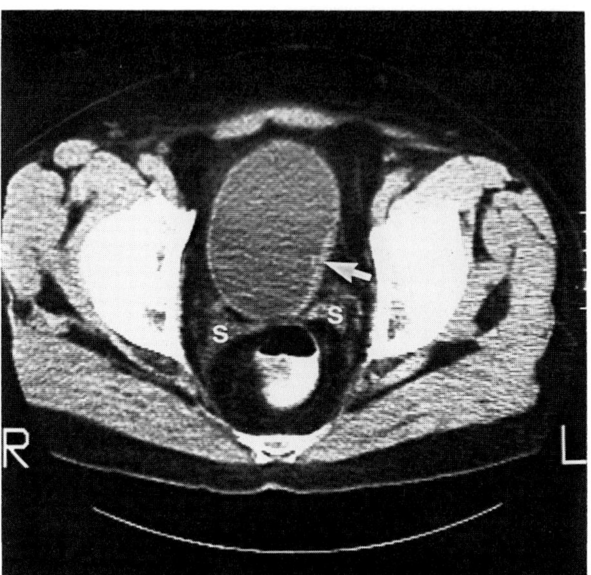

Fig. 5.5 In this patient the only abnormality demonstrated is slight thickening of the left bladder wall (arrowed). The seminal vesicles are clearly shown (s)

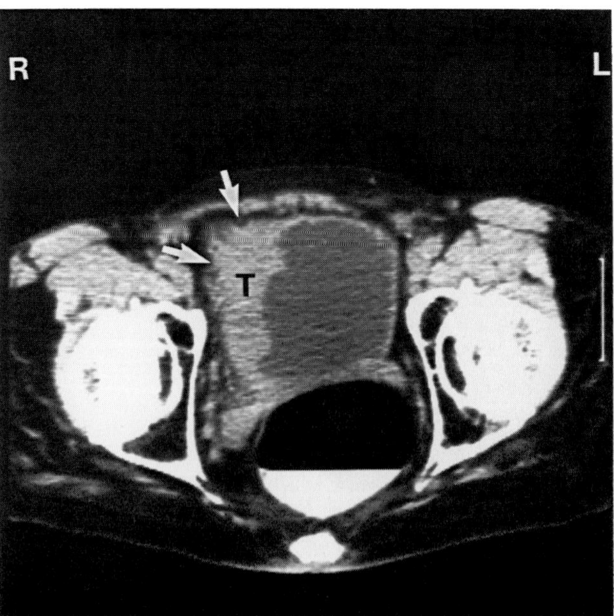

Fig. 5.6 CT scan showing a large tumour occupying the right bladder wall. The tumour (T) clearly extends into the perivesical fat (arrowed)

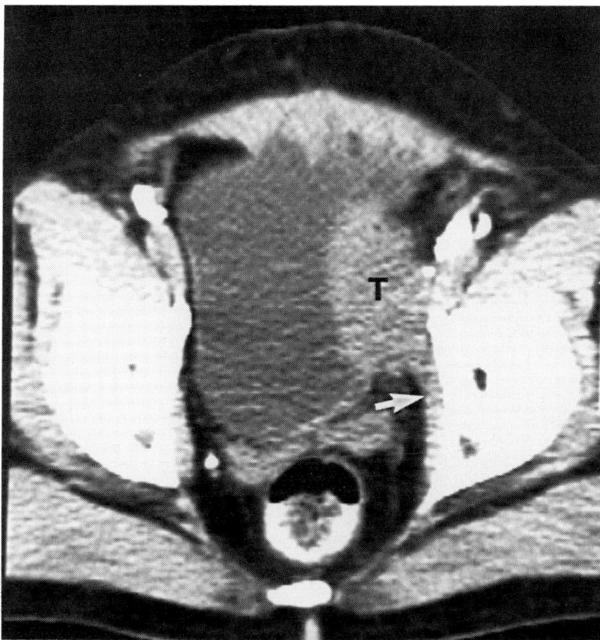

Fig. 5.7 Bladder tumour (T) spreading through the extravesical fat as far as the pelvic side wall where it is continuous with the obturator internus muscle (arrowed)

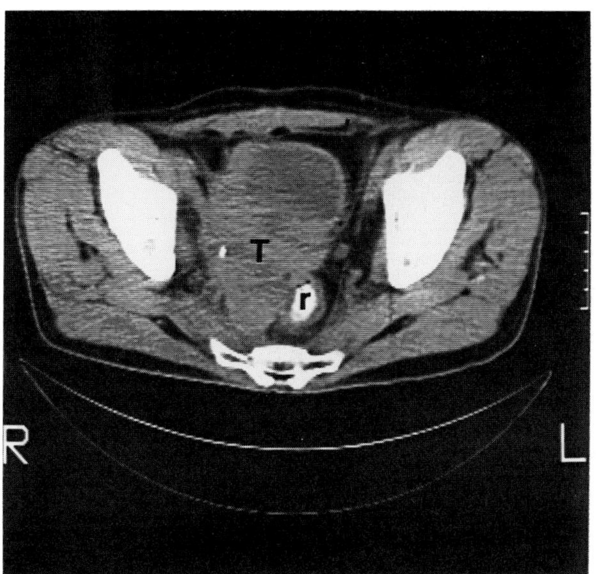

Fig. 5.8 CT scan showing an advanced bladder tumour (T) which has spread posteriorly. The rectum (r) is displaced to the left and is almost certainly invaded by tumour

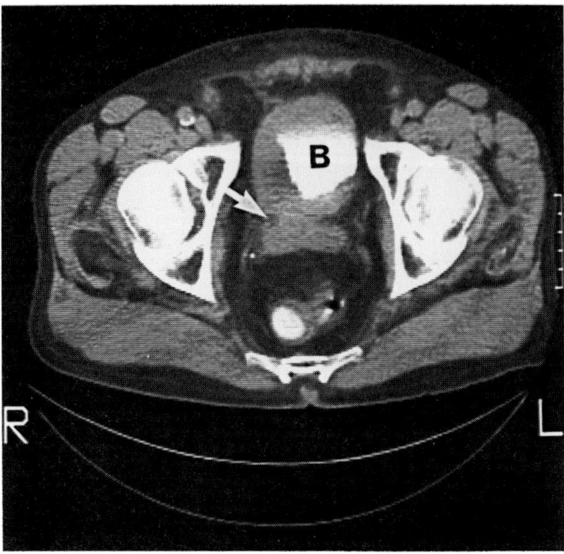

Fig. 5.9 CT scan showing tumour involvement of the right lateral and posterior bladder walls. The seminal vesicle angle on the right is obliterated by tumour extension (arrowed). The bladder (B) is opacified with contrast medium

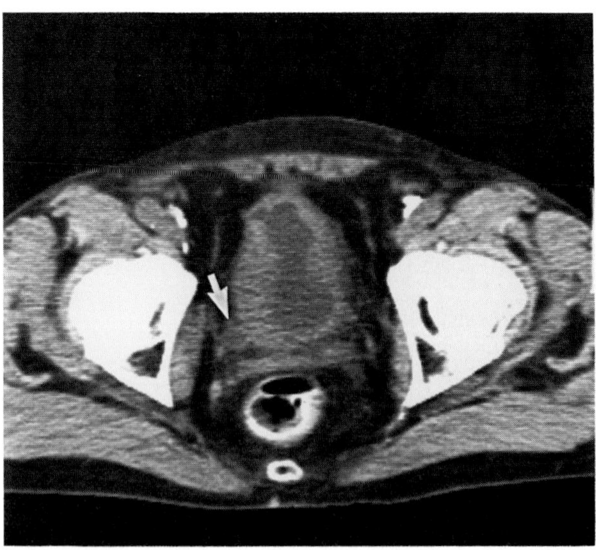

Fig. 5.10 CT scan following radiotherapy. The bladder capacity is reduced and the whole of the bladder wall is irregularly thickened. Note the dilated ureter on the patient's right side (arrowed)

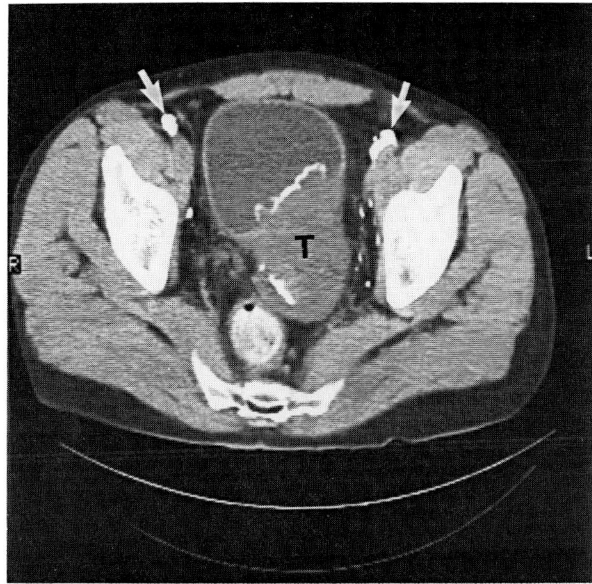

Fig. 5.11 A large tumour (T) arising in a posterior bladder diverticulum. Note calcification encrusted on the intraluminal surface of the tumour and also within the diverticulum. External iliac nodes have been opacified at lymphography (arrowed)

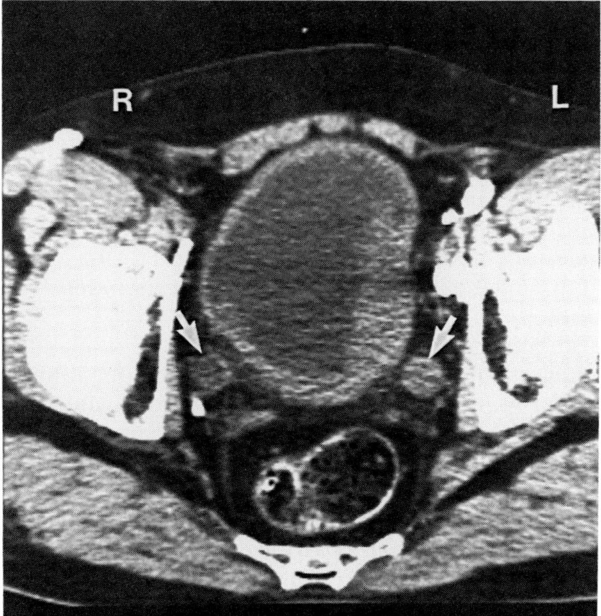

Fig. 5.12 CT scan showing tumour occupying the left lateral and posterior bladder walls. The ureters are dilated (arrowed). The left ureter contains soft-tissue tumour

with CT, minimal degrees of obstruction are better shown at intravenous urography. A bladder tumour extending into the lower ureter may, however, be occasionally identified on CT (Fig. 5.12).

Differential diagnosis
CT is usually used for staging bladder cancer in patients in whom the diagnosis has been proved histologically. However, a diagnostic problem occasionally exists in the distinction of a primary prostatic cancer from a primary bladder tumour. In this situation, CT is usually unhelpful in determining the origin of the tumour because a large prostate cancer invading the bladder may have identical appearances to a bladder cancer invading the prostate. Other primary tumours which involve the bladder, such as carcinoma of the cervix or colon, can usually be distinguished from a primary bladder tumour because the major part of the tumour lies outside the bladder wall. Metastases to the bladder (for example, melanoma) or other rare tumours such as phaeochromocytoma or leiomyosarcoma have identical appearances to a primary bladder cancer (Fig. 5.13). Malacoplakia of the bladder is an uncommon condition representing granulomatous inflammation of the bladder wall. Although this is a benign condition the appearances are also similar to a primary bladder cancer (Fig. 5.14).

Ultrasound

Transabdominal ultrasound is used effectively for staging bladder tumours in several centres (Morley, 1979; Singer et al., 1981). As with CT, meticulous attention to technique is essential and a full bladder is mandatory. One of the main advantages of transabdominal ultrasound compared with CT is that the bladder may be examined in multiple planes, which is particularly helpful for assessing tumours at the bladder dome and bladder base. Recently, transurethral and transrectal ultrasound techniques have been introduced and are considered to be more accurate for superficial tumours than transabdominal ultrasound (Schuller et al., 1982). The main disadvantage of these techniques is that they are invasive, and furthermore transurethral ultrasound must be undertaken at cystoscopy under general anaesthesia. A further limitation of an intraluminal ultrasound probe is that it is of little value for lesions which extend beyond the penetration depth of the ultrasound beam (Schuller et al., 1982).

Using ultrasound techniques the intraluminal portion of a bladder tumour appears as an echogenic lesion projecting into the bladder lumen. The bladder wall has stronger/more intense echoes than tumour tissue, thus permitting detection of early-stage tumour. Thus, in T1 tumours the echogenic bladder wall appears smooth and uninterrupted by tumour (Abu-Youssef et al., 1984). With T2 and T3A tumours the bladder wall is interrupted either partially or completely by the tumour mass. Infiltrating tumours extending into the perivesical fat (T3B) are seen as a relatively echogenic mass spreading through the bladder wall into the adjacent tissues (Fig. 5.15).

The main advantage of ultrasound over CT is the possibility of staging early tumours more accurately (Nakamura and Niijima, 1980; Abu-Youssef et al., 1984). However, several factors lead to errors of staging with

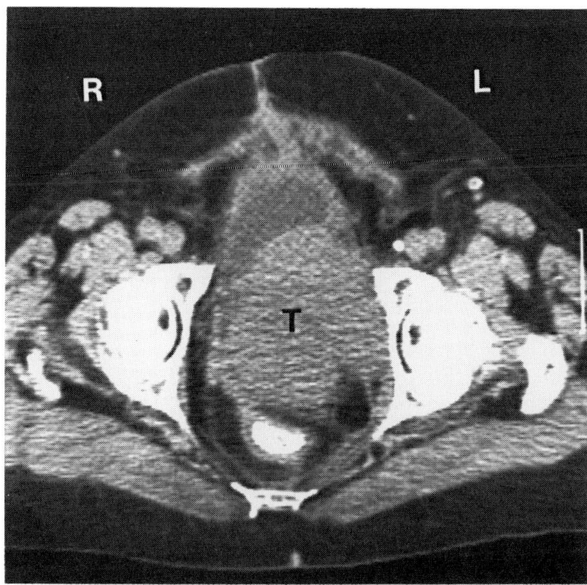

Fig. 5.13 Leiomyosarcoma of the bladder. The tumour (T) is fixed to the left pelvic side wall

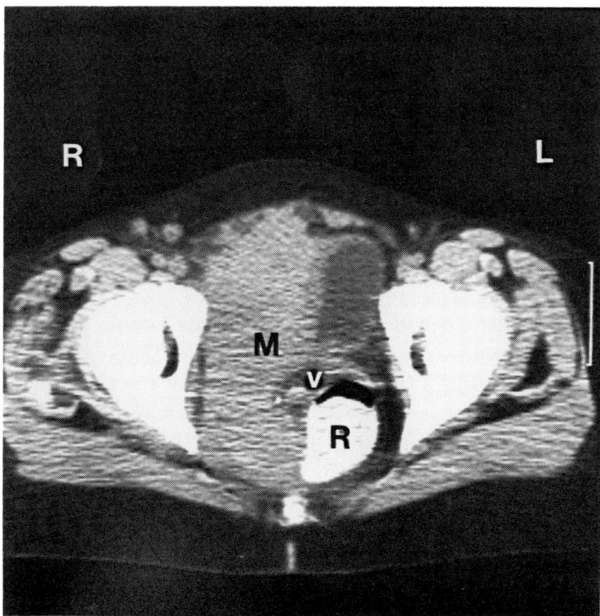

Fig. 5.14 Malacoplakia of the bladder. The mass (M) extends beyond the bladder to the anterior abdominal wall and also displaces the vagina (v) and rectum (R) to the left

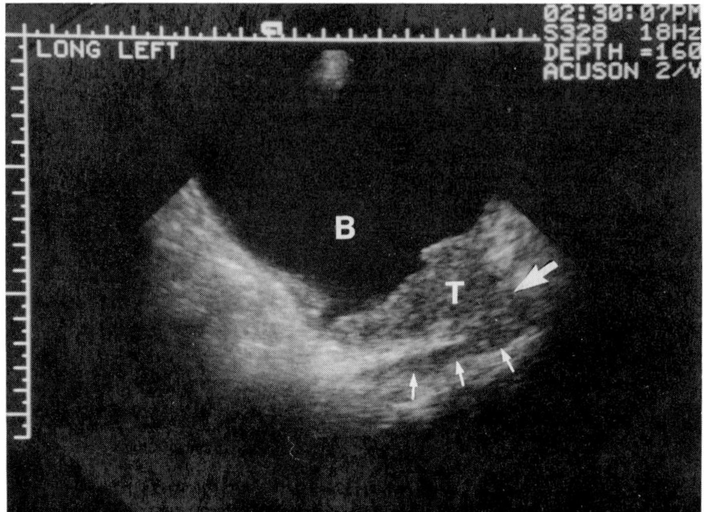

Fig. 5.15 Transabdominal ultrasound (transverse section) showing a large bladder tumour (T) extending through the posterior bladder wall (arrowed) and involving the seminal vesicles (small arrows). Bladder (B)

ultrasound. These include the difficulty of assessment of tumours in obese patients, tumours close to the anterior abdominal wall and those extending into the perivesical tissues close to bone. Similar difficulties are encountered to those with CT in patients who have undergone radiotherapy or have recently undergone transurethral resection (Winger *et al.*, 1981).

With ultrasound the presence of hydronephrosis and ureteric dilatation is readily assessed at the time of staging the primary tumour (Fig. 5.16).

Accuracy

Several studies have reported the accuracy of ultrasound and CT compared with clinical and histopathological staging in carcinoma of the bladder. The overall accuracy of CT ranges from 64 to 92 per cent (Koss *et al.*, 1981; Morgan *et al.*, 1981) and in a series reported by Abu-Youssef *et al.* (1984) the accuracy with transabdominal ultrasound approached 95 per cent. However, there is considerable disparity between results expressed from different centres using the various techniques. For example, in a series reported by Singer *et al.* (1981), a staging accuracy of nearly 100 per cent was achieved with transabdominal ultrasound for deep tumours of the bladder wall or those penetrating into the extravesical tissues, whereas many superficial tumours were overstaged with an accuracy of less than 60 per cent. Using intravesical ultrasound, Schuller *et al.* (1982) found that the technique was more accurate for superficial tumours than for those which have just extended through the bladder wall. It is difficult to make direct comparison between the results of CT and ultrasound—not only does the equipment vary in different studies, but the patient selection also varies. In some series, patients are examined following radiotherapy and this leads to errors of overstaging (Kellett *et al.*, 1980). For example, Vock *et al.* (1982) reported

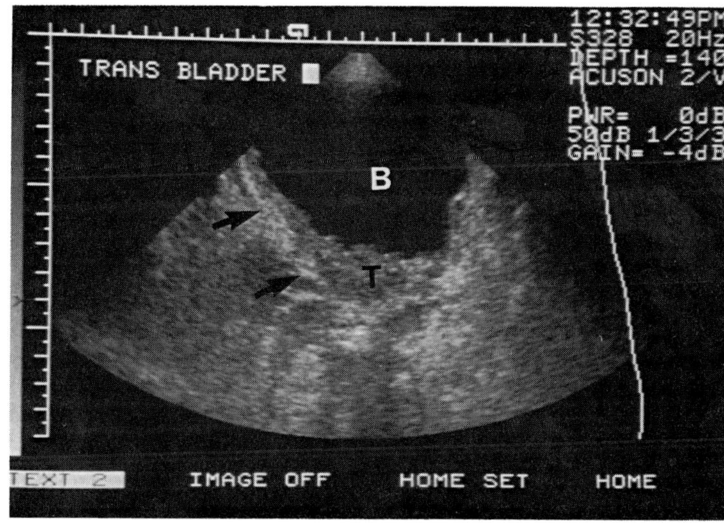

(a)

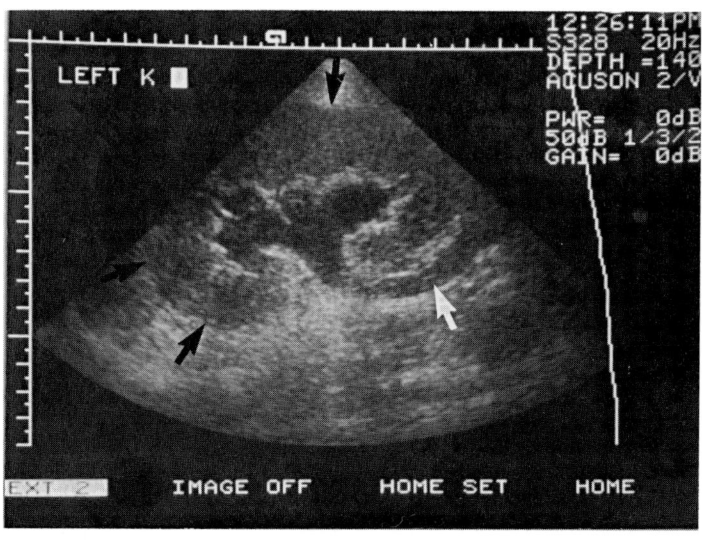

(b)

Fig. 5.16 Transabdominal ultrasound in a patient with bladder cancer. (a) Transverse section through the pelvis shows the bladder (B) and the tumour (T) arising on the posterior bladder wall. There is posterior extension of tumour. The bladder wall (arrowed) is interrupted. (b) Longitudinal section through the right kidney in the same patient showing hydronephrosis and dilatation of the right ureter. Renal outline (black arrow), dilated ureter (white arrow)

that CT overstaged 14 of 77 patients (80 per cent), all of whom had undergone radiotherapy before evaluation. Errors due to understaging are also important and account for many of the incorrect results in untreated patients. These errors occur because neither ultrasound nor CT can detect minimal or microscopic invasion of the perivesical fat. With ultrasound, detection of tumour spread to the anterior abdominal wall and pelvic side walls is less reliable than with CT (Abu-Youssef *et al.*, 1984).

Although errors with both ultrasound and CT are inevitable, these techniques can provide superior information to clinical staging alone. With CT the accuracy increases significantly in advanced disease: Vock *et al.* (1982) found that CT was correct in all 10 cases of stage-4 tumours. With clinical staging it is frequently impossible to distinguish T3A from T3B disease, and even if there is a palpable mass outside the bladder, fixation to the pelvic side wall or involvement of seminal vesicles may not be identified. We compared CT staging with clinical staging in 75 patients and found that CT was able to identify definite extravesical tumour spread in 23 out of 36 patients (64 per cent) with clinical stage T3 tumours (Husband and Hodson, 1981). Thus, in our view, CT should be undertaken in all patients as part of the initial staging investigation, but ultrasound may provide equally accurate results in those centres where appropriate expertise and experience is available.

Lymph node metastases

Carcinoma of the bladder spreads initially to the regional pelvic lymph nodes; those first involved include the anterior and lateral perivesical nodes, the hypogastric, obturator, external iliac and lateral sacral nodes. In more advanced disease, lymph nodes in the common iliac, para-aortic and inguinal chains are involved. The presence of lymph node metastases is rare in superficial tumours (up to T3A). If deep muscle is involved, the incidence of metastases approaches 20–30 per cent and rises to 50–60 per cent in patients with extravesical extension (van der Werf-Messing, 1982). The volume of the primary tumour is also important since the number and size of involved nodes and the risk of haematogenous spread increases with the size of the primary tumour (Dretler *et al.*, 1973).

Until the introduction of CT some twelve years ago, lymphography was the only method of assessing lymph node involvement prior to surgery. However, CT has now challenged the use of lymphography and the results of CT in different tumour types are such that there has been a dramatic reduction in the use of lymphography. In general terms the main drawbacks of lymphography are that it is an invasive procedure, may be time-consuming to perform and difficult to interpret. The internal iliac and obturator nodes are not opacified, and since these are the first nodes to be involved in carcinoma of the bladder lymphography has a further important drawback. In addition, false-negative examinations result from microscopic metastases in normal sized nodes and false-positive examinations from misinterpretation of filling defects in those nodes which are opacified. In lymphography, lymph node metastases are identified by alteration of the architecture of the nodes as well as by enlargement; but with CT, enlargement is the only criterion for involvement. Using CT, enlarged nodes can be detected in the internal iliac, the external iliac and obturator chains, and nodes 1.5 cm in diameter or greater are considered to be enlarged (Fig. 5.17). With CT, metastases in normal or minimally enlarged nodes may be missed and, similar to lymphography, microscopic metastases cannot be identified. It may be impossible to distinguish enlargement due to tumour from other causes of lymphadenopathy such as benign hyperplasia; normal structures (such as vessels or small bowel loops) may be misinterpreted as enlarged nodes on a CT scan.

Overall, the reported accuracy of lymphography in the detection of lymph node metastases from pelvic cancers ranges from 48 to 94 per cent (Cerney *et al.*, 1975; Wajsman *et al.*, 1975; O'Donoghue *et al.*, 1976; Hilaris *et al.*, 1977; Loening *et al.*, 1977; Spellman *et al.*, 1977; Vock *et al.*, 1982) and the accuracy for CT ranges from 70 to 93 per cent (Walsh *et al.*, 1980; Golimbu *et al.*, 1981; Koss *et al.*, 1981; Levine *et al.*, 1981; Morgan *et al.*, 1981; Vock *et al.*, 1982; Weinerman *et al.*, 1982). Thus, in general, both techniques appear to provide similar orders of accuracy in the detection of lymph node metastases, and it is not surprising that there has been much controversy regarding their relative roles in the assessment of pelvic cancers. In the author's view, if CT is being undertaken to assess the primary tumour and multiple enlarged nodes are identified, then lymphography is not required. Histological confirmation may be obtained by percutaneous biopsy under CT control. If the CT examination is negative or equivocal, lymphography may be useful for identifying metastases in normal or only minimally enlarged nodes. However, if the urologist chooses to undertake lymphadenectomy, lymphography may be superfluous. Ultrasound is less reliable than lymphography and CT in the detection of pelvic lymph node metastases, and it is perhaps partly for this reason that CT is more widely used than ultrasound to assess the primary tumour.

Distant metastases

In bladder cancer, haematogenous spread to the lungs, bone and liver is seen quite frequently. Distant metastases occur late and investigation is usually carried out for suspected metastases in a definite site. Bone metastases are detected on conventional radiographs or by radionucleide scanning and CT is rarely required. Occasionally, however, CT is helpful for demonstrating a deposit which may otherwise be difficult to identify, for example in the sacrum or vertebral body (Fig. 5.18).

Lung metastases in bladder cancer are usually diagnosed on the plain chest film, and since their incidence at presentation is low, CT of the lungs is not indicated as an initial staging investigation (unless cystectomy is being considered [Ed.]).

In patients with involved pelvic nodes on the initial CT scan, the study should be extended to include the para-aortic region and the liver. The accuracy of CT for detecting liver metastases is similar to that of ultrasound (Snow *et al.*, 1979; Alderson *et al.*, 1981; Knopf *et al.*,1982). In patients with clinical suspicion of liver metastases during the course of their disease, radionucleide scanning may be performed. Even if multiple lesions are identified, ultrasound or CT is required to determine whether the lesions represent cysts or solid liver tumours (Stanley *et al.*, 1977).

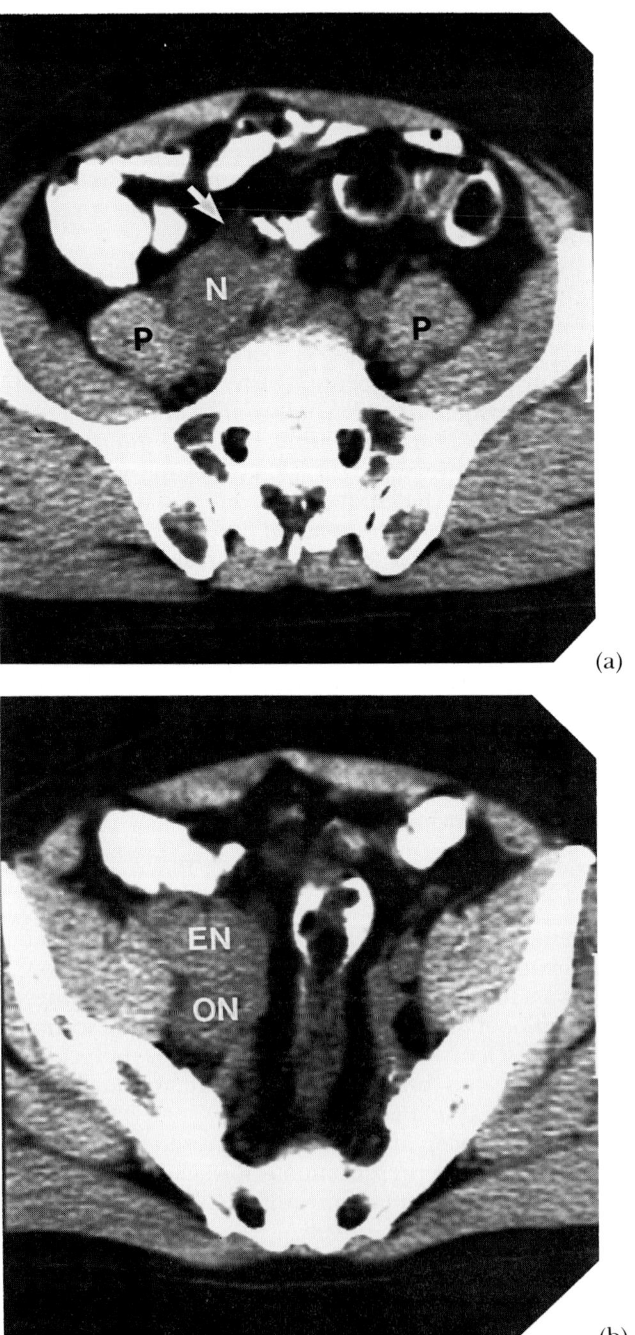

(a)

(b)

Fig. 5.17 CT scan in a patient with carcinoma of the bladder. (a) The right common iliac nodes (N) are enlarged. Note dilated right ureter (arrowed), psoas muscles (P). (b) The external iliac nodes (EN) and the obturator nodes (ON) are also enlarged

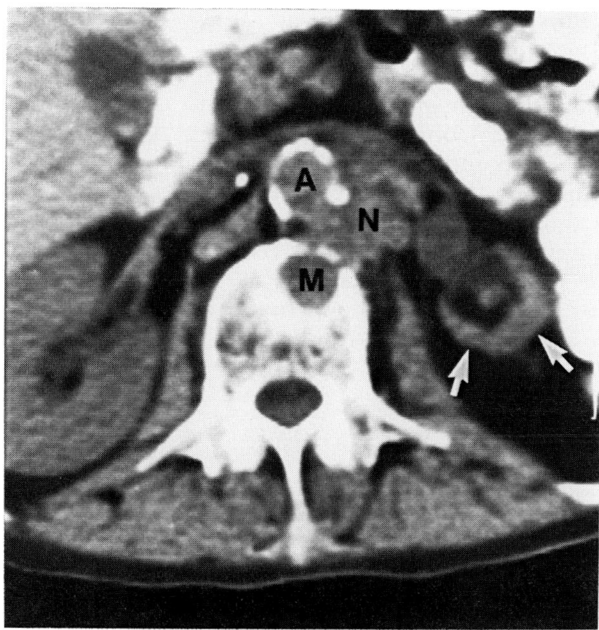

Fig. 5.18 CT scan of a patient with recurrent bladder cancer. The left kidney is atrophic (arrowed). There is enlargement of the para-aortic nodes (N). There is also a metastasis in the anterior aspect of the vertebral body (M). The aorta (A) is calcified

Radiotherapy treatment planning

In those patients selected for external-beam irradiation, CT scanning plays an important role in determining tumour extent and provides an accurate cross-sectional display of the tumour and related normal anatomy. If the whole pelvis is to be treated, CT is not required to define the target volume. The technique is reserved for small-volume treatment planning. Small-volume treatment includes a 1.5–2 cm margin around the bladder and such tumour extension as is detected by CT. The patient empties his bladder before the CT examination and also before treatment on each day to ensure that the tumour remains within the planned treatment volume. A skin tattoo is placed over the symphysis pubis and marked with barium paste with two additional lateral tattoos placed over the iliac crest. The patient is scanned in the treatment position with the bladder full for diagnostic purposes. The bladder is then emptied and the CT examination repeated, ensuring that the whole body contour is contained within the field of view. Using the CT planning integrated system the image through the centre of the tumour/bladder is used to obtain the patient body contour, treatment of volume and localization of the rectum and femoral heads (Fig. 5.19). CT sections at different levels are used to check that the tumour is encompassed within the planned volume throughout its length.

Several studies have compared conventional tumour localization with CT integrated planning (Munzenrider *et al.*, 1977; Ragan and Perez, 1978; Goitein *et al.*, 1979) and have demonstrated that CT has improved the accuracy of tumour localization. In one series, CT led to changes in the treatment volume compared with conventional planning in 33 per cent of patients (Dobbs *et al.*, 1983). Recently, Rothwell *et al.* (1985) have analysed treatment results according to the accuracy of tumour localization for radiotherapy with and without CT. They have shown a significant improvement in survival in those patients whose tumour received 90 per cent or more of the prescribed dose, as delineated by CT. These results are encouraging and support the view that the expense of high technology is justified to provide more accurate tumour localization.

Monitoring treatment response

Following initial investigation and staging with CT the technique may be employed to determine therapeutic response. Immediately following radiotherapy there is oedema of the bladder wall which renders the examination difficult to interpret. It is therefore recommended that CT or ultrasound examination should be carried out approximately six weeks after the completion of radiotherapy, although radiation fibrosis may have already developed with accompanying reduction of bladder capacity. However, if the patient has previously undergone CT or ultrasound, regression or resolution of a tumour can usually be assessed (Fig. 5.20). Although precise volume measurements of bladder tumours is difficult

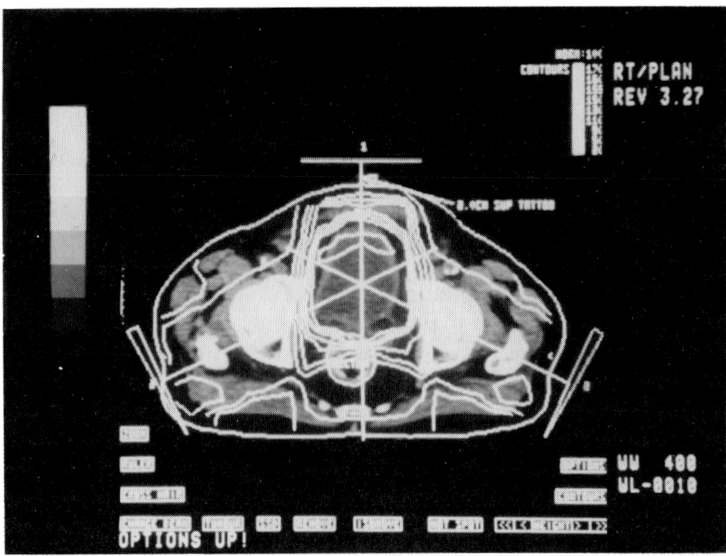

Fig. 5.19 CT scan of a patient with bladder cancer. The treatment volume and position of the beams are superimposed on the CT image

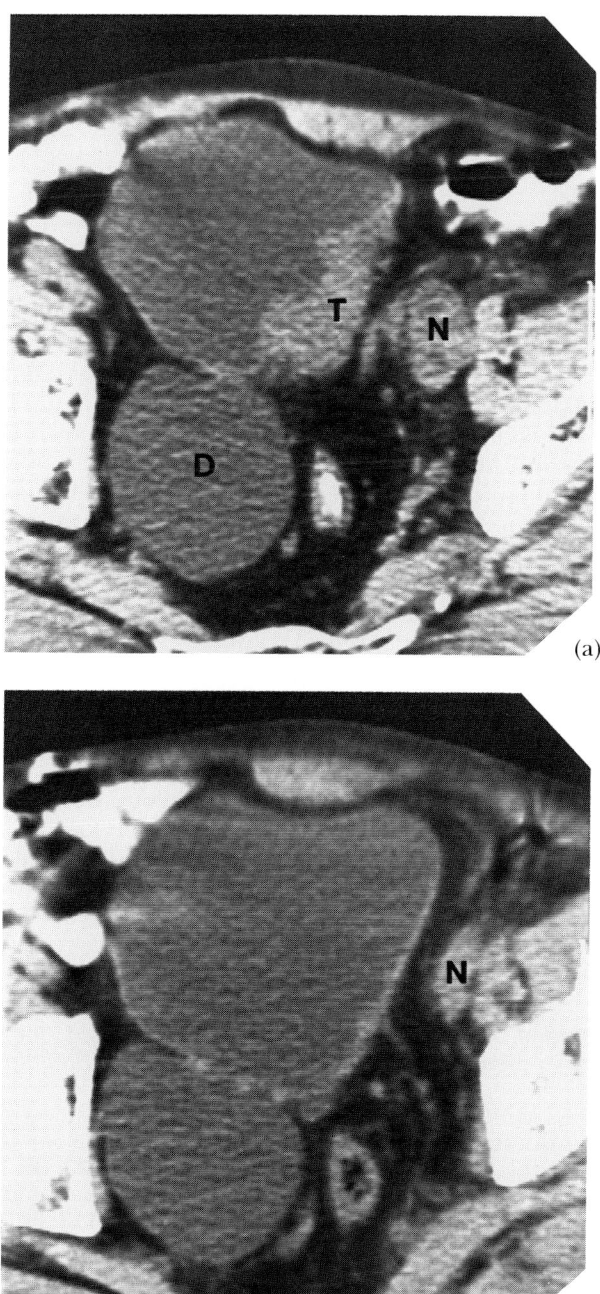

Fig. 5.20 (a) CT scan in a patient with a T3B bladder tumour (T). There is an enlarged external iliac node (N). Note bladder diverticulum (D). (b) A follow-up CT scan three months later shows excellent tumour regression. There is now only minimal thickening of the bladder wall. The enlarged node (N) has also regressed

owing to irregularity of contour and variation of bladder size, it is usually possible to make a qualitative assessment regarding percentage reduction of tumour. Changes in size of lymph node metastases may also be assessed with CT provided the involved nodes are at least 2 cm in diameter on the initial scan.

Conclusions

The introduction of non-invasive imaging is an important advance in the management of patients with bladder cancer. Both ultrasound and CT can achieve highly accurate results for staging disease at presentation and improved delineation of the extent of disease has been shown, in at least one series, to improve local control. The main drawback of these techniques is lack of tissue specificity; for example, tumour cannot be distinguished from radiation fibrosis, oedema and inflammation. In addition, enlarged nodes due to tumour may be indistinguishable from enlarged nodes due to benign hyperplasia. Magnetic resonance imaging may provide more information regarding tumour spread, but as yet there is insufficient information to determine its precise role in clinical practice.

Acknowledgements

I am most grateful to my clinical colleagues for referring patients under their care; to Dr D.O. Cosgrove for his advice and for providing illustrations for the ultrasound section; and to Dr Jane Dobbs for her advice on the 'radiotherapy treatment planning' section. The CRC Radiology Research Group at the Royal Marsden Hospital is funded by the Cancer Research Campaign and the Department of Health and Social Security, and I should like to acknowledge their support.

References

Abu-Youssef, M.M., Narayana, A.S., Brown, R.C. and Franken, E.A. (1984). Urinary bladder tumors studied by cystosonography. II: Staging. *Radiology* **153**: 227.

Alderson, P.O., Adams, D.F., McNeil, B.J. *et al.* (1981). A prospective study of computed tomography, ultrasound and nuclear imaging of the liver in patients with breast or colon cancer. *Journal of Nuclear Medicine* **22**: 35.

Cerney, J.C., Farah, R., Rian, R. and Weckstein, M.L. (1975). An evaluation of lymphangiography in staging carcinoma of the prostate. *Urology* **113**: 367.

Dobbs, H.J., Parker, R.P., Hodson, N.J., Hobday, P. and Husband, J.E. (1983). The use of CT in radiotherapy treatment planning. *Radiotherapy and Oncology* **1**: 133.

Dretler, S.P., Ragsdale, B.D. and Leadbetter, W.F. (1973). The value of pelvic lymphadenectomy in the surgical treatment of bladder cancer. *Journal of Urology* **109**: 414–16

Fisher, M.R., Hricak, H. and Tanagho, E. (1985). Magnetic resonance imaging of bladder neoplasms. *Fourth Annual Meeting of the Society of Magnetic Resonance in Medicine, London*, vol. 1, p. 222 (abstract).

Goitein, M., Wittenberg, J., Mendiondo, M. *et al.* (1979). The value of CT scanning in radiation therapy treatment planning: a prospective study. *International Journal of Radiation Oncology, Biology and Physics* **5**: 1787.

Golimbu, M., Morales, P., Al-Askari, S. and Shulman, Y. (1981). CAT scanning in staging of prostatic cancer. *Urology* **18**: 305.

Hamlin, D.J., Cockett, A.T.K. and Burgener, F.A. (1981). Computed tomography of the pelvis: sagittal and coronal image reconstruction in the evaluation of infiltrative bladder carcinoma. *Journal of Computer Assisted Tomography* **5**: 27.

Hidell, J.G., Nyman, U.R., Norlindh, S.T. *et al.* (1981). New intravesical contrast medium for CT: preliminary studies with arachis (peanut oil). *American Journal of Roentgenology* **137**: 777.

Hilaris, B.S., Whitmore, W.F., Batata, M. and Barzall, W. (1977). Behavioural patterns of prostate adenocarcinoma following an I^{125} implant and pelvic node dissection. *International Journal of Radiation Oncology, Biology and Physics* **2**: 632.

Hodson, N.J., Husband, J.E. and Macdonald, J.S. (1979). The role of computed tomography in the staging of bladder cancer. *Clinical Radiology* **30**: 389.

Hricak, H., Williams, R.D., Spring, D.B. *et al.* (1983). Anatomy and pathology of the male pelvis by magnetic resonance imaging. *American Journal of Roentgenology* **141**: 1101.

Husband, J.E. and Hodson, N.J. (1981). Computerised axial tomography in staging and assessing response to treatment in bladder cancer. In *Bladder Cancer: Principles of Combination Therapy*, pp. 27–36. Edited by Oliver, T.D., Hendry, W.F. and Bloom, H.J.G. Butterworth, London.

Jeffrey, R.B., Palubinskas, A.J. and Federle, M.P. (1981). CT evaluation of invasive lesions of the bladder. *Journal of Computer Assisted Tomography* **5**: 22.

Jewett, H.J. and Strong, G.H. (1946). Infiltrating carcinoma of the bladder. *Journal of Urology* **55**: 365.

Kellett, M.J., Kelsey Fry, I., Husband, J.E. and Oliver, T.D. (1980). CT scanning as an adjunct to bimanual examination for staging of bladder tumours. *British Journal of Urology* **52**: 101.

Koss, J.C., Arger, P.H., Coleman, B.G., Mulhern, C.B., Pollack, H.M. and Wein, A.J. (1981). CT staging of bladder carcinoma *American Journal of Roentgenology* **137**: 359.

Knopf, D.R., Torres, W.E., Fajman, W.J. and Sones, P.J. (1982). Liver lesions: comparative accuracy of scintigraphy and computed tomography. *American Journal of Roentgenology* **138**: 623.

Levine, M.S., Arger, P.H., Coleman, B.G. *et al.* (1981). Detecting lymphatic metastases from prostatic carcinoma: superiority of CT. *American Journal of Roentgenology* **137**: 207.

Loening, S.A., Schmidt, J.D., Brown, R.C. *et al.* (1977). A comparison between lymphangiography and pelvic lymph node dissection in the staging of prostatic cancer. *Journal of Urology* **117**: 752.

Morgan, C.L., Calkins, R.F. and Cavalcanti, E.J. (1981). Computed tomography in the evaluation, staging and therapy of carcinoma of the bladder and prostate. *Radiology* **140**: 751.

Morley, P. (1979). Clinical staging of epithelial bladder tumours by echotomography. In *Ultrasound in Tumor Diagnosis*, pp. 145–61. Edited by Hill, C.R., McCready, V.R. and Cosgrove, D.O. Chicago Year Book Medical Publishers.

Munzenrider, J.E., Pilepich, M., Rene-Ferrero, J.B. *et al.* (1977). Use of body scanner in radiotherapy treatment planning. *Cancer* **40**: 170.

Nakamura, S. and Niijima, T. (1980). Staging of bladder cancer by ultrasonography: a new technique by transurethral intravesical scanning. *Journal of Urology* **124**: 341.

Narayana, A.S., Loening, S.A., Slymen, D.J. and Culp, D.A. (1983). Bladder cancer: factors affecting survival. *Journal of Urology* **130**: 56.

O'Donoghue, E.P.N., Shridhor, P., Sherwood, T. *et al.* (1976). Lymphography and pelvic lymphadenectomy in carcinoma of the prostate. *British Journal of Urology* **48**: 689.

Oliver, R.T.D., Hendry, W.F. and Bloom, H.J.G. (1981). Overview and conclusions. In *Bladder Cancer: Principles of Combination Therapy*, pp. 311–15. Edited by Oliver, T.D., Hendry, W.F. and Bloom, H.J.G. Butterworth, London.

Prout, G.R. (1977). Bladder carcinoma and a TNM system of classification. *Journal of Urology* **117**: 583.

Ragan, D.P. and Perez, C.A. (1978). Efficacy of CT-assisted two-dimensional treatment planning: analysis of 45 patients. *American Journal of Roentgenology* **131**: 75.

Richie, J.P., Skinner, D.G. and Kaufman, J.J. (1975). Carcinoma of the bladder: treatment by radical cystectomy. *Journal of Surgical Research* **18**: 271.

Rothwell, R.I., Ash, D.V. and Thorogood, J. (1985). An analysis of the contribution of computed tomography to the treatment outcome in bladder cancer. *Clinical Radiology* **36**: 369.

Sager, E.M., Talle, K., Fossa, S. *et al.* (1983). The role of CT in demonstrating perivesical tumor growth in the preoperative staging of carcinoma of the urinary bladder. *Radiology* **146**: 443.

Schmidt, J.D. and Weinstein, S.H. (1976). Pitfalls in clinical staging of bladder tumours. *Urologic Clinics in North America* **3**: 107.

Schuller, J., Walther, V., Schmiedt, E., Staehler, G., Bauer, H.W. and Schilling, A. (1982). Intravesical ultrasound tomography in staging bladder carcinoma. *Journal of Urology* **128**: 264.

Seidelmann, F.E., Cohen, W.N., Bryan, *et al.* (1978). Accuracy of CT staging of bladder neoplasms using the gas-filled method: report of 21 patients with surgical confirmation. *American Journal of Roentgenology* **130**: 735.

Singer, D. Itzchak, Y. and Fischelovitch, Y. (1981). Ultrasonographic assessment of bladder tumors. II. Clinical staging. *Journal of Urology* **126**: 34.

Snow, J.H., Goldstein, H.M. and Wallace, S. (1979). Comparison of scintigraphy, sonography and computed tomography in the evaluation of hepatic neoplasms. *American Journal of Roentgenology* **132**: 915.

Spellman, M.C., Castellino, R.A., Ray, G.R. *et al.* (1977). An evaluation of lymphography in localized carcinoma of the prostate. *Radiology* **125**: 637.

Stanley, R.J., Sagel, S.S. and Levitt, R.G. (1977). Computed tomography of the liver. *Radiologic Clinics of North America* **15**: 331.

UICC (1978). *TNM Classification of Malignant Tumours*, 3rd edn. Edited by Harmer, M.H. International Union Against Cancer, Geneva.

van der Werf-Messing, B., Schroeder, F.H. and Bush, H. (1982). Bladder. In *Textbook of Cancer*, p. 457. Edited by Halnan, K.E. Chapman and Hall, London.

Vock, P., Haertel, M., Fuchs, W.A., Karrer, P., Bishop, M.C. and Zingg, E.J. (1982). Computed tomography in staging of carcinoma of the urinary bladder. *British Journal of Urology* **54**: 158.

Wajsman, Z., Baumgartner, G., Murphy, G.P. *et al.* (1975). Evaluation of lymphangiography for clinical staging of bladder tumors. *Journal of Urology* **114**: 712.

Walsh, J.W., Amendola, M.A., Konerding, K.F. *et al.* (1980). Computed tomographic detection of pelvic and inguinal lymph node metastases from primary and recurrent pelvic malignant disease. *Radiology* **137**: 157.
Weinerman, P.M., Arger, P.H. and Pollack, H.M. (1982). CT evaluation of bladder and prostate neoplasms. *Urologic Radiology* **4**: 105.

6

The management of superficial bladder cancer, with emphasis on intravesical chemotherapy*

Mark S. Soloway

Introduction

The subject of this chapter is the management of the two-thirds of the patient population with bladder cancer who present with tumours of various grades (I–III) which are confined to the urothelium (Ta) or which have invaded into the lamina propria (T1) but not into the muscle. Although only 10–15 per cent of this group will subsequently develop tumours which invade into the muscle, approximately one-half will develop a subsequent tumour following endoscopic removal of initial tumours. Intravesical therapy is designed to· reduce the incidence of new occurrences or true recurrences. Patients with extensive superficial disease at presentation, particularly those with carcinoma-in-situ (CIS), will require intravesical chemotherapy as part of a treatment schedule since it is unlikely that all the tumour can be endoscopically removed at the initial endoscopic session.

Before reviewing the various drugs used for intravesical chemotherapy, it is important to outline the steps the urologist must perform during the initial evaluation.

Initial evaluation in patients with superficial bladder cancer

The initial diagnosis of bladder cancer may be made during an outpatient cystoscopy performed using topical anaesthesia. The definitive evaluation, however, which includes endoscopic resection of tumour, should be performed when complete bladder relaxation can be assured. This allows the urologist adequately to remove the tumour and to obtain sufficient mucosal biopsies to determine whether tumour is unifocal or multifocal (i.e. to detect areas of severe dysplasia or carcinoma-in-situ). It is the author's personal preference to use spinal or epidural anaesthesia since this provides excellent relaxation of the bladder with minimal cardiovascular risk to the patient. In the USA, most of these procedures are performed in the outpatient surgery suite (see Table 6.1).

* The work reported in this chapter was supported by PHS grants CA 15934 and CA 18643 awarded by the National Cancer Institute, and by research funds from the US Veterans Administration.

Table 6.1 Steps in thorough evaluation of patients with suspected superficial bladder cancer

1.	Adequate bladder relaxation
2.	Bimanual examination
3.	Cystoscopic urine plus bladder washing; combine and send for cytology
4.	View all areas of the bladder and urethra; use several lenses
5.	Use bladder diagram to document location, size, number and configuration of obvious tumour as well as location of suspicious urothelium
6.	Resect or biopsy tumour as indicated by extent of tumour; obtain muscle in specimen if invasion suspected
7.	Consider selected mucosal biopsies to determine likelihood of new occurrence
8.	Biopsy prostatic urethra if known or suspected CIS of bladder or suspicious appearance

A bimanual examination is an integral part of the initial evaluation. One hand is placed suprapubically, and the other provides counter-pressure with a finger in the rectum or two fingers in the vagina depending upon the patient's sex. This procedure should be performed both before and after resection of a bladder tumour and is particularly important if invasion is suspected since the presence of a mass following resection will usually indicate tumour invasion into deep muscle or serosa. A bimanual examination is also necessary in the male since the urologist must thoroughly examine the prostate. Should any suspicious alteration in the size or configuration of the prostate be detected one should readily perform a biopsy or aspiration for cytology.

At the beginning of the endoscopic procedure, the urine obtained following introduction of the cystoscope is collected and combined with a bladder washing. The specimen is sent for cytological analysis. The bladder washing specimen is obtained by repeated barbotage with 50–100 ml of saline through the cystoscope or resectoscope. The millipore filter technique is used to prepare the slides, and this provides superb cytology specimens. An improved yield of tumour cells is obtained by performing both the cystoscopic urine and bladder washing (Murphy *et al.*, 1981). Cytology material should be submitted to the laboratory as soon as possible, although it is possible to refrigerate specimens overnight with little loss of cellular detail.

Endoscopic equipment has improved greatly over the last few years, so that with the variety of lenses available one can thoroughly evaluate the entire bladder, prostatic urethra, and even the upper urinary tract. The examination can be begun with either a 45° or 70° lens to evaluate the bladder thoroughly. A 120° lens, if available, is useful to visualize the anterior bladder wall. A 0, 5 or 12° lens is used to look once again at the trigone and examine the urethra with particular attention to the prostatic urethra.

A ureteroscope has been developed which provides access to the entire ureter and a part of the renal collecting system. Although there may be some trauma to the ureterovesical junction, this may be an important step in patients suspected of having an upper tract tumour. This is particularly helpful in patients with a positive cytology but no evident urothelial abnormality.

The clinician should document the location, appearance (papillary or sessile), size and number of all tumours. This can be done with a bladder diagram. The diagram should be an integral part of the patient's chart.

Another way of recording the urologist's findings is by endoscopic photography. Although this is particularly useful in teaching and for communication in conferences, it is also an excellent way to monitor serially the tumour status in a given patient. Most manufacturers produce an automatic light source which can be integrated with the endoscope and a specially designed 35 mm single-lens-reflex camera. This system provides the appropriate amount of high-intensity light when the shutter of the camera is depressed.

Cold-cup mucosal biopsies may be useful in some instances and aid in determining appropriate therapy. Since the presence of carcinoma-in-situ may alter the urologist's treatment plan, such mucosal biopsies should be obtained to determine if CIS is present. These biopsies are usually obtained from selected sites: lateral to each ureteral orifice, the posterior mid-line, and the dome. The author's preference is to perform a biopsy from the prostatic urethra in patients with a positive cytology but lacking an obvious tumour, carcinoma-in-situ anywhere in the bladder, and in patients with tumour(s) located near the bladder neck. In addition to selected-site biopsies, any raised, granular or erythematous area should be biopsied. Biopsies can be obtained with either the cold-cup or with a resectoscope using minimal coagulation current.

When the urologist suspects pathology in the prostate, he must obtain sufficient material to document whether the neoplasm is confined to the prostatic urethra, the prostatic ducts, or has invaded into the prostatic stroma. This can usually be documented by transurethral biopsies; however, a perineal or transrectal biopsy may be required.

The predictive value of severe dysplasia or carcinoma-in-situ in selected-mucosal biopsies has been shown by numerous investigators (Schade and Swinney, 1983; Soloway *et al.*, 1978; Murphy *et al.*, 1979). Selected mucosal biopsies performed both on initial evaluation and subsequently during endoscopic follow-up in a number of patients demonstrated a significantly higher likelihood of recurrence in those with urothelial abnormalities (Soloway *et al.*, 1978; Murphy *et al.*, 1979). Wolf and Hojgaard (1983) have confirmed these results in patients with T1 or T2 bladder cancers. They found that 13 of 15 patients (87 per cent) who had urothelial dysplasia or carcinoma-in-situ in these biopsies developed new occurrences, compared with only 7 of 27 patients (26 per cent) who had negative mucosal biopsies. Most of these subsequent tumours appeared within six months from initial diagnosis.

A continuous-flow resectoscope is quite helpful in performing endoscopic bladder tumour resection. This enables the bladder to be maintained at approximately one-third capacity and, with the aid of suprapubic pressure, tumours can be readily resected even if they are located on the dome, posterior wall, or even in the anterior wall. A patient's initial tumour can usually be removed in its entirety if it is superficial. Mucosa and lamina propria are included in the specimen. If there is concern about muscle invasion, then muscle must be incorporated in the specimen submitted to the pathologist. The pathologist's report should indicate whether there is muscle present in the submitted material. If the tumour, however, is clearly low-grade and exophytic it may be unnecessary to resect into the muscle and fulguration may be adequate. This will be most pertinent during follow-up examinations for patients whose prior tumours have always been low-grade and confined to the mucosa.

Following endoscopic resection of tumours the 45 or 70° lens should be reinserted to re-evaluate whether all tumour has been resected. Follow-up cytology within a week is an excellent way to document further whether all tumour has been removed. This will establish whether subsequent intravesical therapy is being used for treatment or prophylaxis. If the cytology is still positive, one is dealing with persistent tumour and a treatment schedule is in order.

There is some controversy concerning the resection of an enlarged prostate at the same setting as resection of a bladder tumour. Although most evidence indicates that there is no substantial increase in the incidence of subsequent tumour either in the bladder or in the prostatic urethra when these procedures are done at the same time (compared with when they are performed as two procedures), these reports do indicate a 20 per cent incidence of subsequent tumour in the prostatic urethra or bladder neck (Green and Yalowitz, 1972; Laor *et al.*, 1981). Possibly these are true recurrences. These studies do not eliminate the possibility that seeding has occurred and is a factor in this relatively high incidence of tumour at these sites. If a high-grade tumour is present in the bladder, resection of the prostate at the same time might lead to implantation into the prostatic bed, resulting in a lethal situation.

Patient monitoring following initial evaluation

Following the initial endoscopic resection, the frequency of monitoring patients can be individualized. The author performs a flexible cystourethroscopy utilizing an Olympus flexible cystourethroscope in most patients every three months for two years, then every six months. This can be performed in a clinic without intravenous sedation. The flexible 'scope' passes over the median lobe by deflecting the distal tip with the hand control. The 15F size helps to reduce trauma to the urethra. All areas of the bladder can be carefully observed with this instrument. The 250° deflection of the tip will even allow the urologist to view the bladder neck in a retrograde manner.

Urinary cytology is inexpensive and can be repeated often, with the results obtained within 24 hours. Ninety-five per cent of high-grade (III) tumours should be identified by cytology (Murphy *et al.*, 1984). The likelihood of a grade-II tumour being identified by cytology is approximately 75 per cent. Thus, if a voided and/or cystoscopic urine or bladder washing fails to reveal tumour cells, the clinician can be reasonably confident that a high-grade tumour is not present. The purpose of intensive endoscopic monitoring following initial tumour resection is to detect potentially lethal new tumours. Therefore, if one delays treatment of a grade-I tumour, little harm results.

We feel that patients with a grade-I stage-Ta lesions may be primarily monitored by cytology, which will detect a high-grade 'recurrence', and less frequently by the more traumatic endoscopy.

An analysis of 36 patients with initial grade-I stage-Ta transitional cell carcinoma has been reported, with particular emphasis on the correlation between urinary cytology and the development of subsequent tumour (Morrison *et al.*, 1984). These patients were followed for an average of 64 months with a range of 6–144 months. Ten patients had a subsequent tumour and eight of these were detected by cytology when there was an increase in grade or stage. In the two patients not detected, the grade increased from I to II and subsequent tumours were grade I. All patients are alive. This supports the view that cytology can be used to monitor patients with grade-I stage-Ta lesions, with endoscopy used more sparingly (e.g. every 9–12 months). An experienced cytopathologist is essential to this form of monitoring. A prospective study must be performed to confirm this approach.

Risk factors and intravesical therapy

A number of predictive factors based on the initial evaluation can be used to direct the clinician as to the intensity of proposed additional treatment. The stage, grade and multicentricity are important factors. Individuals whose tumour has invaded the lamina propria are at greater likelihood of progression in stage than are those whose tumour is confined to the urothelium. This was underscored by Anderstrom *et al.* (1980) in their survival analysis of patients with Ta or T1 tumours. Only three of 78 patients whose tumour did not invade through the basement membrane (Ta) died of bladder cancer, in contrast to 24 of 99 with invasion into lamina propria (T1). The surveillance study performed by the US National Bladder Cancer Group (Cutler *et al.*, 1982) indicated that only 4 per cent of those with Ta tumours progressed, compared with 30 per cent with T1 lesions. The low risk of progression is even more dramatic for those with an initial grade-I stage-Ta lesion. Three hundred and seven patients with an initial grade-I Ta tumour have been analysed by the multi-institutional National Bladder Cancer Group (G.R. Prout, personal communication, 1985). Only 10 per cent of the patients progressed in grade, while 3 per cent had a subsequent T1 lesion and only 2 per cent developed a subsequent tumour which invaded into the muscle.

The presence of severe dysplasia in biopsies of normal-appearing mucosa was re-emphasized by Wolf *et al.* (1985). They followed 27 patients with newly diagnosed bladder cancer who had dysplasia. Twenty (74 per cent) had a subsequent tumour within two years, in contrast to 47 per cent of patients without dysplasia. The likelihood of developing an invasive lesion was higher (15 per cent) in those who had dysplasia—compared with none of the 145 patients without dysplasia. The authors conclude that the finding of dysplasia in normal-appearing urothelium requires a more rigorous follow-up.

Patients with invasion into the lamina propria (T1) are at higher risk of progression to T2 or greater, in part because of understaging and in part because of the aggressive nature of these tumours despite apparent initial complete endoscopic resection. Some suggest that transurethral management plus intensive intravesical therapy is not appropriate. They feel that these patients should have a cystectomy. The author analysed a select group of 18 patients with initial stage-T1 TCC who were given mitomycin C after biopsy; in no case was all tumour resected during the initial endoscopy. Only 2 of the 18 (11 per cent) died of bladder cancer. Neither patient was an operative candidate and they were given radiation therapy. They died of cancer at 15 and 31 months after radiation. Four of the 18 patients have not had a 'recurrence' and are alive with an average follow-up of 39 months. Two are alive and have a positive cytology; an additional two have had superficial recurrences. Three patients had a cystectomy and are free of disease with an average interval of 46 months. Of the remaining patients, three have died of other causes and two were lost to follow-up. I believe that this small series indicates that virtually all patients with superficial bladder cancer can be initially treated with endoscopic resection and intravesical therapy. Only a small subgroup will require removal of the bladder (see also Chapter 4).

Intravesical chemotherapy

Whether subsequent tumours following initial endoscopic resection are due to new occurrences or true recurrences of the initial tumour (implantation or failure to resect the initial lesion), between 50 and 80 per cent will have another tumour at follow-up endoscopic examinations. This fact clearly shows the need for additional treatment in most patients as a supplement to endoscopic resection. Topical or intravesical therapy offers the advantage of instilling an agent which would affect virtually the entire urothelial surface and thus inhibit the growth of pre-neoplastic lesions and eradicate viable tumour cells remaining in contact with the urothelium following resection (assuming the agent is delivered within a relatively short interval following resection). Toxicity is minimized by instilling the agent into the bladder.

A number of factors influence the amount of drug absorbed through the urothelium. These include the drug's molecular weight, concentration, pH, the volume of solution, the duration of contact, and the extent of alteration of the urothelial surface. The degree to which each of these contributes to drug absorption and local toxicity has not been established.

The influence of pH has only recently been explored by Eksborg *et al.* (1980). They have performed studies using doxorubicin (Adriamycin) which indicate that absorption can be minimized if the pH is maintained below 8 utilizing a phosphate buffer.

The clinician should emphasize to the patient the need to rotate during the one to two hour instillation time in an effort to have the drug contact as much of the urothelial surface as possible. A relative state of dehydration is also helpful to minimize the dilution of the drug during the contact interval. Extensive endoscopic resection of a tumour will allow more of the drug to be absorbed and may also affect the degree of local toxicity.

Treatment or prophylaxis?

There are certain indications for intensive intravesical therapy: if the cytology is positive following tumour resection; if mucosal biopsies contain carcinoma-in-situ; or if the urologist feels that the tumour was not entirely resected one has a marker which can be evaluated (see Table 6.2). On the other hand, if the cytology following resection of a bladder tumour does not contain tumour cells, the mucosal biopsies do not contain carcinoma-in-situ, and all tumour was probably resected, the clinician may decide not to initiate intravesical therapy or to utilize only a prophylaxis schedule. A treatment schedule usually consists of drug instillation on a weekly basis for 8 weeks with evaluation of efficacy 4 weeks later—at the 12-week interval. A prophylaxis schedule will usually consist of weekly instillation for 4 weeks and then monthly. If at the 12-week evaluation there is no tumour present, the drug may be continued for up to one year.

Table 6.2 Treatment or prophylaxis?

Treatment schedule
1.   Tumour remaining following biopsy or resection
2.   Cytology remains positive after endoscopic resection
3.   Mucosal biopsy from normal-appearing urothelium indicates
       carcinoma-in-situ

No treatment or prophylaxis schedule
1.   All obvious tumour resected
2.   Cytology following resection is negative
3.   No CIS in mucosal biopsies

In reviewing the result of intravesical chemotherapy it is important for the reader to be keenly aware that there is no uniformity of pathological interpretation between centres. This is particularly important in the diagnosis of carcinoma-in-situ. If the urologists at one centre are treating dysplasia found in mucosal biopsies and another group reports on their results in patients with symptomatic CIS, the results are likely to be quite different. The use of a reference pathologist using a generally accepted terminology may avoid this. Authors should publish examples of their histological material, particularly for CIS. Finally, cytology is critical for monitoring patients with high-grade tumours.

Thiotepa (N^1, N^{11}, N^{111}-triethylene thiophosphoramide)

Until a few years ago thiotepa was the only agent used for intravesical chemotherapy in the USA and probably still remains the most widely used intravesical therapeutic agent. Thiotepa is an alkylating agent. The usual dose is 30–60 mg and it is usually delivered in a concentration of 1 mg/ml. The treatment schedule has varied somewhat; however, one of the more standard regimens is to deliver the drug weekly for 4–8 weeks followed by monthly instillations. Therapy is usually discontinued after one year. The standard contact time for thiotepa as well as all other agents is two hours and this is mainly based on the convenience of the patient.

The major side effect of thiotepa is myelosuppression and is primarily related to its relatively low molecular weight of 189. Because of this a leucocyte and platelet count should be performed prior to each instillation.

The response rate when thiotepa has been used for treatment of an existing lesion is between 45 and 80 per cent, and this includes both complete and partial responses (Soloway, 1980). A recent trial conducted by the US National Bladder Cancer Group with thiotepa used as treatment for superficial bladder cancer found a complete response rate of 43 per cent when the drug was used at a dose of 30 mg weekly for 8 weeks (Koontz *et al.*, 1981).

Most studies with thiotepa have used it as prophylaxis. The dose, administration schedule, and the timing of the first dose following endoscopic resection have varied widely. Until recently the concern over absorption of the drug with the attendant potential for myelosuppression prevented urologists from initiating therapy within a few days after resection; however, the likelihood of severe myelosuppression is sufficiently low that therapy is now being initiated within 48 hours of resection.

Burnand *et al.* (1976) were among the first to employ a high dose of thiotepa immediately following endoscopic resection. They used a dose of 90 mg with an instillation time of 30 minutes, and this was initiated immediately following surgery. Patients who received thiotepa had a much lower incidence of subsequent tumour (8 of 19 free of tumour at one year) compared with only one of 31 patients who did not receive intravesical thiotepa after endoscopic resection. Leucopenia was not a problem.

The National Bladder Cancer Group performed a multi-institutional study evaluating two doses of thiotepa, 30 and 60 mg, used as prophylaxis (Koontz *et al.*, 1981). Patients who received thiotepa had a statistically significant reduction in the subsequent tumour incidence compared with a control group who received no intravesical therapy. Importantly, there was no difference between those who received 30 or 60 mg. Sixty-six per cent of the patients who received thiotepa were free of tumour at one year compared with only 40 per cent of those who received no instillations. This difference was significant ($p = 0.02$).

Prout *et al.* (1985) recently reviewed the follow-up of these patients treated with thiotepa. The purpose of this report was to determine whether the likelihood of tumour progression or cystectomy correlated with an initial response to thiotepa. Progression was defined as muscle invasion or cancer beyond the confines of the bladder, including the prostatic urethra, prostatic ducts or prostatic substance.

Follow-up data for 5 years or to death was available in 64 of the 78 patients. Fourteen patients were successfully treated with thiotepa and were randomized to receive prophylaxis. Some patients received other intravesical agents following thiotepa.

The likelihood of progression was not associated with the number of visible tumours at entry, the size of the largest tumour, or whether the patient had a positive or negative cytology. On the other hand, a positive cytology after thiotepa and a grade-II or grade-III tumour initially were associated with disease progression or cystectomy.

In the 78 patients who were followed, 34 failed thiotepa. Twenty-two did not have either progression or cystectomy in the follow-up interval. Eight patients had a cystectomy and four had progression but did not have a cystectomy. Only six patients died of bladder cancer during the follow-up period. Two of 44 were treatment successes and four of 34 were treatment failures.

Although this study did not provide evidence that initial benefit with thiotepa indicated long-term prevention of progression, a multi-institutional trial performed in Europe did suggest long-term benefit from intravesical therapy (Schulman *et al.*, 1982). In this study patients received either thiotepa (30 mg in 30 ml), VM-26 (50 mg in 30 ml) or no treatment following endoscopic resection. Treatment was continued weekly for 4 weeks and then monthly for 11 months. Forty-nine per cent of those receiving thiotepa had a subsequent tumour compared with 62 per cent in the group receiving VM-26. The control group had a tumour incidence of 52 per cent. There was no significant difference among the groups in regard to the recurrence rate. However, when the analysis was performed for the number of tumours per 100 patient months, there was a significant benefit for those receiving thiotepa. When one treatment centre analysed the long-term follow-up of this group of patients, the likelihood of dying from bladder cancer was lower for those who received either of the intravesical chemotherapeutic agents when compared with the control group (Green *et al.*, 1984). The difference was not statistically significant.

England *et al.* (1981) reviewed their experience with the use of thiotepa as prophylaxis. Forty-five patients entered this trial and most had a long history of prior transitional cell carcinoma of the bladder. The dose (30 mg in 50 ml) was given on days one, three and five following resection. Thiotepa was continued even in those patients in whom there was tumour present at the first 3-month endoscopy. Patients were judged to have 'responded' if the bladder was tumour-free or if the number of subsequent tumours was dramatically reduced compared with the patient's prior tumour recurrence pattern. Most of the patients had multifocal disease.

Seventeen of 21 patients (81 per cent) with Ta lesions and 14 of 24 (63 per cent) with T1 tumours had a 'response'. The overall response rate was 71 per cent. Seven of the 45 patients died of urothelial cancer; one of these from a primary in the renal pelvis. Despite initiation of thiotepa within 24 hours there was no significant toxicity.

Experience with myelosuppression has been reviewed in patients who received thiotepa in doses of 30–60 mg (Soloway and Ford, 1983); 670 consecutive installations were analysed, 50 of which were given within 48 hours of endoscopic resection. Twenty-six (3.9 per cent) installations were associated with some myelosuppression (WBC<4000). Eighteen per cent of the patients had myelosuppression at some time during their course which may have lasted up to 5 years. Importantly, no patient experienced myelosuppression with the initial dose of thiotepa, and in no case was myelosuppression associated with sepsis or bleeding.

Jones and Swinney (1961) estimated that approximately one-third of an administered dose of thiotepa is absorbed and correlates with the amount of tumour resected. A survey of the literature indicates that the incidence of myelosuppression ranges from 2–25 per cent (England *et al.*, 1981). There are isolated reports of profound and prolonged myelosuppression. Mukamel *et al.* (1982) evaluated whether the presence of vesicoureteral reflux was related to thiotepa administration and also to myelosuppression. In a group of patients who had had a prior transurethral resection of bladder tumours, 43 per cent had unilateral reflux. In 61 patients who had both a TUR and thiotepa, 25 (41 per cent) had reflux. In half of the ureters involved with reflux there was no tumour at the site of the orifice, and it was felt that reflux could be attributed to the intravesical chemotherapy and its effect on the mucosa.

These workers also analysed the likelihood of myelosuppression related to reflux (Nissenkorn *et al.*, 1985). Thirty-three patients had reflux, 28 of which was unilateral and 5 bilateral. Transient myelosuppression was found in 15 per cent of the patients. This is the same as in most studies with or without reflux. Thus, reflux is not a contraindication to the use of thiotepa.

Thiotepa is currently the standard to which other agents are compared. It is not expensive. Local toxicity (i.e. bladder irritative symptoms) occurs, but infrequently requires discontinuation of therapy. Myelosuppression is a potentially major problem but is quite unusual; monitoring of the white blood cell and platelet count is mandatory, however.

Mitomycin C

Mitomycin C (MMC) is an antitumour antibiotic whose primary mechanism of action is believed to be inhibition of DNA synthesis. MMC is used as an intravenous antitumour agent and is active in a number of tumour sites. Myelosuppression is the major toxicity associated with the systemic administration of this agent. The molecular weight of MMC is 329 and thus absorption from the bladder is quite low, obviating this side effect. Van Oosterom *et al.* (1984) analysed the serum levels of mitomycin C in 15 patients after they had received a 60 mg intravesical dose: they found that the level of absorption was extremely low, varying from 0.1 to 1.1 per cent of the administered drug.

A number of single- and, more recently, multi-institutional studies have established the activity of mitomycin C both for treatment as well as for prophylaxis of superficial TCC. Although thiotepa has been primarily used for prophylaxis, the efficacy of mitomycin C has largely been examined in treatment studies in which a tumour marker is present.

The only dose-response study using mitomycin C was performed by Bracken *et al.* (1980). Forty-three patients with Ta or T1 TCCs were treated with doses ranging from 20 to 60 mg weekly for 8 weeks. Response was evaluated at week 12. The overall response rate was 84 per cent: 49 per cent complete responses, 30 per cent partial responses, and an additional 5 per cent who were listed as 'improved'. Unfortunately, there were insufficient numbers of patients in each dose category to make any statistical comparison and evaluation of the optimal dose; however, it appeared that the response rate was higher with doses above 25 mg. Following this study, 40 mg per treatment has been generally used in the USA.

The author has treated 70 patients with stages TIS, Ta and T1 transitional cell carcinoma with mitomycin C. The first six received 30 mg weekly for 8 consecutive weeks; subsequent patients received 40 mg in 40 ml (see Table 6.3). The drug was used as treatment in all of these instances. There was always biopsy-documented tumour which was confined to the mucosa or lamina propria and tumour remained in the bladder prior to initiation of therapy. The mean follow-up in this group was 28 months with a range of 6–63 months. Sixty-two of the 70 patients were followed for a minimum of one year.

Table 6.3 MMC for treatment of Ta and T1 TCCs (Soloway, unpublished data)

70 patients: 19 grade-I, 26 grade-II, 25 grade-III
40 mg weekly ×8 weeks
Response monitored by endoscopy, cytology, biopsy at week 12

CR = 39%
PR = 39%
Failure = 22%

Nineteen patients had a grade-I tumour, 26 grade-II and 25 grade-III. Twelve patients with grade-III TCC had only carcinoma-in-situ. Thirty-nine patients clearly failed thiotepa as they developed tumours while on a regular maintenance schedule of this agent.

At the time of the first 12-week evaluation, 27 of the 70 patients (39 per cent) had no visible tumour at endoscopy, the mucosal biopsies did not contain severe dysplasia or carcinoma-in-situ, and no tumour cells were identified on the cytology. These patients thus had a complete response. An additional 27 patients (39 per cent) were thought to have had a partial response since they had either a 50 per cent reduction in the amount of tumour remaining in the bladder compared with the pretreatment tumour volume, or more likely they had a positive cytology despite the fact that on endoscopy no tumour was evident. Sixteen patients (22 per cent) failed intravesical mitomycin C. Among the 12 patients with carcinoma-in-situ, five (42 per cent) had a complete response indicating that their cytology converted to negative.

An important aspect of this personal series is the long-term follow-up. Of the 27 patients who had a complete response at the first 12-week interval, only 44 per cent have had a subsequent tumour with a mean follow-up of 30 months. This contrasts with the partial responders; 78 per cent have had a subsequent tumour. Only 7 per cent of the complete responders and 15 per cent of the partial responders have developed a tumour which has invaded muscle. Twenty-five per cent of those who failed mitomycin C (4 of 16) subsequently had a T2 tumour.

Another way of analysing the results is to look at the likelihood of requiring a cystectomy. Two of the 27 complete responders (7 per cent) had a cystectomy. One developed a tumour in the prostatic urethra which invaded the stroma and the other developed a muscle-invasive tumour. Nine of the partial responders (33 per cent) had a cystectomy during a mean follow-up of 27 months. The indications for cystectomy were a positive cytology in one patient, carcinoma-in-situ in the bladder or prostatic urethra in five, and muscle invasion in two.

In the entire group of 70 patients treated with mitomycin C, only seven have died of bladder cancer. I believe this indicates that even in this high-risk group of patients with superficial bladder cancer a trial of intensive intravesical chemotherapy is warranted.

Koontz *et al.* (1985) recently reported the results of a National Bladder Cancer Group study in which mitomycin C was used for patients who failed thiotepa. The dose and treatment regimen were the same as those used in the foregoing study. One hundred and seventeen patients were entered and

32 (27 per cent) had a negative endoscopy, biopsies, and importantly a negative cytology, i.e. complete response. An additional 11 patients (9 per cent) met all of the criteria for a complete response with the exception that a biopsy of the index lesion was not performed. Thus, 36 per cent of the patients had a complete response as defined by failure to detect the original remaining lesion(s) by endoscopy or cytology. An additional 14 patients (12 per cent) had absence of tumour on the follow-up study as indicated by biopsy and endoscopy, although the cytology remained positive, i.e. partial response.

Patients with an initial Ta lesion(s) had a 29 per cent complete response rate compared with 18 per cent for those with T1 lesions. Forty-five per cent (9 of 20) with CIS as the indicator lesion had a complete response.

The National Bladder Cancer Group has also completed one of the few trials comparing mitomycin with thiotepa (Heney, 1985). Eighty-eight patients have been analysed for response. Thirty-five had carcinoma-in-situ as the only lesion in the bladder. After initial evaluation, patients were randomized to receive either 30 mg of thiotepa or 40 mg of mitomycin C in a concentration of 1 mg/ml. The agents were given weekly for 8 weeks. Response was evaluated at week 12. At the initial 3-month evaluation, the complete response rate for mitomycin C was 50 per cent (23/46) and it was 43 per cent (18/42) for those who received thiotepa.

A few studies have evaluated MMC as prophylaxis following endoscopic resection of all evident tumour. Huland *et al.* (1984) used a long-term intensive course of MMC and reported one of the lowest incidences of subsequent tumour. Patients received 20 mg of MMC in 20 ml beginning 4 weeks after transurethral resection of all tumour (Ta or T1). This dose was continued every 2 weeks for one year followed every 4 weeks for the second and third years. Initially, they performed a randomized study in which patients received either MMC or no intravesical therapy. Importantly, all patients were documented to have a negative cytology before entry on to this protocol. Those with initial T1 lesions were re-evaluated before entry.

Only 10 per cent of the patients treated with MMC had a subsequent tumour compared with 51 per cent of those who received no intravesical chemotherapy. Five of the controls subsequently died of bladder cancer and none of the patients treated with MMC died as a result of carcinoma of the bladder.

Jacobi *et al.* (1985), reviewed their 5-year follow-up of a prospective randomized trial comparing doxorubicin with mitomycin C following endoscopic resection of all evident tumour in patients with Ta–T1 bladder cancer. Twenty-eight of 35 (80 per cent) in the doxorubicin group and 21 of 38 (35 per cent) in the mitomycin group had prior tumour before initiation on to this prophylaxis study. Patients were treated with either Adriamycin (50 mg in 30 ml) or mitomycin C (10 mg in 30 ml) every other week for 6 months.

Five years after initiation of the study, 82 per cent of the patients who received Adriamycin and 50 per cent of those who received mitomycin C had a subsequent tumour. The number of recurrences per patient was 2.0 in the Adriamycin group and 1.2 in the mitomycin group, providing a recurrence rate of 6.9 for Adriamycin and 4.9 for mitomycin C. The interval between the recurrences was 14.3 months for the Adriamycin group and

20.2 months for the mitomycin group. This difference was statistically significant.

Side effects related to MMC differ from those associated with thiotepa. Myelosuppression is rarely observed and the author no longer obtains routine blood studies. The side effect that, although infrequent, can be a nuisance is a palmar or even occasionally a generalized rash. This may be a contact dermatitis. The patient should avoid contact with mitomycin C-urine solution. The patients should be asked to wash their hands and genitalia thoroughly for the first 24 hours after treatment. A chemical cystitis is seen with mitomycin as with all of the intravesical agents but is rarely a cause for discontinuation of therapy. Long-term administration may result in a reduction in the bladder capacity but will rarely lead to urinary diversion.

The endoscopic appearance of the bladder following MMC, as well as some of the other intravesical agents, may be significantly altered and, in fact, may mimic a neoplasm. Areas of tumour resection or biopsy sites have superficial necrosis and it may be difficult to biopsy these areas owing to intense fibrosis created by the initial biopsy and the intravesical therapeutic agent. This emphasizes the importance of urinary cytology which is critical for monitoring these patients. Urinary cytology is also an integral part of monitoring carcinoma-in-situ of the prostatic urethra and prostatic ducts.

Doxorubicin hydrochloride (Adriamycin)

Adriamycin has been used by the intravenous route for the treatment of metastatic bladder cancer. It has also been used for intravesical therapy in the treatment of superficial bladder cancer. In most studies it has been used as prophylaxis following endoscopic resection rather than as an intensive treatment course.

Garnick *et al.* (1984) used Adriamycin as prophylaxis in 45 patients following endoscopic resection of all obvious tumours. The dose ranged from 60 to 90 mg in a volume of 50 ml with an instillation time of one hour. Treatment was repeated every 3 weeks for 8 treatments, every 6 weeks for 2, and every 12 for 2 further instillations. Fifty-three percent of the 45 patients were free of tumour with a median duration of 18 months. However, seven of the patients (16 per cent) developed a muscle-invasive tumour within a relatively short period.

Jakse *et al.* (1984) have used doses of 40 or 80 mg diluted in 20 or 40 ml of saline, respectively. The drug was given bi-weekly when the lower dose was used or monthly for the 80 mg dose. This was continued for one year at this interval and every one or two months during the subsequent year. Patients were divided into three categories:

1. Fourteen patients had primary CIS, i.e. no prior or concurrent bladder cancer. All were symptomatic. Two of these patients were treated with mitomycin C, 40 mg in 40 ml, rather than doxorubicin. Ten of 14 patients (71 per cent) had a complete response. In two that had failed doxorubicin a complete response was achieved with mitomycin C. In two patients CIS of the prostatic urethra developed and was successfully treated conservatively. Only one of these 14 patients died of bladder cancer. The average follow-up was 29 months (range 6–69 months).

2. Jakse *et al.* treated 17 patients with secondary CIS. These patients had a

prior superficial bladder cancer and CIS was found during follow-up. All received doxorubicin; the follow-up averaged 42 months. Thirteen (67 per cent) had a good response to this treatment. Only one patient had a radical cystectomy and two died of bladder cancer.

3. A third group of 15 patients had carcinoma-in-situ detected at the time of transurethral resection of a superficial tumour. Twelve received doxorubicin and three MMC. Eleven (73 per cent) had a complete response with a follow-up of 28 months. None died of bladder cancer.

One of the pertinent facts about this series with carcinoma-in-situ is that only one of the 46 patients died of bladder cancer. The mean follow-up was 33 months.

Kurth *et al.* (1984) reported a prospective randomized trial conducted by the European Organization for the Research and Treatment of Cancer (EORTC) Genitourinary Group. They compared the use of intravesical doxorubicin, ethoglucid (Epodyl) or no treatment following endoscopic resection of all evident tumour. There was a statistically significant decrease in the recurrence rate per 100 patient months for those who received either one of the intravesical agents compared with those in the control group (9.17 tumours versus 2.91). The mean interval between recurrences was 34 months for those receiving chemotherapy, compared with 11 months for the control group. There was no significant difference between patients treated with doxorubicin and Epodyl.

The Southwest Oncology Group in the United States recently compared doxorubicin with BCG for prophylaxis (Crawford *et al.*, 1985). The recurrence rate was significantly lower in those receiving BCG compared with doxorubicin: 23 per cent versus 65 per cent.

This cooperative group also looked at these two agents in 58 patients with carcinoma-in-situ. The complete response rate at the first 3-month evaluation was 73 per cent for those receiving BCG compared with 29 per cent for doxorubicin, a significant difference.

An interesting study was performed by Ek *et al.* (1984) using doxorubicin in 22 patients with either primary (7) or secondary carcinoma-in-situ (15). None of the patients had received prior intravesical chemotherapy. Four of the patients had severe symptoms attributed to CIS. Doxorubicin was instilled in an amount dependent on the bladder volume, and the dose ranged from 20 to 160 mg (mean 80) in a volume of 30–500 ml (mean 220). Patients received the drug monthly and had an average of 12 instillations. Only 2 of the 22 patients experienced a long-term complete response, although the authors indicated that 10 had some benefit from this therapy. Five of the 22 patients required a radical cystectomy; four for an invasive tumour and one for persistent CIS. One other patient had radiation therapy.

The molecular weight of doxorubicin is 580 and thus absorption of the drug is low. Leucopenia has not been reported. Most of the side effects are related to irritative bladder symptoms and this occurs in up to 25 per cent of patients and is more likely in patients with prior radiation therapy.

Crawford (personal communication, 1985) observed six patients who had a systemic allergic reaction following intravesical doxorubicin. All of these patients received multiple instillations of this agent.

One of the few investigations into the incorporation of an intravesical therapeutic agent into the normal and abnormal urothelium was performed by Nakada *et al.* (1985). Patients received 50 mg of doxorubicin hydrochloride in 30 ml saline for a 2-hour period prior to bladder biopsies. Doxorubicin in tissue was measured by high-performance liquid chromatography. Concentrations of doxorubicin were between 2.5 and 3.5 times greater in neoplastic than in normal bladder. Biopsies obtained from the dome had a significantly lower level of doxorubicin compared with either the bladder neck, the fundus, or the lateral walls. This may explain why patients have more 'recurrence' in the dome than in other locations. Larger tumours had a lower concentration of doxorubicin than tumours less than 1 cm.

Bacillus Calmette–Guerin (BCG)

With the intention of inducing an inflammatory reaction, a specific immunologic response to the tumour or a non-specific response, BCG (an attenuated mycobacterium) has been instilled into the bladder. Several strains of BCG have been used: Montreal, Tice and Connaught. BCG consists of freeze-dried living organisms. Each ampoule contains $(5-8\pm4)\times10^8$ colony-forming units. There is increasing evidence that an immunologic reaction is central to BCG's activity.

The number of viable organisms per vial varies and this may be clinically significant (see Table 6.4). Bennett *et al.* (1983) found that the ability of different batches of Tice-strain BCG to protect mice against circulating tumour cells correlated with the benefit received by patients who were given these same vials of BCG intrapleurally as adjuvant therapy in surgically resected lung cancer. This is not surprising since BCG is a living organism and subject to genetic changes inherent in rapidly dividing organisms.

Table 6.4 Important aspects related to BCG

1.	Tice and Montreal (Institute Armand Frappier) strains appear equally effective
2.	Number of organisms per vial varies and may be clinically important
3.	Local toxicity variable; may be prevented with oral INH

Herr *et al.* (1985) performed a prospective randomized study evaluating BCG as prophylaxis in patients at 'high risk for recurrent tumours'. A control group had transurethral resection alone. Eighty-six patients were entered in this study, 43 assigned to each group. All patients had papillary tumours resected and 57 per cent also had associated multifocal carcinoma-in-situ. Approximately half in each group had a T1 lesion and half had received intravesical chemotherapy.

Following endoscopic resection of all obvious tumour, patients received BCG, 120 mg in 50 ml of the Institute Armand Frappier (Montreal) strain weekly for 6 weeks.

The minimum follow-up in the two groups of patients was more than two years, with a median of 30 months. Using each patient as his own control there was a reduction from the pretreatment tumour frequency only in the group receiving BCG: 3.6 tumours per patient to 0.7 tumours. Only 27 patients in the non-treated control group had a significant reduction in the number of tumours at the first two endoscopic follow-up visits, compared with all 43 patients who received BCG. This difference was highly significant, as was the time to first recurrence, which was prolonged in the BCG-treated group with a median time to recurrence of 18 months compared with only 3 months in the TUR-alone group.

Pretreatment positive urinary cytology converted to negative in only 3 of the 34 TUR patients, compared with 22 of 33 who received BCG. All patients did not have cytology monitored.

The authors changed the treatment plan in 27 of 43 (63 per cent) control patients compared with 14 of 43 (33 per cent) of the TUR plus BCG group. This included a cystectomy in 15 of the group receiving TUR alone but only in 3 of those who had BCG.

Treatment-related side effects were observed frequently and consisted of dysuria (88 per cent), haematuria (58 per cent), urinary frequency (51 per cent), fever (44 per cent), chills (28 per cent) and lethargy or malaise (26 per cent).

Lamm (1985) recently reviewed his experience in a variety of groups of patients with superficial bladder cancer who received intravesical as well as intradermal BCG. This was a heterogeneous group of patients, many of whom had only had one or two recurrent tumours prior to initiation of BCG. The BCG used was the Pasteur strain, given in a dose of 120 mg dissolved in 50 ml of saline. In addition to the intravesical treatment which was given weekly for 6 weeks, patients received percutaneous BCG in a dose of 5 mg in 0.5 ml delivered to the upper thigh with a Heaf gun. Many patients received a maintenance regimen consisting of intravesical and intradermal BCG delivered every 3 months for 2 years and then every 6 months for a subsequent 2-year period.

In one controlled study, the control group had a 52 per cent recurrence rate (14/27) compared with a 20 per cent incidence of subsequent tumour in those treated with BCG (6/30). This difference was significant ($p<0.008$). Lamm also compared a relatively small cohort of patients in an attempt to determine if maintenance BCG provided an improvement in the disease-free interval, and concluded that there was an advantage although the difference only approached statistical significant ($p=0.053$).

It was also suggested that if a patient's skin test converted from negative to positive, only rarely was there a subsequent tumour. Patients whose skin tests were positive before initiation of BCG or who failed to convert following treatment had a 32 per cent incidence of recurrence (Lamm, 1985).

Kelley *et al.* (1985) reviewed their results with intravesical BCG. Forty patients were divided into three treatment groups. A prophylaxis group (17 patients) had a TUR and all obvious tumour resected. A group with residual carcinoma included four who did not have all tumour removed, three with persistent positive cytology, and four who had tumour in selected mucosal biopsies. There were 12 patients with carcinoma-in-situ.

Patients received 120 mg or one ampoule of the Pasteur strain of BCG in 50 ml saline weekly for 6 weeks. The instillation time was 2 hours. Intradermal BCG was not given. Some patients were given another course of treatment if they had persistent tumour. The mean follow-up for most of the patients was less than one year.

Of the 17 patients treated with prophylaxis, six had a recurrent tumour. The PPD skin test failed to convert in five of the six failures. These patients were retreated with a second course of BCG and five of the six remained free of tumour for an interval less than 6 months. In the group of patients with residual bladder carcinoma, 6 of 11 had a complete response. Two of the five failures responded to a second course of BCG. Six of the 12 patients with CIS had a complete response after the first 6-week course. Three patients responded to a second course of BCG.

Analysis of the PPD skin test conversion and correlation with clinical response indicated a recurrence rate of 3 of 16 (19 per cent) for PPD converters and 14 of 20 (70 per cent) for non-converters. A further analysis looked at the number of colony-forming units per ampoule and correlated this with the likelihood of converting the PPD skin test. Of 14 patients treated with vials containing 6 million colonies per ampoule, 10 had recurrent tumour and only a third had conversion of the PPD skin test. In contrast, only 3 of 12 patients treated with vials containing 300 billion colonies per ampoule had recurrent tumour and the majority had conversion of the PPD skin test to positive. Thus, the viability and the number of colony-forming units seems to be important, correlating with PPD conversion and response to BCG.

Brosman (1985) recently analysed results of 33 patients treated with the Tice strain of bacillus Calmette–Guerin for carcinoma-in-situ. Eighteen patients had a transurethral resection of concomitant superficial bladder cancer; random biopsies detected the carcinoma-in-situ. Twenty-seven of the 33 patients had received at least one course of intravesical chemotherapy prior to initiation of BCG. Only 12 had severe irritative symptoms. Seven had carcinoma-in-situ involving the prostatic urethra. Patients were given an induction phase of 12 weekly instillations and if they had no evidence of tumour they received BCG every other week for 3 months and monthly for 18 months. Therapy was stopped at 24 months.

Twenty-seven patients tolerated the 12-week induction regimen and nine still had CIS. They continued the weekly instillation. After 18 weeks of BCG, three patients still had carcinoma-in-situ and received 24 weeks of BCG. Thus, although one-third of the patients still had CIS after the 12-week induction phase, by 24 weeks all of the 27 patients who tolerated the agent were rendered tumour-free and were placed on the maintenance regimen. Six patients did not tolerate BCG for the full 12 weeks, and four still became tumour-free.

Thirty-one of 33 patients (94 per cent) who were entered on to this protocol were rendered free of disease. Only four of 31 (13 per cent) later had a recurrent tumour with average follow-up of 4 years.

The predominant side effect was bladder irritative symptoms, and Brosman noted that patients were improved with isoniazid, 300 mg daily, beginning on the day of instillation and continuing for two more days.

Of note, the seven patients who had CIS into the prostatic urethra had resection of the bladder neck to allow the BCG to enter the prostatic urethra and all were rendered free of disease.

The present author has treated 26 patients with the Tice strain. All patients had tumour remaining in the bladder prior to BCG. Twenty had failed thiotepa (77 per cent), 17 had failed mitomycin C (65 per cent), and 12 (46 per cent) had failed both thiotepa and mitomycin C.

The present author has treated 26 patients with the Tice strain. Some of these patients had tumour remaining in the bladder prior to BCG. Twenty had failed thiotepa (77 per cent), 17 had failed mitomycin C (65 per cent), and 12 (46 per cent) had failed both thiotepa and mitomycin C. complete response. Thus, 11 of 26 patients (42 per cent) with superficial bladder cancer who failed at least one prior intravesical agent had a complete response at the initial 3-month evaluation.

The follow-up corresponds to the author's studies with mitomycin C. None of the complete responders have required alternative treatment, i.e. cystectomy, radiation or other chemotherapy. Only one of the 11 complete responders has had a 'recurrence' in the mean follow-up of 11 months (3–24). Of the 15 patients who failed BCG, six (40 per cent) had a cystectomy. This was usually performed within 6 months of failing BCG. The initial pathology in these six patients was carcinoma-in-situ in three; grade-II Ta in one; grade-II T1 in one; and grade-III Ta in one. Two of the three with carcinoma-in-situ had extension into the prostatic ducts. The cystectomy specimen in three patients contained grade-III tumours, two had muscle invasion.

Nine patients failed BCG at the first 3-month evaluation but still had disease confined to the bladder. Six have not been followed for more than 6 months while the remaining three have been followed for an average of 20 months. It is too early to determine the outcome of this group of patients.

Summary

The clinician treating patients with superficial bladder cancer must have sufficient information to make a decision regarding therapy. This will include biopsy and/or resection of tumour (with a careful review of the histological material with the pathologist), mucosal biopsies from normal-appearing urothelium when indicated, and urinary cytology. The clinician integrates this information with the patient's tumour history to determine whether it is appropriate to use intravesical chemotherapy and, if so, whether it should be used as prophylaxis or treatment. Many situations are straightforward, such as the patient with an easily resected grade-I stage-Ta transitional cell tumour with negative cytology, no prior history of tumour, and a normal cytology following endoscopic resection. Such a patient is unlikely to develop a subsequent invasive tumour. Since he has only a 50 per cent chance of 'recurrence', one might seriously question whether any prophylaxis is indicated. Alternatively, a patient who has carcinoma-in-situ found on mucosal biopsies is a candidate for a treatment schedule which might be intensive and long-term. If the patient has irritative symptoms related to the carcinoma-in-situ, their presence will aid in monitoring the tumour status since an excellent response usually correlates with a diminution in symptoms.

The follow-up schedule can also be tailored to the individual patient's tumour diathesis. The patient with a low-grade non-invasive tumour can be followed primarily in the office with infrequent endoscopy and frequent cytology. Development of a higher-grade tumour (II or III) should be detected by cytology. If the patient has a low-grade non-invasive 'recurrence' a delay in diagnosis will not pose a risk to the patient. On the other hand, a patient with a positive cytology or known residual tumour following trans-urethral resection must be followed closely, particularly if there is a suggestion of invasion or extension into the prostatic urethra.

The optimal agent to be used for intravesical chemotherapy has not been determined (see Table 6.5). The essential comparative studies to determine which agent or agents are most effective are in progress. It appears that both mitomycin C and BCG are more effective than thiotepa. However, in some countries the cost of mitomycin C limits its use.

Table 6.5 Areas for investigation

1.	Do intravesical therapeutic agents merely delay or do they prevent subsequent tumour?
2.	What is the relative efficacy of agents in preventing cystectomy/radiation/death from TCC?
3.	What is the optimal volume, concentration, dose of most agents?
4.	Does treatment more proximate to endoscopic tumour resection offer an advantage?
5.	Which agent is most effective for prophylaxis?
6.	Which agent is best for treatment?
7.	Is there a role for combination or alternating intravesical agents?

Do these intravesical agents merely delay the development of subsequent tumour and, if so, for how long? Do they prevent 'recurrences' in a proportion of patients? Our current data indicate that if patients have complete responses following treatment, they have a dramatic lengthening in the interval between recurrences.

The optimal volume, concentration, duration of contact, and even the dose of many agents needs to be addressed. Such studies may require large numbers of patients. A drug such as mitomycin C might be equally effica-cious at a lower dose than the one currently used and thus reduce cost as a major factor.

The importance, if any, of instillation of drug soon after tumour resection needs clarification. Side effects are reduced if healing takes place prior to initiation of intravesical chemotherapy. Does this allow implantation to occur and reduce effectiveness?

The concept of combining intravesical chemotherapeutic agents or an immunomodulator (e.g. BCG) with chemotherapy is attractive. These ques-tions require prospective randomized studies with large numbers of pa-tients.

Intravesical chemotherapeutic and immunotherapeutic agents are cur-rently an integral aspect of the treatment of many patients with superficial bladder cancer. Many questions remain and appropriate studies designed to answer some of these questions are in progress.

References

Anderstrom, C., Johansson, S. and Nilsson, S. (1980). The significance of lamina propria invasion on the prognosis of patients with bladder tumors. *Journal of Urology* **124**: 23–6.

Bennett, J.A., Gruft, H., McKneally, M.F., Zelterman, D. and Crispen, R.G. (1983). Differences in biological activity among batches of lyophilized Tice bacillus Calmette–Guerin and their association with clinical course in stage-I lung cancer. *Cancer Research* **43**: 4184–90.

Bracken, R.B., Johnson, D.E., Von Echenbach, A.C., Swanson, D.A., DeFuria, D. and Crooke, S. (1980). Role of intravesical mitomycin C in management of superficial bladder tumors. *Urology* **16**: 11–15.

Brosman, S.A. (1985). The use of bacillus Calmette–Guerin in the therapy of bladder carcinoma-in-situ. *Journal of Urology* **134**: 36–9.

Burnand, K.G., Boyd, P.J.R., Mayo, M.E., Shuttleworth, K.E.D. and Lloyd-Davies, R.W. (1976). Intravesical thiotepa as an adjuvant to cystodiathermy in the treatment of transitional cell bladder cancer. *British Journal of Urology* **48**: 55–9.

Crawford, E.D., Lamm, D.L., Monti, J.E., Scardino, P.T., Grossman, B., Stanisik, T., Smith, J.A. and Sullivan, J.W. (1985). Intravesical Adriamycin for recurrent superficial bladder cancer: a Southwest Oncology Group protocol. *Journal of Urology* **133**: 213A.

Cutler, S.J., Heney, N.M. and Friedell, G.H.L. (1982). Longitudinal study of patients with bladder cancer: factors associated with disease recurrence and progression. In *Bladder Cancer*, pp. 35–46. Edited by Bonney, W.W. and Prout, G.R. Williams and Wilkins, Baltimore.

Ek, A., Hellsten, S., Henrikson, H., Edwall, I., Lindholm, C.E., Lindholm, K., Mikulowski, P. and Mansson, W. (1984). Intravesical Adriamycin therapy in carcinoma-in-situ of the urinary bladder. *Scandinavian Journal of Urology and Nephrology* **18**: 131–4.

Eksborg, S., Nillson, S. and Edsmyr, F. (1980). Intravesical instillation of Adriamycin: a model for standardization of the chemotherapy. *European Urology* **6**: 218–20.

England, H.R., Flynn, J.T., Paris, A.M.I. and Blandy, J.P. (1981). Early multiple-dose adjuvant thio-tepa in the control of multiple and rapid T1 tumour neogenesis. *British Journal of Urology* **53**: 588–92.

Garnick, M.D., Schade, D., Israel, M., Maxwell, B. and Richie, J.P. (1984). Intravesical doxorubicin for prophylaxis in the management of recurrent superficial bladder cancer. *Journal of Urology* **131**: 43–6.

Green, D.F., Robinson, M.R.G., Glashan, R., Newling, D., Dalesio, O. and Smith, P.H. (1984). Does intravesical chemotherapy prevent invasive bladder cancer? *Journal of Urology* **131**: 33–5.

Green, L.F. and Yalowitz, P.A. (1972). The advisability of concomitant transurethral excision of vesical neoplasm and prostatic hyperplasia. *Journal of Urology* **107**: 445–7.

Heney, N.M. (1985). First line chemotherapy of superficial bladder cancer—mitomycin versus thio-tepa. *Urology* **26** (Suppl.): 27–9.

Herr, H., Pinsky, C.M., Whitmore, W.F., Sogani, P.G., Oettgen, H.F. and Melamed, M.R. (1985). Experience with intravesical bacillus Calmette–Guerin therapy of superficial bladder tumors. *Urology* **25**: 119–23.

Huland, H., Otto, U., Droese, M. and Kloppel, G. (1984). Long-term mitomycin C instillation after transurethral resection of superficial bladder carcinoma: influence on recurrence, progression, and survival. *Journal of Urology* **132**: 27–9.

Jacobi, G.H., Engelmann, U., Frohneberg, D., Wilbert, D., Thuroff, J.W. and

Alken, P. (1985). Short-term chemoprophylaxis of adriamycin versus mitomycin C in superficial bladder cancer: a five year follow-up. Presented at the 20th Annual Meeting of the Society International D'Urologie, Vienna, Austria.

Jakse, G., Hofstadter, F. and Marberger, H. (1984). Topical doxorubicin hydrochloride therapy for carcinoma-in-situ of the bladder: a follow-up. *Journal of Urology* **131**: 41–6.

Jones, H.C. and Swinney, J. (1961). Thiotepa in the treatment of tumors of the bladder. *Lancet* **2**: 615.

Kelley, D.R., Ratliff, T.L., Catalona, W.J., Shapiro, A., Lage, J.M., Bauer, W.C., Haaff, E.O. and Dresner, S.J. (1985). Intravesical bacillus Calmette–Guerin therapy for superficial bladder cancer: effect of bacillus Calmette–Guerin viability on treatment results. *Journal of Urology* **134**: 48–53.

Koontz, W.W., Grout, G.R., Smith, W., Frable, W.J. and Minnis, J.E. (1981). The use of intravesical thiotepa in the management of non-invasive carcinoma of the bladder. *Journal of Urology* **125**: 307–12.

Koontz, W., Jr., Heney, N.M., Soloway, M.S., Platz, C., Hazra, T.A. and Trump, D.L. (1985). Mitomycin C for patients who have failed on thio-tepa. *Urology*.

Kurth, K.H., Schroder, F.H., Tunn, U., Ay, R. and Members of the EORTC Genitourinary Tract Cancer Cooperative Group (1984). Adjuvant chemotherapy of superficial transitional cell bladder carcinoma: preliminary results of a European Organization for Research on Treatment of Cancer randomized trial comparing doxorubicin, hydrochloride, ethylglucide, and transurethral resection alone. *Journal of Urology* **132**: 258–62.

Lamm, D.L. (1985). Bacillus Calmette–Guerin immunotherapy for bladder cancer. *Journal of Urology* **134**: 40–47.

Laor, E., Grabstald, H. and Whitmore, W.F. (1981). The influence of simultaneous resection of bladder tumors and prostate on the occurrence of prostatic urethral tumors. *Journal of Urology* **126**: 171–2.

Morrison, D.A., Murphy, W.M., Ford, K.S. and Soloway, M.S. (1984). Surveillance of stage 0, grade I bladder cancer by cytology alone—Is it acceptable? *Journal of Urology* **132**: 672–4.

Mukamel, E., Glanz, I., Nissenkorn, I., Cytron, S. and Servadio, C. (1982). Unanticipated vesicoureteral reflux: a possible sequela of long-term thiotepa instillations to the bladder. *Journal of Urology* **127**: 245.

Murphy, W.M., Crabtree, W.N., Jukkola, A.F. and Soloway, M.S. (1981). Diagnostic value of urine versus bladder washing in patients with bladder cancer. *Journal of Urology* **126**: 320–22.

Murphy, W.M., Nagy, G.K., Rao, M.K., Soloway, M.S., Pariji, G.C., Cox, C.E. and Friedell, G.H. (1979). 'Normal' urothelium in patients with bladder cancer. *Cancer* **44**: 1050–58.

Murphy, W.M., Soloway, M.S., Jukkola, A.F., Crabtree, W.N. and Ford, K.S. (1984). Urinary cytology and bladder cancer: the cellular features of transitional cell neoplasms. *Cancer* **53**: 1555–65.

Nakada, T., Akiya, T., Yoshikawa, M., Koike, H. and Kayayama, T. (1985). Intravesical instillation of doxorubicin hydrochloride and its incorporation into bladder tumors. *Journal of Urology* **134**: 54–7.

Nissenkorn, I., Servadio, C., Vilikowski, E. and Glanz, I. (1985). Long-term intravesical thio-tepa treatment in patients with superficial bladder tumors and vesicoureteral reflux. *Journal of Urology* **133**: 198–9.

Prout, G.R., Coombs, L.J., Frable, W., Showel, J. and Hafermann, M. for the National Bladder Cancer Group (1985). The comparison of the fates of patients with bladder cancer who were treated with thiotepa successfully and unsuccessfully. *Journal of Urology*.

Schade, R.O.K. and Swinney, J. (1983). The association of urothelial abnormalities with neoplasia: a 10-year follow-up. *Journal of Urology* **129**: 1125–6.

Schulman, C.C., Robinson, M., Denis, L., Smith, P., Viggiano, G., dePauw, M., Dalesio, O. and Sylvester, R. (1982). Prophylactic chemotherapy of superficial transitional cell carcinoma; an EORTC randomized trial comparing thio-tepa, VM-26 and TUR alone. *European Urology* **8**: 207–12.

Soloway, M.S. (1980). Rationale for intensive intravesical chemotherapy for superficial bladder cancer. *Journal of Urology* **123**: 461–6.

Soloway, M.S. and Ford, K.S. (1983). Thio-tepa-induced myelosuppression: review of 670 bladder instillations. *Journal of Urology* **130**: 889–91.

Soloway, M.S., Murphy, W.M., Rao, M.K. and Cox, C.E. (1978). Serial multiple-site biopsies in patients with bladder cancer. *Journal of Urology* **120**: 57–9.

Van Oosterom, A.T., de Bruijam, E.A., Dan, D.N., Hartigh, J., Van Oort, W.J., Pienedo, H.M. and Jaden, U.R. (1984). The pharmokinetics of intravenous, intrahepatic, and intravesical administration of mitomycin C. In *Aktuelle Rondologie*. Eb. g. Nagel Zuchschwerdt-Verlag.

Wolf, H. and Hojgaard, K. (1983). Urothelial dysplasia concomitant with bladder tumors as a determinate factor for future new occurrences. *Lancet* **1**: 134–6.

Wolf, H., Olsen, P.R. and Hojgaard, K. (1985). The clinical significance of the presence of urothelial dysplasia grade II concomitant with a newly detected bladder tumor. Presented at the 20th Annual Meeting of the Society International D'Urologie, Vienna, Austria.

7

Radical cystectomy: innovations and results

Jerome P. Richie

Introduction

In the United States the mainstay of therapy for patients with bladder cancer that is no longer confined to the superficial layers of the bladder has been surgical extirpation by removal of the urinary bladder. This once formidable procedure has become more acceptable as developments in technique, anaesthesia, intraoperative and postoperative monitoring, and newer forms of urinary diversion, have been developed. In this chapter, the developments leading up to the current state of the art for dealing with invasive transitional cell carcinoma of the bladder will be detailed and analysed.

Traditionally, management of carcinoma of the bladder has been the responsibility predominantly of the urological surgeon. Today, however, appropriate treatment of the patient with carcinoma of the bladder requires the expertise of a group of specialists, including the urologist, the medical oncologist, the radiologist, the pathologist, and radiotherapist, working together as a cohesive unit. Transitional cell carcinoma of the bladder may be manifest by tumour heterogeneity, a factor which makes therapeutic decisions for a given individual patient somewhat difficult. In this chapter, consideration will be given to attempting to decide when major therapeutic intervention is indicated, the extent of the intervention, and the need to incorporate cooperative ventures with other specialists.

Historical aspects

Tumours of the urinary bladder were first described in the early seventeenth century as an outgrowth of the removal of stones by lithotomists. Early observations of bladder tumour were reviewed by Albarran in the 1890s. During the latter part of the nineteenth century, instruments designed to grasp calculi were used to try to remove bladder tumours. The first suprapubic removal of a vesical neoplasm was performed by Billroth in 1874. The first total cystectomy for tumour of the bladder was carried out by Bardenheuer in 1887. While these advances in surgery were taking place, cystoscopic methods of evaluation and therapy were also being developed.

The invention of the cystoscope revolutionized the investigation of bladder tumours. In 1889, Nitze published a paper on the cystoscopic diagnosis of bladder tumours. The introduction of cystography in the early 1900s proved a useful adjunct, and intravenous pyelography proved to be of major value in assessing the effect of bladder tumours on the upper urinary tract and the planning of surgical procedures.

Perineal urethrotomy and extirpation of bladder tumours

Digital exploration of the bladder through a perineal urethrotomy was first advocated by Henry Thompson in 1880. Various types of forceps and curettes were used. The perineal approach, however, never proved popular and was soon abandoned.

Suprapubic cystotomy and removal of bladder tumours

A suprapubic approach for the extirpation of bladder tumours was advocated in the 1880s by French surgeons such as Bazy, Pousson and Albarran. This technique rapidly became the accepted method of dealing with bladder tumours on the continent and spread to America and to England. The use of the wide transverse incision advocated by Trendelenburg allowed for better exposure, along with symphysectomy as advocated by Guyon and Albarran. In 1892, Albarran reviewed 100 suprapubic operations for bladder tumour and stressed the importance of removing both the tumour and a margin of normal mucosa (Albarran, 1892).

Partial cystectomy

The first partial cystectomy was carried out in 1884 via an intraperitoneal approach. Supporters of both the intraperitoneal and extraperitoneal approach created significant controversy. In 1905, Rafin reviewed 96 partial cystectomies, with a mortality rate of 21 per cent (Rafin, 1905).

Total cystectomy

Total cystectomy was first performed in 1887 in Cologne for a tumour of the bladder involving both ureters. Although the intention was to implant both ureters into the bowel, the surgeon was unable to localize one ureter and thus left both draining into the pelvis; the patient succumbed 2 weeks postoperatively. In 1888, Pawlick carried out the first successful cystectomy with an anastomosis of the ureter to the vagina. The patient was alive and well 16 years later. The technique of total cystectomy included freeing the anterior and posterior surfaces as far as the bladder neck, then the vascular pedicles of the bladder, then the ureter on each side. The bladder neck was divided and the prostate was usually not removed en bloc with the specimen. The operation was technically difficult and Hugh Young maintained that the high mortality rate and rarity of success rendered the operation unjustifiable. The morbidity and mortality ranged up to 60 per cent by the early 1920s. Urinary diversion was resolved in numerous ways, including suturing of the ureters to the urethra, cutaneous ureterostomy, and ureterosigmoidostomy. The first successful ureterointestinal anastomosis for bladder cancer was reported in 1899 by Kraus. Advances in anaesthesia during the 1940s as well as the development of antibiotics decreased the hazards of major extirpative surgery, although long-term survivals were still relatively poor. In attempts to achieve more complete local removal, the extent of the operation was increased to include an anterior pelvic exenteration or occasionally a total pelvic exenteration (Whitmore and Marshall, 1956). Jewett and Lewis (1948) found no cures when the bladder wall was deeply infiltrated, but a higher proportion of cures when the tumours infiltrated less than halfway through the muscularis. Other surgeons, disappointed with the results of total cystectomy, resorted to transurethral resection for all patients with carcinoma (Barnes *et al.*, 1955).

The operation of cystectomy has had proponents and opponents throughout the decades, representing a polarization of urologists based upon the difficulty of the operation itself as well as the morbidity and mortality associated with the operation. The attitude of many urologists has been that the high mortality incident to the operation precluded its frequent use. Indeed, Fishel, in 1925, spoke of radical cystectomy as fascinating but obsolete. Problems with development of urinary diversion also dampened enthusiasm towards routine use of cystectomy. Operative mortality from early single-stage cystectomy and urinary diversion was between 25 and 60 per cent. Part of the problem related to blood loss, but a significant portion of the morbidity and mortality related to ascending infections and sepsis, especially with the use of ureterosigmoidostomy. Coffey's anti-reflux technique reduced somewhat the risk of mortality and sepsis; however, ascending infections still remained a significant problem. Bricker's technique of an isolated ureteroileal segment, in 1950, significantly reduced dangers of ascending infections and led to more widespread acceptance of cystectomy.

Staging

Classification

The current staging systems for clinical evaluation of patients with carcinoma of the bladder evolved almost 40 years ago when Denoix (1978) and Jewett and Strong (1946) independently described systems for classification of bladder cancer. The TNM system, adopted by the Union International Contre le Cancer (UICC), was based upon Denoix's description and classifies tumours based on assessment of the extent of the primary tumour (T), the status of regional nodal involvement (N), and the presence or absence of metastases (M).

The other system began in the early 1940s when Dr Hugh Jewett, a resident under the tutelage of Dr Hugh Hampton Young at Johns Hopkins University, analysed a large series of cases of bladder cancer to determine management guidelines for its treatment. Dr Jewett, along with Dr George Strong, a resident in pathology, initially analysed 100 autopsy cases of patients with carcinoma of the bladder (Jewett and Strong, 1946). Jewett suggested that bladder tumours be divided into three pathological stages, with invasion of submucosa (A), muscularis (B), or perivesical tissue (C). In that study, metastases were found in 0 per cent of patients with tumours confined to the submucosa, 13 per cent of patients with tumours involving the muscularis, and 74 per cent of patients with tumours involving the perivesical fat. In a subsequent study, Jewett suggested subdividing muscle-invasive (B) tumours into those involving the superficial muscle layers (B1) and those involving the deep muscle layers (B2). Unfortunately, however, the separation of survival for stage-B patients was based on 18 patients, 4 of 5 with B1 disease who survived 5 years compared with only 1 of 13 of stage B2 who survived 5 years (Jewett, 1952).

In 1952, Victor Marshall presented a modification of the Jewett and Strong staging system and added stage 0 to include tumours confined to the mucosa and not invading into the lamina propria (Marshall, 1952). A subsequent category of stage D was defined to include tumours with evident metastatic disease and subdivided into stage-D1 lesions, still confined within the bony pelvis, and stage-D2 lesions, extending beyond the limits of the true pelvis. Thus, both a TNM pathologic staging system and the current American Marshall modification of the Jewett and Strong system now exist for staging of carcinoma of the bladder (see Table 7.1).

Errors in staging

Prior to discussion of the indications for radical cystectomy, it is worthwhile to consider the problems associated with preoperative estimation of the pathological stage of bladder cancer. The traditional staging methods, discussed in Chapters 4 and 5, include cystoscopic biopsy, bimanual examination, ultrasonography, computed tomography scan, and possibly lymphangiography, with magnetic resonance imaging still in its infancy. One should recognize that clinical staging systems are only as good as the techniques available to assess the pathological extent of disease. The National Cooperative Bladder Cancer Study, in 1976, reported an error rate as high as 50 per cent between clinical and pathological stages for patients with stage-B and stage-C disease, with an understaging error for patients treated with surgery alone of 42 per cent, and an overstaging error of 21 per cent (Slack *et al.*, 1977). Understaging for all patients with pathological stage-B cancers of the bladder ranges from 31 to 46 per cent, and overstaging varies between 20 and 50 per cent. Several other series have also borne out the shortcoming of the clinician in accurately predicting the extent of involvement. Skinner *et al.* (1982) reported a 40 per cent understaging and 23 per cent overstaging error in T1 to T3 bladder cancers, with agreement of the clinical and pathological stage in only 36 per cent of patients. Chisholm and associates, using the TNM system, felt that it was impossible to distinguish TA from T1 tumours and also lumped T2 and T3 tumours into a single category (Chisholm *et al.*, 1980). These errors in estimation of stage make the clinical decision for management of patients with bladder cancer somewhat an art rather than a science, and should be recognized as such.

Definition of cystectomy

Surgical extirpation of the bladder for cancer has evolved through three basic stages, that of simple cystectomy, total cystectomy, and radical cystectomy. Simple cystectomy denotes removal of the bladder alone, usually

Table 7.1 American versus TNM classifications

Jewett and Strong (1946)	Jewett (1952)	Marshall (1952)	TNM (1978) Clinical	TNM (1978) Pathological	Features
		0	T0	P0	No tumour definitive specimen
			TIS	PIS	Carcinoma-in-situ
			Ta	Pa	Papillary tumour without invasion
A	A	A	T1	P1	Invasion of lamina propria
B	B1	B1	T2	P2	Superficial muscle invasion
	B2	B2	T3A	P3A	Deep muscle invasion
C	C	C	T3B	P3B	Invasion of perivesical fat
				P4A	Invasion of prostate, vagina or uterus
		D1	T4	P4B	Fixed to pelvic or abdominal wall
			N1–3		Pelvic nodes
			M1		Distant metastases
		D2	M4		Nodes above aortic bifurcation

performed by excision close to the bladder wall. The prostate remains intact. This procedure is now usually performed for benign diseases such as pyocystis or interstitial cystitis, although a simple cystectomy was used for removal of bladder cancers at an earlier time. Total cystectomy encompasses removal of the bladder, prostate and seminal vesicles in the male but usually with a margin close to the bladder. The term radical cystectomy usually implies removal of the bladder with contiguous organs and tissues en bloc. Thus, radical cystectomy in the male would include removal of the urinary bladder, prostate, and seminal vesicles with a margin of surrounding adipose tissue as well as the overlying pelvic peritoneum. The proximal vas deferens and 1 or 2 cm of the proximal urethra are also resected. In the female patient, radical cystectomy consists of an anterior exenteration, with removal of the bladder, urethra and surrounding fascia, en bloc with the uterus, fallopian tubes, ovaries and a segment of the anterior vaginal wall.

A regional bilateral pelvic lymph node dissection is usually, but not always, included at the time of radical cystectomy. This involves removal of nodal tissue from the aortic bifurcation and corresponding levels at the inferior vena cava encompassing common iliac, external iliac, hypogastric, and obturator nodal tissue. The limits of dissection are, laterally, the geni- tofemoral nerve, and inferiorly, the inguinal ligament and node of Cloquet.

Partial cystectomy is an attractive alternative to radical cystectomy in very selected individuals because of its lower operative morbidity and mortality. Potency can be preserved and there is no need for an external urinary collecting device. Survival figures reported for selected patients approach those achieved with more radical forms of therapy. However, it should be emphasized that partial cystectomy is indicated only in a select patient population. In the Mayo Clinic experience, partial cystectomy was applicable for only 199 patients out of a total of some 3000 individuals (Utz *et al.*, 1973).

Because carcinoma of the bladder is a field disease, partial cystectomy has no place in the management of patients with carcinoma-in-situ or with multiple cancers occurring synchronously or metachronously. The location and size of the tumours is extremely important in consideration for partial cystectomy. Tumours should be located well away from the trigone and bladder neck so that at least a 2 cm surgical margin can be achieved. In selected patients, with localized lesions preferably in the dome, well away from the ureteral orifices and bladder neck, and without presence of associated carcinoma-in-situ, partial cystectomy represents a reasonable alternative. The perivesical fat should be removed en bloc with the bladder specimen and unilateral or bilateral pelvic node dissection, as described above, should be performed as well. In patients in whom partial cystectomy is contemplated, preoperative radiation therapy is important to prevent spillage of tumour cells. A minimum of 1500 cGy can reliably prevent wound contamination (Van der Werf-Messing, 1969). Preoperative radia- tion therapy is important because partial cystectomy inherently represents a relatively poor cancer operation. There is no isolation of the venous and lymphatic drainage, and the potential for vascular and lymphatic dissemina- tion as well as tumour cell spillage exists.

The necessity for rigid patient selection makes segmental resection appropriate for only 5 per cent of patients with bladder cancer. Five-year survival rates in patients with stage 0, A or B bladder cancer treated by partial cystectomy range from 65 to 81 per cent (Novick and Stewart, 1976; Utz *et al.*, 1980).

Surgical technique

The patient is best approached through an incision slightly to the left of the midline. An inverted V incision is then made into the anterior peritoneum beginning at the umbilicus and continuing bilaterally to the internal rings. The lateral margins of this incision should be the inferior epigastric vasculature. The inferior portion of the peritoneal envelope is incised and the incision is carried cephalad in the posterior peritoneum using the testicular vasculature as the lateral margin of dissection. This defines the limits of the dissection and exposes the pelvic vasculature, lymphatics and ureters. Pelvic lymphadenectomy should begin at the level of the aortic bifurcation and include the node-bearing tissue surrounding the common and external iliac vessels, obturator nerves, and hypogastric vasculature. After completion of the lymphadenectomy, the lateral pedicles, based on the hypogastric artery, are doubly clipped and divided. The posterior peritoneum is divided at the retrovesical pouch, and the posterior layer of Denonvillier's fascia is dissected bluntly from the serosa of the rectum. The posterior pedicles are ligated and the bladder and surrounding structures removed. The pelvic floor, at the completion of the procedure, contains only the intact rectal serosa, external iliac vessels, obturator nerve, and urethra at the level of the urogenital diaphragm.

Radical cystectomy requires institution of an acceptable method of urinary diversion. The enteric conduit is preferred by most as it effectively separates the urinary and faecal streams. The primary consideration in construction of an enteric conduit is that the bowel tube created be sufficiently short to function merely as a conduit and not as a repository for urine. This will keep absorption of excretory products to a minimum and prevent the electrolytic disturbances which accompany the absorption of urine.

The distal ileum is the preferred bowel segment. A segment approximately 15 cm in length should be isolated and the continuity of the bowel re-established with a two-layer ileo-ileostomy. The proximal end of the isolated segment is closed with an inverted running absorption suture. The left ureter is led through a tunnel beneath the sigmoid mesocolon to lie in the right retroperitoneum alongside the right distal ureter. Both ureters are spatulated and are anastomosed to the proximal end of the isolated ileal segment on the antimesenteric border using a mucosal-to-mucosal anastomosis with absorbable suture. Both distal ureters are optimally spatulated to prevent postoperative stricture.

The distal end of the isolated ileal segment is led out through a defect in the right lower abdominal wall, usually placed one-half of the distance between the anterior superior iliac spine and the umbilicus. An inverted mucocutaneous anastomosis is established with absorbable suture material.

The necessity for simultaneous urethrectomy in all males undergoing radical cystectomy remains in debate. Only 7 per cent of all patients subjected to radical cystectomy will subsequently develop urethral malignancy. However, this figure will double when diffuse *in situ* changes exist within the bladder or prostatic urethra, or when the primary tumour is at the level of the bladder neck. These patients should undergo simultaneous in-continuity urethrectomy (Richie and Skinner, 1978). Patients in whom the urethra is not removed should be followed with urethral cytologies obtained by washing or by direct swabbing of the retained urethra.

Indications

The decision as to when to perform radical cystectomy in a patient with carcinoma of the bladder is based on a combination of factors, with consideration of the polychronotopism of bladder tumour as well as the individual medical condition of the patient. Basically, patients are considered for radical cystectomy when the threat of aggressiveness of the primary bladder tumour, and the likelihood of spread into the deeper layers of the bladder and especially into the lymphatic or vascular spaces, heralding metastases, outweighs the risk to the patient in undergoing a major operative procedure. Because of the relatively protracted time course of bladder cancers in some patients, many patients are followed conservatively with periodic endoscopic resections unless a change occurs in the status of the bladder cancer—either increasing grade of tumour, increasing frequency of recurrences, presence of carcinoma-in-situ, increasing irritative symptoms, or increasing stage of the tumour leading to consideration of radical cystectomy.

Once the urothelial malignancy has penetrated through the submucosa into the muscularis, radical cystoprostatectomy is the preferred treatment. This operation can satisfy the treatment of field changes that are common in urothelial malignancy and results in a reasonable potential for cure if the cancer is still confined within the bladder wall. Unfortunately, as described earlier, tumours may already have progressed beyond the point of curability by means of local therapy with radical cystectomy alone. Survival rate for patients with superficial muscle invasion is approximately 50 per cent, whereas with deeper muscle penetration the survival rate is similar, 40–50 per cent. Failures in patients managed by radical cystectomy alone are usually due to distant metastases, with approximately 10 per cent of patients failing locally.

Prior to the mid-1970s, bladder tumours were subdivided, based on the work of Jewett, into superficial tumours (stages 0, A and B1) and deep tumours (stages B2 and C, T3A and T3B). This distinction was based on the original work of Jewett in which patients with superficial muscle invasion had a survival advantage (4 out of 5 survived five years) whereas patients with deep-muscle invasion had less of a survival advantage (1 out of 13 survived 5 years) (Jewett, 1952). This preliminary information was incorporated into staging systems and into the TNM system, with stage B1 being a T2 and stage B2 being a T3A (Table 7.1). In the mid-1970s, a review of 113 patients who had undergone radical cystectomy from 1956 to 1971 disclosed 5-year survival rates of 70–75 per cent for patients with pathological stage 0 or A, 40 per cent with pathological stage B1, 40 per cent for patients with pathological stage B2, and 20 per cent for patients with pathological stage C (Richie *et al.*, 1975; Table 7.2). Subsequent reviews of several series in the literature, encompassing approximately 1400 patients, have borne out this

Table 7.2 Pathological stage and 5-year survival for 140 patients treated by cystectomy (Richie *et al.*, 1975)

Stage	5-year survival (%)	
0–A	78.6	
B1	39.9	
B2	40.4	All B, 40.0 ($p<0.01$)
C	19.7	
D	6.2	

Note the nearly identical survival for stage B1 and stage B2 and the statistical significance between survival of those patients with tumour confined to the mucosa compared with those with muscle invasion ($p<0.01$)

significant difference in survival rates, with patients with stage-0 and stage-A cancers having a 5-year survival rate of approximately 67 per cent, all stage-B patients having a survival rate of 40 per cent, and Stage C's having a survival rate of 18 per cent. Thus, the depth of muscle invasion becomes far less significant than the infiltration in the muscle wall, a feature that can be ascertained with far greater accuracy than the clinician's or pathologist's ability to assess depth into the muscle wall. In support of this, Barnes found that it was impossible to distinguish superficial from deep-muscle penetration with any degree of accuracy.

In addition to depth of infiltration, the presence and natural history of carcinoma-in-situ have become important in understanding the field-change defect and its implications for therapy. The presence of carcinoma-in-situ, certainly in association with overt bladder cancer, is ominous and should encourage the use of more aggressive therapy (e.g. cystectomy). Althausen and associates reported an 83 per cent incidence of progression to muscle-wall invasion in patients with an overt bladder tumour and associated carcinoma-in-situ (Althausen *et al.*, 1976). Because of this associated feature, random biopsies are necessary in the assessment of patients with high-grade bladder cancer. Newer methodologies may become useful in predicting patterns of recurrence and progression to invasion, as discussed in Chapters 1 and 2.

Prognosis

Prognosis in patients with carcinoma of the bladder who have undergone cystectomy has traditionally been reported on the basis of 5-year survival rates. Originally, this was based on observed survival data, with all patients followed at least 5 years. Beginning in the 1970s, however, actuarial survival rates using statistical correlation, such as Kaplan Meyer curves, have been used to present projected 5-year survival rates. This technique allows incorporation of patients followed for less than 5 years but considered at risk for the interval in which they have been followed. One problem with reports of survival are that most 5-year survivals have been based on the pathological stage, which may be at significant variance from the clinical stage.

Until the 1950s, survival rates had little meaning since the operative mortality varied from 25 to 60 per cent. In 1966, Glantz reported a mortality rate of 20 per cent in patients who underwent total cystectomy in the 1950s and early 1960s (Glantz, 1966). Whitmore and Marshall (1962) reported a mortality rate of 14 per cent in radical cystectomies done between 1945 and 1955. Richie and associates reported a 15 per cent overall operative mortality from 1955 to 1971, but a 2 per cent operative mortality in the most recent 50 patients done in the early 1970s (Richie *et al.*, 1975). Johnson and Lamy (1977) reported a 3.3 per cent mortality rate in 214 radical cystectomies done between 1969 and 1975. More recently, Skinner reported a less than 1 per cent operative mortality in 128 radical cystectomies from 1971 to 1977 (Skinner, 1980).

With the improvement in postoperative mortality rate, survival data have become more meaningful. Prior to 1975, most survival rates were broken down into patients with superficial (0, A and B1; T_0, Ta, T1) and deep (B2, C or T3A, T3B) pathologically staged lesions. Whitmore and associates reported a 63 per cent 5-year survival for superficial and a 20 per cent 5-year survival for deep lesions in 137 patients who underwent radical cystectomy alone between 1949 and 1958. With preoperative radiation therapy of 4500 cGy, and with improved surgical techniques, 5-year survivals for 119 patients operated on between 1959 and 1966 were 58 per cent for the superficial group and 48 per cent for the deep group. Eighty-six patients who received a short course (2000 cGy) to the bladder and true pelvis and then radical cystectomy, between 1966 and 1970, had a 5-year survival of 56 per cent for the superficial lesions and 58 per cent for the deep lesions (Whitmore *et al.*, 1977). Although this series suggests improvement in survival rates related to preoperative radiation, an equally plausible alternative explanation relates to improved survival rates from improved techniques of surgical approach, anaesthetic management and better patient monitoring.

The fallacy of dividing patients into superficial and deep groups can be shown by the figures in Table 7.2. These results, based on a 16-year study, show statistically significant survival differences for patients with stage 0 and A, all stage-B patients and patients with stage-C disease. More recent data by Skinner and associates have shown that the 5-year survival of patients with P2 and P3A tumours (stages B1 and B2) was not statistically different, either when analysed separately or combined, implying that the presence or absence of muscle invasion is the seminal event concerning the need for

Table 7.3 5-year survival in relation to depth of bladder-wall invasion at the time of cystectomy (Skinner, 1980)

Pathological stage	Number of patients	5-year survival (%)
P0, P1, PIS	61	81
P2	20	53
P3A	13	39
P3B	28	39
P4	8	25
P2 + 3A	33	50
P3A + P3b	41	41
N+	34	36

All patients received 1600 cGy preoperative radiation + radical cystectomy and pelvic node dissection.

Table 7.4 Bladder carcinoma: 5-year survival rates

Reference	Number of patients	P0/P1/ PIS (0, A)	P2 (B1)	P3a (B2)	P3b (C)	P4 or N+
Bowles and Cordonier (1963)	50		63	50	20	0
Jewett et al. (1964)	61		50	16	12	
Pearse *et al.* (1978)	52		50	42	13	0
Mathur *et al.* (1981)	58	71	88	57	40	29
Skinner and Lieskovsky (1984)	197	75	64	44		36

aggressive therapy (see Table 7.3) (compare with Chapter 8). Even though survival rates have improved with contemporary surgical techniques (see Table 7.4), the majority of patients with bladder cancers invasive deep into the muscle wall or through into the perivesical tissue will succumb to their disease within a 5-year period. More than 50 per cent of such patients will develop distant metastases, usually within one or two years after cystectomy. The future, therefore, undoubtedly lies in the coordination of adjuvant systemic therapy, which would appear at this point in time to be some combination of chemotherapy. It is important to learn from the past and to recognize that carefully controlled and randomized studies will be essential to delineate the beneficial effects of combination therapy.

Combination therapy

In an effort to improve on patient survival, various combinations of radiation therapy along with radical cystectomy have been advocated. Much of this is covered elsewhere in this volume. Radiation therapy prior to radical cystectomy seems to result in a definite although small increase in survival when compared with surgery alone (see Chapters 4, 8 and 15). However, most of these studies have been flawed by the use of historical controls or lack of randomized studies. Even when considering randomized studies of cystectomy versus preoperative radiation followed by cystectomy, the combined treatment results in a significant survival advantage only in those patients who are downstaged to P0, with no viable tumour remaining after radiation therapy. In addition, two non-randomized concurrent series without historical controls have shown no survival advantage to preoperative radiation therapy versus current surgical cystectomy (Montie *et al.*, 1984; Skinner and Lieskovsky, 1984). Because of the persistent systemic failure rate with combined therapies of radiation and cystectomy, coupled with the effectiveness of systemic chemotherapy for patients with disseminated disease, newer approaches using up-front or neoadjuvant chemotherapy followed by cystectomy are now being evaluated and seem to show promise (Pearson and Raghavan, 1985). Active agents include methotrexate, cisplatinum, vinblastine, and doxorubicin in various combinations. Randomized studies are now under way to determine if a significant survival advantage can be achieved by this combination of therapies (see Chapter 17).

New approaches

Potency-preserving technique for radical cystectomy

Prior to the early 1980s, virtually all patients who had undergone radical cystectomy were impotent postoperatively. Following the pioneering work by Walsh and associates for delineation of the anatomy of Santorini's plexus (Reiner and Walsh, 1979), as well as description of the anatomical relationships between the nerves supplying the corpora cavernosum and the apex of the prostate (Walsh and Donker, 1982), anatomical approaches have been described for radical prostatectomy and radical cystectomy that can preserve potency in a high percentage of patients. Radical cystectomy proceeds as described in the section on surgical techniques, including bilateral pelvic lymph node dissection and division of the lateral pedicles to the prostate. A plane is developed between the bladder and rectum by incising the peritoneum and using gentle blunt dissection to free the rectum from the prostate at Denonvilliers' fascia. Dissection is stopped prior to encountering lateral pedicles of the bladder near the pelvic fascia. Attention is then turned to the dorsal-venous complex and plexus of Santorini as for radical retropubic prostatectomy. Isolation of the dorsal venous complex is achieved and the membranous urethra is transected with division of the lateral pelvic fascia and pedicles to the prostate. The seminal vesicals are then dissected away from the neurovascular bundle on each side and the remainder of the lateral bladder pedicles are ligated.

Utilizing these principles, radical removal of bladder cancer can be performed with preservation of the neurovascular bundles and therefore preservation of potency. Indeed, approximately two-thirds of patients who were potent preoperatively will recover potency from 6 months to one year following radical cystectomy using this modified technique.

Urinary diversion

The standard method of urinary diversion following cystectomy remains the ileal conduit. However, newer techniques have been described to include continent forms of urinary diversion, such as the Kock pouch or Camey procedure or ileocecal segment. These techniques involve innovative use of bowel segments brought either to the skin or sutured to the urethra, allowing the patient to void in a normal fashion or be catheterized intermittently on a periodic basis rather than wearing an external collecting device. The Kock pouch involves utilization of a long segment of ileum and creation of an internal pouch with antirefluxing intersusscepted nipple connected to both ureters and a second nipple to preserve continence. The pouch is usually brought to the abdominal wall but may, on rare occasions, be placed down to the urethra (Kock, 1982). The Camey procedure involves utilization of a long segment of ileum hooked to the end of the urethra in an end-to-side anastomotic fashion (Lillien and Camey, 1984). Each ureter is implanted into one end of the upper portion of the U using an antirefluxing ureteroileal anastomosis. The patients void normally during the daytime but have problems with nocturnal enuresis. The ileocecal segment can be used with the ileocecal valve as an antireflux mechanism and the cecum brought to the skin for intermittent catheterization or a cecoileal segment can be anastomosed directly to the urethra for normal voiding. All of these techniques are somewhat experimental and should be used in selected patients only. Urinary diversion continues to evolve through a variety of new techniques, all of which will require long-term follow-up to be certain that complications not yet suspected do not arise.

References

Albarran, J. (1892). *Les Tumeurs de la Vessie*. G. Steinhall, Paris.

Althausen, A.F., Prout, J.R. and Daly, J.J. (1976). Non-invasive papillary carcinoma of the bladder associated with carcinoma-in-situ. *Journal of Urology* **116**: 575.

Barnes, R.W., Hadley, H.L., Bergman, R.T. and Turner, R. (1955). Conservative versus radical treatment of bladder tumours. *Medical Journal of Australia* **1**: 197.

Bowles, W.T. and Cordonnier, J.J. (1963). Total cystectomy for carcinoma of the bladder. *Journal of Urology* **90**: 731.

Chisholm, G.D., Hindmarsh, J.R. and Howatson, A.G. (1980). TNM (1978) in bladder cancer: use and abuse. *British Journal of Urology* **52**: 500.

Denoix, P.F. (1978). *TNM Classification of Malignant Tumors*, 3rd edn. International Union Against Cancer, Geneva.

Glantz, G.N. (1966). Cystectomy and urinary diversion. *Journal of Urology* **96**: 714.

Jewett, H.J. (1958). The carcinoma of the bladder: influence of depth of infiltration on the 5 year results following extirpation of the primary growth. *Journal of Urology* **67**: 672.

Jewett, H.J., King, L.R. and Shelley, W.M. (1964). A study of 365 cases of infiltrating bladder cancer: relation of certain pathological characteristics to prognosis after extirpation. *Journal of Urology* **92**: 668.

Jewett, H.J. and Lewis, E.L. (1948). Infiltrating carcinoma of bladder: curability by total cystectomy. *Journal of Urology* **60**: 107.

Jewett, H.J. and Strong, G.H. (1946). Infiltrating carcinoma of the bladder: relation of depth of penetration of the bladder wall to incidence of local extention and metastases. *Journal of Urology* **55**: 366.

Johnson, D.E. and Lamy, S.M. (1977). Complications of a single stage radical cystectomy and ileal conduit diversion: review of 214 cases. *Journal of Urology* **117**: 171.

Kock, N.G., Nilson, A.E., Nilsson, L.O., Norlen, L.J., Philipson, B.M. (1982). Urinary diversion via a continent ileal reservoir: clinical results in 12 patients. *Journal of Urology* **128**: 469.

Lilien, O.M. and Camey, M. (1984). 25-year experience with replacement of the human bladder (Camey procedure). *Journal of Urology* **132**: 4886.

Marshall, V.F. (1952). The relation of the pre-operative estimate to the pathologic demonstration of the extent of vesical neoplasms. *Journal of Urology* **68**: 714.

Mathur, V.K., Krahn, H.P. and Ramsey, E.W. (1981). Total cystectomy for bladder cancer. *Journal of Urology* **125**: 784.

Montie, J.E., Straffon, R.A. and Stewart, B.H. (1984). Radical cystectomy without radiation therapy for carcinoma of the bladder. *Journal of Urology* **131**: 477.

Novick, A.C. and Stewart, B.H. (1976). Partial cystectomy in the treatment of primary and secondary carcinoma of the bladder. *Journal of Urology* **116**: 570.

Pearse, H.D., Reed, R.R. and Hodges, C.V. (1978). Radical cystectomy for bladder cancer. *Journal of Urology* **119**: 216.

Pearson, B.S. and Raghavan, D. (1985). First-line intravenous cisplatin for deeply invasive bladder cancer: update on 70 cases. *British Journal of Urology* **57**: 690.

Rafin, M. (1905). Indications et resultats du traitement des tumeurs de la vessie. *Ass. Franc. Urol.* **9**: 1.

Reiner, W.G. and Walsh, P.C. (1979). An anatomical approach to the surgical management of the dorsal vein and Santorini's plexus during radical retropubic surgery. *Journal of Urology* **121**: 998.

Richie, J.P. and Skinner, D.G. (1978). Carcinoma-in-situ of the urethra in association with bladder carcinoma: the role of urethrectomy. *Journal of Urology* **119**: 80.

Richie, J.P., Skinner, D.G. and Kaufman, J.J. (1975). Radical cystectomy for carcinoma of the bladder: 16 years experience. *Journal of Urology* **113**: 186.

Skinner, D.G. (1980). Current perspectives in the management of high-grade invasive bladder cancer. *Cancer* **45**: 1866.

Skinner, D.G. and Lieskovsky, G. (1984). Contemporary cystectomy with pelvic node dissection compared to preoperative radiation therapy plus cystectomy in management of invasive bladder cancer. *Journal of Urology* **131**: 1069.

Skinner, D.G., Tift, J.P. and Kaufman, J.J. (1982). High dose, short course preoperative radiation therapy and immediate single stage radical cystectomy with pelvic node dissection in the management of bladder cancer. *Journal of Urology* **127**: 671.

Slack, N.H., Bross, I.D.J. and Prout, G.R. (1977). Five-year follow-up results of a collaborative study of therapies for carcinoma of the bladder. *Journal of Surgical Oncology* **9**: 393.

Utz, D.C., Farrow, G.M., Rife, C.C. *et al.* (1980). Carcinoma-in-situ of the bladder. *Cancer* **45**: 1842.

Utz, D.C., Schmitz, S.E., Fugelso, P.D. *et al.* (1973). A clinical pathologic evaluation of partial cystectomy for carcinoma of the urinary bladder. *Cancer* **32**: 1075.

van der Werf-Messing, B. (1969). Carcinoma of the bladder treated by suprapubic radium implants: the value of additional external irradiation. *European Journal of Cancer* **5**: 227.

Walsh, P.C. and Donker, P.J. (1982). Impotence following radical prostatectomy: insight into etiology and prevention. *Journal of Urology* **128**: 492.

Whitmore, W.F. and Marshall, V.F. (1956). Radical surgery for carcinoma of the urinary bladder. In *Bladder Tumours*. J.B. Lippincott, Philadelphia.

Whitmore, W.F. and Marshall, V.F. (1962). Radical total cystectomy for cancer of the bladder: 230 consecutive cases five years later. *Journal of Urology* **87**: 853.

Whitmore, W.F., Batata, M.A., Ghoneim, M.A. *et al.* (1977). Radical cystectomy with or without prior radiation in the treatment of bladder cancer. *Journal of Urology* **118**: 184.

8

Radiation therapy in invasive bladder cancer: principles, results, patient selection and innovations

Mary Ann Rose and William U. Shipley

Introduction

In the last decade, many institutions have reported that modern megavoltage radiation therapy can be curative for patients with muscle-invasive bladder cancer. Data have been accumulated from large numbers of patients, through prospective randomized trials and retrospective reviews, which indicate a 17–39 per cent overall 5-year survival with preservation of a functioning bladder (Goffinet *et al.*, 1975; Morrison 1975; Miller, 1977; Greiner *et al.*, 1977; Blandy *et al.*, 1980; Madsen *et al.*, 1980; Goodman *et al.*, 1981; Bloom *et al.*, 1982; Gospodarowicz *et al.*, 1984; Shipley *et al.*, 1985). In the United States, radical cystectomy has been the standard method of treatment for invasive bladder cancer (see Chapter 7), creating an unfavourable bias in many radiation series where patients have been older, medically inoperable, or technically unresectable. Recent observations on prognostic indicators in this disease—including pathological subtypes, radiographical studies, clinical stage and radiation responsiveness (Chapters 1 and 2)—may allow the careful selection of patients for full-dose radiation therapy, reserving cystectomy for salvage of local failures.

The purpose of this chapter is four-fold: first, to describe the technical considerations in pelvic external-beam irradiation and interstitial radiation therapy; second, to review the results of important clinical trials and the complications of therapy; third, to delineate prognostic factors and possible criteria for patient selection for full-dose radiation therapy; and finally, to explore innovative approaches to bladder cancer, such as intraoperative radiation therapy, radiation sensitizers, and combinations of radiation and chemotherapy.

Technical considerations

The techniques used to deliver curative irradiation to the bladder tumour volume while sparing normal tissue will vary from institution to institution, depending on the availability and energy of radiation therapy machines, the quality of physics and computer support and the skill and experience of the radiation therapist in treating bladder cancer.

At the Massachusetts General Hospital, most patients with bladder cancer have been treated with external-beam irradiation using a 10 MV or 25 MV linear accelerator. For the initial course of treatment a 'four-field box' technique is used with contoured paired anterior–posterior and lateral fields (Fig. 8.1). The fields are designed to treat the entire bladder, perivesical tissues and draining lymph nodes to a total dose of 5040 cGy (rads) given in daily doses of 180 cGy fractions, five times a week. This dose can be reasonably expected to be effective in sterilizing microscopic tumour deposits in lymph nodes and microscopic extension of the primary (Fletcher, 1984). A cone down 'boost' is delivered to the clinically evident tumour to a total dose of 6840 cGy, using the same fractionation schedule as in the initial course. The boost may be delivered through paired lateral fields (Fig. 8.2) or through rotational fields, depending on the size of the tumour and its location within the bladder. Fig. 8.3 demonstrates a representative treatment plan. The tumour volume is carefully mapped out by the urologist and radiotherapist at the time of initial cystoscopy and transurethral resection of the bladder tumour (TURB). Diagnostic techniques such as the cystogram or occasionally CAT scanning and ultrasound may be useful in the final stages of treatment planning if they are performed prior to transurethral resection and irradiation (Hodson *et al.*, 1979; Nakamura and Niijima, 1980). Preservation of a functioning bladder is more likely if a portion of the bladder can safely be excluded from the high dose of radiation needed to the bladder tumour itself. Treatment of the entire bladder with high doses per fraction, or a high total dose, will more likely result in scarring and contracture with intolerable urinary frequency. Similarly, care must be taken to observe known tolerance of other structures within the radiation portals, including the rectum, femoral heads and small bowel, particularly if the patient has had a history of previous abdominal surgery, colitis, diverticular disease or pelvic infection.

Considerable experience in the use of radium needle interstitial implantation to 'boost' the bladder tumour volume has been accumulated by Brigit Van der Werf Messing *et al.* (1980, 1983). This technique affords the advantage of delivering a high dose of radiation in a short time to a localized area implanted under direct visualization, thus maximizing tumour dose while minimizing the risk of damage to other pelvic structures. Tumours treated in this fashion must be under 5 cm in diameter for optimum dose distribution. In addition, the patient's medical condition must allow the risks of general anaesthesia and surgical intervention. In this procedure, the bladder is opened and threaded radium needles are placed through the tumour. The bladder is closed in two or three layers. After the calculated dose has been delivered, the needles are removed without re-exposing the bladder. This is done by traction on sutures that were attached to each needle and brought out through a separate site. The implant delivers a dose of 3500 cGy to the tumour, which also receives an additional 4000 cGy through a combination of pre- and postoperative external-beam irradiation. Thus, the total dose to the bladder cancer is 7500 cGy (Van der Werf Messing *et al.*, 1983). Other centres have attempted to use similar techniques substituting after-loading iridium[192] for radium in an effort to reduce the radiation risk to therapy and operating-room personnel (Strauss *et al.*, 1985). Intraoperative radiation therapy, to be discussed later in this chapter, affords the same advantage of delivering a high dose of radiation under direct visualization.

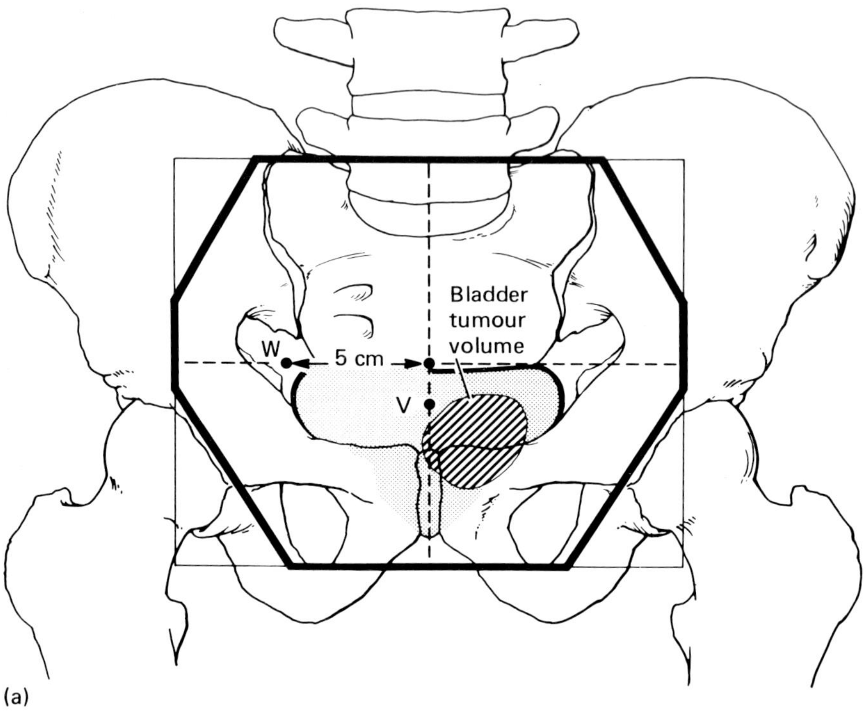

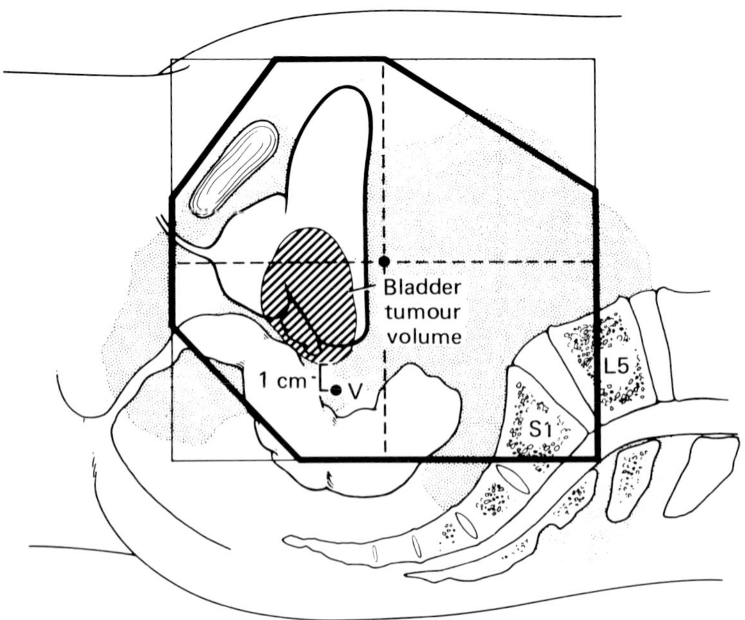

Fig. 8.1 (a) AP pelvis field. (b) Lateral pelvis field

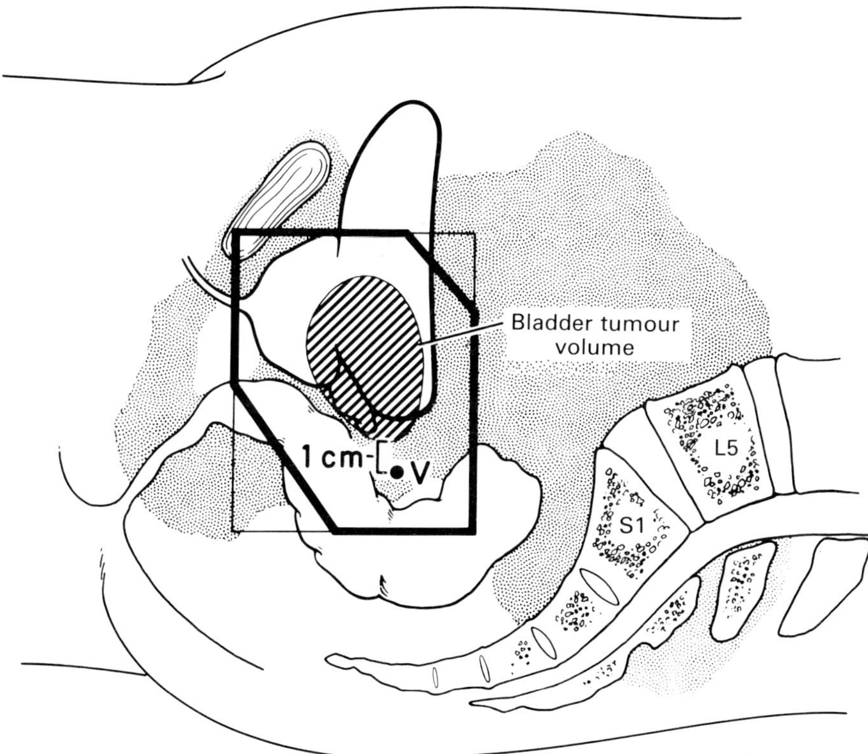

Fig. 8.2 Lateral boost field

Results of treatment

External-beam irradiation

Many patients who present with muscle-invasive bladder cancer will ultimately succumb to distant metastatic disease, either alone or in combination
with local tumour recurrence, regardless of the treatment modality employed. The major issue, then, facing urologists and radiation therapists is
whether certain patients can predictably be managed with full-dose radiation therapy, thus sparing them both the risk of major surgery and the
management of a stoma and bag without compromising their survival. The
relative merits of cystectomy with or without preoperative irradiation over
radiation therapy alone have been addressed in a small number of prospective randomized trials (Miller, 1977; Madsen *et al.*, 1980; Bloom *et al.*, 1982),
while the variables related to radiation response and likelihood of local
control have been most closely scrutinized in retrospective reviews where
analysis of large numbers of patients was possible.

Prospective studies (Table 8.1)
Of three published prospective randomized trials of preoperative radiation
and cystectomy versus cystectomy alone, only the study from the M.D.

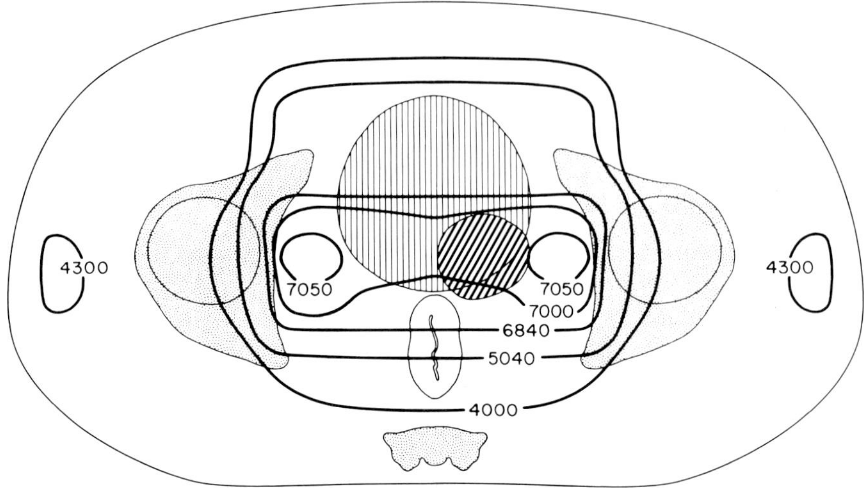

Fig. 8.3 Definitive XRT plan for T2–T3 bladder carcinoma. 10 MV x-rays are used. Whole pelvis: 5040 cGy; lateral tumour boost: 1800 cGy; AP–PA/lateral=20/8

Anderson Hospital (Miller, 1977), ironically the one with the smallest total number of patients entered, demonstrated a survival advantage on removal of the bladder. The 5-year survival of the 35 patients randomized to 5000 cGy preoperative radiation and cystectomy was 46 per cent compared with the statistically significantly poorer results in the 32 patients randomized to receive 7000 cGy by external megavoltage radiation where 22 per cent survived, including two patients who underwent salvage cystectomy. The results of this trial were analysed only with respect to treatment assigned, whether completed or not, with death as the end-point (whether due to tumour, treatment or intercurrent disease).

A second small prospective randomized trial was reported by Madsen *et al.* in 1980. This was an eight-institution three-armed study comparing radiation only versus preoperative irradiation plus partial or total cystectomy versus cystectomy alone. The radiation doses used in the radiotherapy-only

Table 8.1 Treatment of invasive bladder cancer: randomized trials

Series	*TUR and XRT*		*XRT and cystectomy*	
	Number	5-year survival (%)	Number	5-year survival (%)
M.D. Anderson Hospital (Miller, 1977)	32	22	35	46
Veterans Administration (Madsen *et al.*, 1980)	27	31	23	32
London Institute of Urology (Bloom *et al.*, 1982)	91	25	98	34

arm were low, 5000 cGy in 4–5 weeks to 6000 cGy in 5–6 weeks; however, no significant differences in survival were noted in any of the three groups.

The most comprehensive prospective randomized trial was mounted in 1966 in England by Wallace and Bloom of the Institute of Urology and the Royal Marsden Hospital (Bloom *et al.*, 1982). One hundred and ninety-nine patients were randomized from 1966 to 1975. Selection criteria included technical resectability and the fitness of the patients to undergo either radical irradiation or surgery. Patients received either 4000 cGy preoperatively followed by radical cystectomy in 4 weeks or 6000 cGy to the bladder followed by salvage cystectomy at the time of failure. Although the early report of the results of this trial indicated a trend in favour of the preoperative radiation-plus-cystectomy group, the differences failed to achieve statistical significance. The 5-year survivals, corrected for intercurrent deaths, were reported as 38 per cent in the preoperative radiation/cystectomy group and 29 per cent in the radiation-alone group ($p = 0.2$). Only in patients less than 60 years of age did elective cystectomy afford a statistically significant survival advantage, where 5-year survival for the combined treatment group was 49 per cent versus only 25 per cent for radical radiotherapy ($p < 0.05$). On the contrary, in patients aged 65–70, there appeared to be better survival, though not statistically significant, for the radiation-alone group. In both treatment arms, patients who had tumours which were responsive to radiation, either by pathological downstaging or by complete clinical response, had improved survivals. This study has been assessed in greater detail in Chapter 4.

A fourth prospective trial was begun at Stanford University Medical Center in 1970, randomizing between 5000 cGy preoperative radiation plus cystectomy versus 7000 cGy radiation alone (Goffinet *et al.*, 1975). The trial was designed such that an initial staging laparotomy including lymph node biopsy was required for randomization. The trial was stopped after accession of only sixteen patients following two deaths due to complications in the combined treatment arm.

In summary, prospective randomized trials have not yielded incontrovertible evidence that initial surgery with or without preoperative radiation confers a significant survival benefit for most patients, although it certainly may benefit certain selected subsets. Radiation therapy alone, however, is successful in controlling local disease only 50 per cent of the time (see Table 8.4). Several large retrospective series have been reported, which give data for both local control and long-term survival, and which critically analyse factors which may have influenced the results of the treatment.

Retrospective studies (Tables 8.2 and 8.3)

Most large retrospective studies from American institutions on the efficacy of external-beam irradiation in the treatment of bladder cancer must be interpreted in light of the fact that selection for radiation therapy was largely 'negative'. Most patients were either too old or too ill to undergo radical surgery, or their tumours had been evaluated and found to be unresectable. Nonetheless, up to 39 per cent of patients with documented muscle invasion survived 5 years (Shipley *et al.*, 1985). Table 8.2 presents a summary of treatment, numbers of patients treated and percentage 5-year

Table 8.2 Results of retrospective studies: stages T2 and T3

Series	Treatment* (cGy)	Clinical stage	Numbers of patients	5-year survival (%)
Miller and Johnson	7000	T3	109	20
Goffinet *et al.*	7000	T3	218	28†
Morrison	5000 (20×250)	T3	40	33†
Greiner *et al.*	7000	T2, T3	195	28
Blandy *et al.*	5000 (20×250)	T2, T3	352	34
Goodman *et al.*	5000 (15×333)	T2, T3	450	38
Shipley *et al.*	6840 (38×180)	T2, T3	37	39†

*Usually 200 cGy per fraction; salvage cystectomy in selected patients.
†Actuarial calculation.

survivals in stages T2 and T3—i.e. otherwise technically resectable patients. Doses ranged from 5000 to 7000 cGy, and most patients received whole pelvic irradiation for at least some of their therapy. The results of external-beam irradiation for otherwise resectable bladder cancers can be compared with results using radiation alone in the stage T4, or unresectable cancers (Table 8.3). The outcome in these patients is quite poor, with only 7–13 per cent surviving 5 years. Intercurrent deaths in all series ranged from 10 to 18 per cent (Goffinet *et al.*, 1975; Shipley *et al.*, 1985), emphasizing the fact that this is an elderly and ill population.

Just as survival rates were fairly consistent between the different retrospective studies, the ability of full-dose radiation to control local disease in the bladder was likewise comparable. The rate of local control in the bladder ranged from 40 per cent (Gospodarowicz *et al.*, 1984) to 58 per cent (Shipley *et al.*, 1985) (see Table 8.1). Of interest, there was a subset of 61 patients within the M.D. Anderson Hospital series (Miller, 1977) categorized as having 'postoperative irradiation'. Forty-three of these patients' operations consisted of transurethral resections of bladder (TURB) followed by full-dose irradiation, and only 2 of 61 had total cystectomy. In this group of 61 patients (59 with intact bladders) where all gross tumour had been removed, local failure was only 33 per cent (67 per cent local control). 'Debulking' of tumour prior to radiation therapy may prove important.

Bladder function following full-dose external beam irradiation is clearly an issue of major concern, with opponents of definitive irradiation claiming that bladder function following treatment is so poor that the bladder does

Table 8.3 Results of retrospective studies: stage T4 (cf. Table 8.2)

Series	Clinical stage	Numbers of patients	5-year survival (%)
Miller and Johnson	T4	128	13
Goffinet *et al.*	T4	65	8
Greiner *et al.*	T4	30	10
Blandy *et al.*	T4	258	9†
Goodman *et al.*	T4	110	7
Shipley *et al.*	T4	18	6†

†Actuarial calculation.

not merit saving. In patients who survive without initial urinary diversion for obstruction or salvage cystectomy for radiation failure, the contrary is generally true. Gospodarowicz *et al.* (1984) reported that small contracted bladders with bleeding as a manifestation of radiation cystitis were rare. Although Miller (1977) reported that the bladder itself was the site of major complications in 42 of 533 patients, the nature of the complications is not stated and the complication rate is only 8 per cent. Goodman *et al.* (1981) reported that 65–70 per cent of the survivors of definitive radiation lived with healthy functioning bladders to at least 10 years after treatment. Shipley *et al.* (1985) confirmed that 80 per cent of patients with retained bladders characterized their function as 'good' or 'fair', and only two patients required urinary diversion for cystitis or bleeding. Raghavan and his colleagues have used questionnaires to assess the quality of life in long-term survivors after combined chemotherapy and radiotherapy and have demonstrated only a small proportion with chronic bladder dysfunction (see Chapters 9 and 15).

Complications of external-beam therapy

Complications of full-dose external-beam irradiation are closely related to radiation doses delivered to normal tissue which must be traversed in prescribing a defined dose to the bladder tumour itself: namely the rectum, the sigmoid colon, the small bowel and the head and neck of the femurs. Small-bowel obstruction should occur in fewer than 5 per cent of patients where the total pelvic dose is limited to 5000 cGy at 180 cGy per fraction, and there is no pre-existing bowel disease or prior abdominal surgery. Severe radiation proctitis is uncommon when the dose to the posterior portion of the rectum is limited to less than 6000 cGy. Goffinet *et al.* (1975) analysed bowel complications in the Stanford series in detail and found an overall incidence of bowel complications of varying severity of 8 per cent (31/384 patients). Miller (1977) also gave details on bowel complications with an overall rate of 5.8 per cent, including 13/533 patients with rectal damage, 8/533 with small-bowel damage and an additional 10 patients with a combination of complications. Shipley *et al.* (1985) reported two patients who had hip fractures following radiation doses calculated at 4000 and 4600 cGy. Calculation of dose to the femurs is particularly important when the cone down 'boost' to the bladder tumour is delivered through lateral fields.

Acute toxicity of radiation treatment will occur in 50–90 per cent of patients treated (Goffinet *et al.*, 1975). Urinary symptoms include frequency, urgency and burning on urination. Fluid intake should be encouraged and symptoms can usually be controlled with urinary anaesthetics and antispasmodics. Bowel symptoms include cramping, flatulence, tenesmus, and frank diarrhoea. Again, antispasmodics and antimotility drugs may yield symptomatic benefit. Symptoms usually resolve spontaneously within a few weeks to a few months of completion of radiation therapy.

Interstitial radium implantation

The work of Van der Werf Messing deserves special attention since she has consistently reported better local control rates of bladder cancer with this technique than have been documented using external-beam irradiation alone. She first reported her results on 615 patients with bladder cancer, staged T1–3, N_{x-1}, M_0 in 1978 and updated these results, concentrating on 41 stage-T3 patients in 1983 (Van der Werf Messing *et al.*, 1978, 1983). These latter patients were treated in a uniform fashion with 250 cGy in three fractions (a total of 1050 cGy) preoperatively to prevent scar recurrence, radium needle implantation as previously described, and 3000 cGy external-beam irradiation to the true pelvis 3 weeks following implant. Selection criteria included medical fitness of the patient for pelvic surgery and tumour size less than 5 cm. Minimum follow-up at the time of the second report was one year, with 31 patients followed for more than 2 years. The 5-year uncorrected actuarial survival of the 41 patients was 57 per cent, with a corrected actuarial survival of 74 per cent. At the time of this report there were only three local recurrences within the bladder in these patients treated with combination external beam and implant. In the earlier report using predominantly implants without external beam, local recurrence rates ranged from 8 per cent in T1 patients to 36 per cent in T3 patients.

Complications of interstitial implants

Complication rates from radium implantation were reported as 9 per cent in the initial Rotterdam series with ureteric deviation (11 patients), lithotrypsy (17 patients), and symptomatic necrosis (8 patients) as the most common complaints. Complications occurred in 8/41 patients (19.5 per cent) in the second report (Van der Werf Messing *et al.*, 1983) where patients all received external-beam irradiation in addition to their implants. Given the success of this technique in controlling the disease, it is not surprising that there is an attendant increased risk of complications.

Patient selection and prognostic factors

In the last ten years, through the publication of both prospective and retrospective trials of full-dose radiation therapy for bladder cancer, several important clinical and pathological determinants of radiation responsiveness and survival have emerged. Identification of these factors should eventually aid clinicians in deciding on the optimum therapeutic option. This section will review these prognostic factors.

Clinical stage

Clinical staging in the reviewed series was generally based on endoscopy, transurethral biopsy (±fulguration), bimanual examination under anaesthesia, chest x-ray, excretory urogram, and histological evaluation of the tumour for depth of invasion. Although clinical staging has an intrinsic inaccuracy of understaging approximately one-third of patients (Prout, 1977), it nonetheless undoubtedly reflects the probability of survival (see Chapters 4 and 7).

In Tables 8.2 and 8.3 the survival differences between the stage T2 and T3 tumours versus the T4 lesions have already been demonstrated. It is clear that conventional methods of radiation treatment in the inoperable subset of patients afford very little chance of cure and it is these patients who might most benefit from experimental treatment modalities. Most authors have reported survival differences between T2 and T3 patients as well (compare Chapter 7), indicating decreased likelihood of both local control and ultimate survival with increasing depth of invasion.

Radiation dose (Table 8.4)

In vitro testing of radiation sensitivity of a human transitional cell carcinoma line suggests that these tumour cells have a radiosensitivity similar to other mammalian normal and tumour cell lines grown in culture (Tannock *et al.*, 1984). On review of both randomized and non-randomized series, there is a suggestion of a relationship between total radiation dose delivered to the primary bladder tumour and its local control. The randomized trial of total radiation dose by Morrison (1975) showed an apparent benefit from the higher dose in local control and in survival, although this was not statistically significant. Miller (1977) reviewed his series carefully with regard to total dose and fractionation time versus local control and found a positive correlation similar to that reported by Morrison. Parsons and colleagues (1980) found a good correlation between total radiation dose (but not overall treatment time) and local control. With doses from 6200 to 6800 cGy, 15 (48 per cent) of 31 patients with locally advanced tumour achieved local control, while none of 15 patients who received less than 6000 cGy was controlled. In Van der Werf Messing's most recent series, the total dose to the bladder tumour was 7500 cGy, a dose which exceeds that given by conventional external-beam irradiation and which may account for the dramatic improvement in local control and survival. The relationship between tumour dose and survival should be further pursued through development of techniques to deliver higher doses safely without sacrificing bladder function.

Table 8.4 Total irradiation dose versus local tumour control

Series	Clinical stage	Total dose* (cGy)	Numbers of patients	Local control (%)
Morrison	T3	4250 (20×212)	38	38
	T3	5000 (20×250)	40	55
Parsons *et al.*	T3, T4	6000	15	0
	T3, T4	6800	31	48
Miller and Johnson	T3, T4	7000	152	44
Van der Werf Messing	T3 (5 cm)	7500†	40	92

*Usually as 200 cGy per fraction.
†4050 cGy external beam plus 3500 cGy by interstitial radium needle implant at 50–80 cGy/hour.

Excretory urogram

Greiner *et al.* (1977) and Shipley *et al.* (1985) have reported that the finding of ureteral obstruction on IVP is a poor prognostic sign. In Greiner's series for patients with T2 tumours, the 5-year survival was 42 per cent for those without ureteral obstruction and 12 per cent for those with obstruction. For T3 patients, the difference was 23 per cent without and 4 per cent with obstruction. In the Massachusetts General Hospital series, corrected 5-year survival was 47 per cent in T2–3 patients without ureteral obstruction versus 14 per cent in patients with obstruction (Shipley *et al.*, 1985). Local control rate was similarly influenced, with 52 per cent control in patients with no obstruction and 22 per cent where obstruction was present (see Fig. 8.4). Although tumour size may be the main determinant of ureteral obstruction, the effects of the obstruction on survival may result from complicating factors such as sepsis and renal failure.

Extent of transurethral resection

There is some evidence that a complete transurethral resection of the

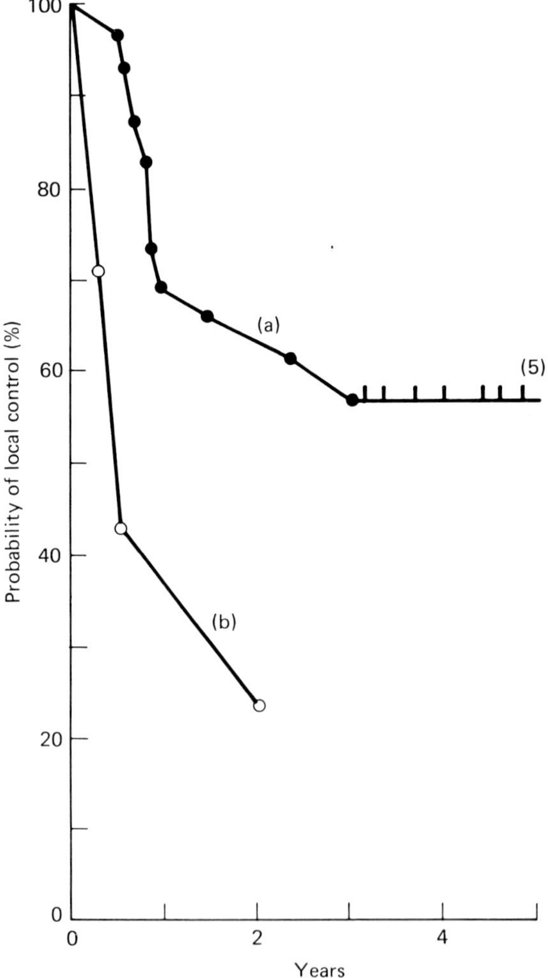

Fig. 8.4 Effect of ureteral obstruction on local control by full-dose XRT for stages T2 and T3. (a) No obstruction, $N=30$; (b) obstruction, $N=7$. $p=0.02$

bladder cancer prior to irradiation may favourably influence local control and survival. As previously mentioned, in the M.D. Anderson Hospital series where 61 patients were listed as having postoperative radiation, 43 of these patients had complete TURB; their overall survival of 40 per cent at 5 years is somewhat better than that of patients who had biopsy only, where overall survival was only 16 per cent (Miller, 1977). In addition, this group had better local control with only 33 per cent local failure. In the MGH series of T2 and T3 patients, when the urologist judged that a 'complete' transurethral resection had been accomplished, the local control rate at 5 years was 68 per cent versus 10 per cent in patients who had biopsy only of incomplete transurethral resection ($p = 0.003$) (see Fig. 8.5). The corrected 5-year survival in the group who underwent 'complete' resection was 54 per

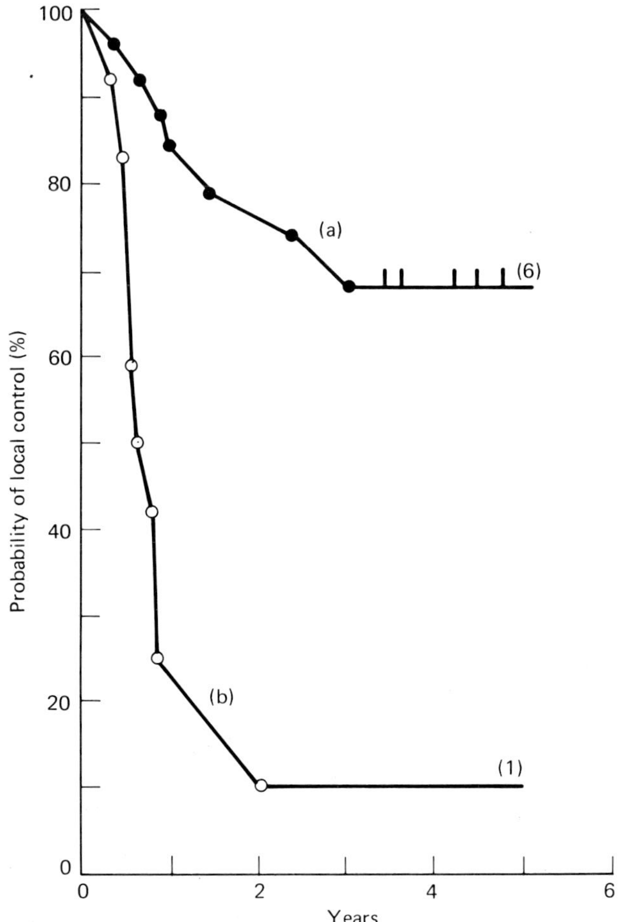

Fig. 8.5 Effect of extent of transurethral resection on local control by full-dose XRT for stages T2 and T3. (a) 'Complete' TURB, $N=25$; (b) incomplete TURB or biopsy only, $N=12$. $p=0.003$

cent versus 17 per cent in the group who did not ($p = 0.009$). As in other tumour types and sites, radiation may prove to be most effective following surgical 'debulking'.

Response to radiation

Permanent local control and a complete response of the local tumour to full-dose radiation therapy are favourable prognostic indicators with regard to 5-year survival. In the London Hospital series, 43 per cent of the 220 clinical stage-T3 patients were recorded as complete responders (Blandy *et al.*, 1980). The actuarial 5-year survival of these patients was 72 per cent. The survival was only 17 per cent for partial or non-responders. In the Institute of Urology trial, 40 per cent of 85 T3 patients showed a complete response following 6000 cGy in 6 weeks. The projected 5-year survival for the complete responders was 49 per cent compared with 20 per cent for the partial or non-responders (Bloom *et al.*, 1982). In the Massachusetts General series, of clinical stage T2 and T3 patients treated with full-dose radiation therapy, the probability of survival from bladder carcinoma in the 19 patients who did not develop or have not developed a local recurrence is 79 per cent compared with 11 per cent for the 18 patients who have developed a local recurrence (Shipley *et al.*, 1985) (see Fig. 8.6). Thus, the predictors of the tumours which will respond to radiotherapy will most certainly predict those patients who will have a higher cure rate.

Pathological predictors

The series from the Massachusetts General Hospital is unique in that pathological material from each patient was reviewed by one pathologist in order to document clearly muscle invasion and to be able to define pathological predictors of improved survival (Shipley *et al.*, 1985). In 21 patients whose microscopic tumour surface showed papillary histology, local control by irradiation alone was 63 per cent compared with 20 per cent local control in the 16 patients whose tumours were classified as solid or flat ($p = 0.01$). Corrected survival was similarly affected, with 62 per cent of patients with papillary tumours surviving 5 years and *no* patient with a flat or solid tumour surviving at 5 years ($p = 0.002$) see Figs. 8.7 and 8.8). Improved survival in the papillary subtype corroborates previously reported data from the Surgical Adjuvant Bladder Group Phase-III trial (Prout, 1984) (comparing cystectomy with and without 4500 cGy preoperative radiation), where survival benefit from preoperative radiation therapy compared with an unirradiated control group only reached statistical significance in those patients having papillary tumours. The 5-year survival in this subset of patients was 71 per cent with preoperative radiation therapy versus 35 per cent without it ($p < 0.05$). Previous pathological studies indicated that papillary tumours may be of less malignant potential than solid tumours, invading more superficially on a broad front, while solid tumours invaded more deeply in a tentacular fashion (Soto *et al.*, 1977). Indeed, in the cystectomy series from the MGH, papillary tumours had a 12 per cent incidence of positive pelvic lymph nodes while those with solid tumours had a 31 per cent incidence of nodal metastases (Heney *et al.*, 1983).

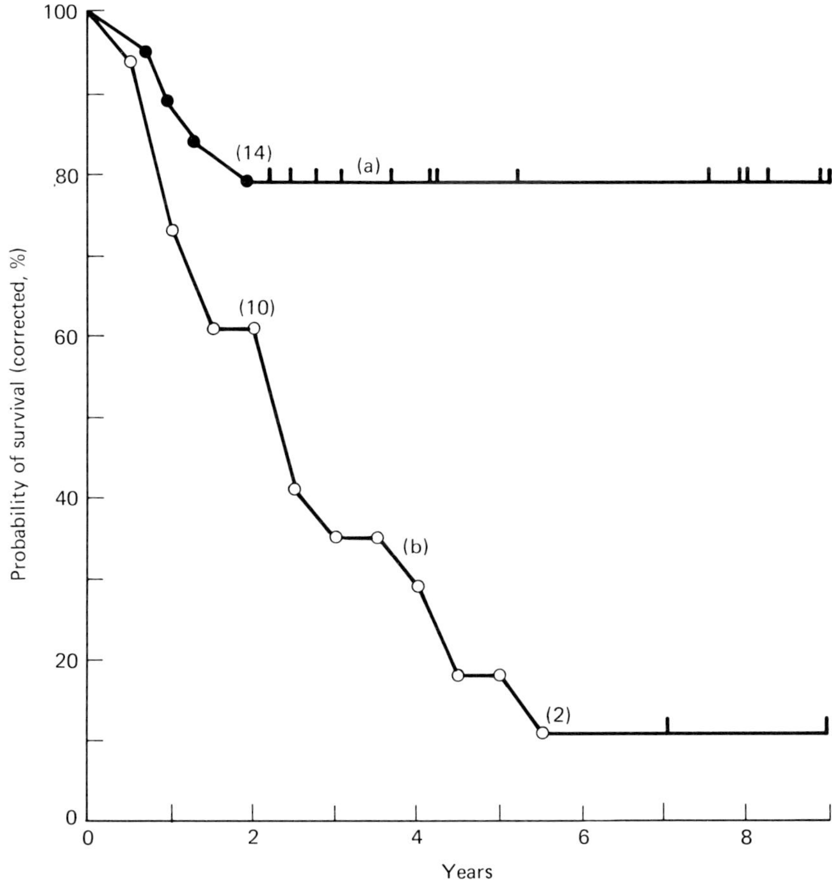

Fig. 8.6 Effect on survival rate of local tumour control by full-dose XRT for stages T2 and T3. (a) Local control, $N=19$; (b) local recurrence, $N=18$. $p=0.001$

Vessel invasion may also be an important pathological predictor. Heney and his colleagues and Batata *et al.* (1981) demonstrated superior survival where tumours showed no evidence of small-vessel invasion in patients undergoing radical cystectomy with or without preoperative irradiation. Van der Werf Messing (1983) confirmed the prognostic significance of vascular invasion in her T3 implant series: 85 per cent of patients without vessel invasion survived 3 years versus 46 per cent of patients with vessel invasion ($p<0.02$). In the series from Massachusetts General Hospital, vascular invasion did not, however, predict for poorer outcome, but the results based on transurethral biopsy may have been biased by sampling error (Heney *et al.*, 1983).

Future considerations and innovative approaches

From our review of available data it has been demonstrated that full-dose irradiation is curative for the minority of patients, particularly for those who

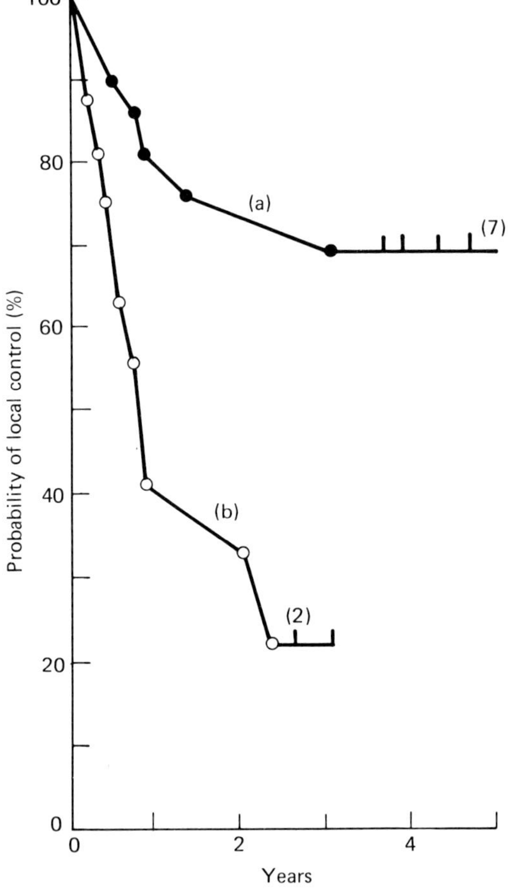

Fig. 8.7 Effect of histology on local tumour control. (a) Papillary histology, $N=21$; (b) solid or flat, $N=16$. $p=0.01$

are inoperable at the outset. The final section of this chapter will review innovative approaches to the patient with muscle-invasive, non-metastatic bladder cancer.

Intraoperative radiation

Intraoperative radiation therapy (IORT) for bladder cancer has been used most extensively by the Japanese. Matsumoto *et al.* reported their early results in 1981. A total of 116 patients were treated, including 50 patients with muscle-invading tumours, using a single electron dose of 2500–3000 cGy to the tumour plus a 1.5 cm margin at the time of surgery. Most patients received additional external-beam irradiation of 3000–4000 cGy to cover the whole bladder. Five-year survival rates in the stage-T2 patients was 61.6 per cent, but for stages T3–T4 combined the 5-year survival was only 7.3 per cent. The numbers of T3 and T4 patients were small, and the authors did not speculate over the reasons for their poor survival. Presum-

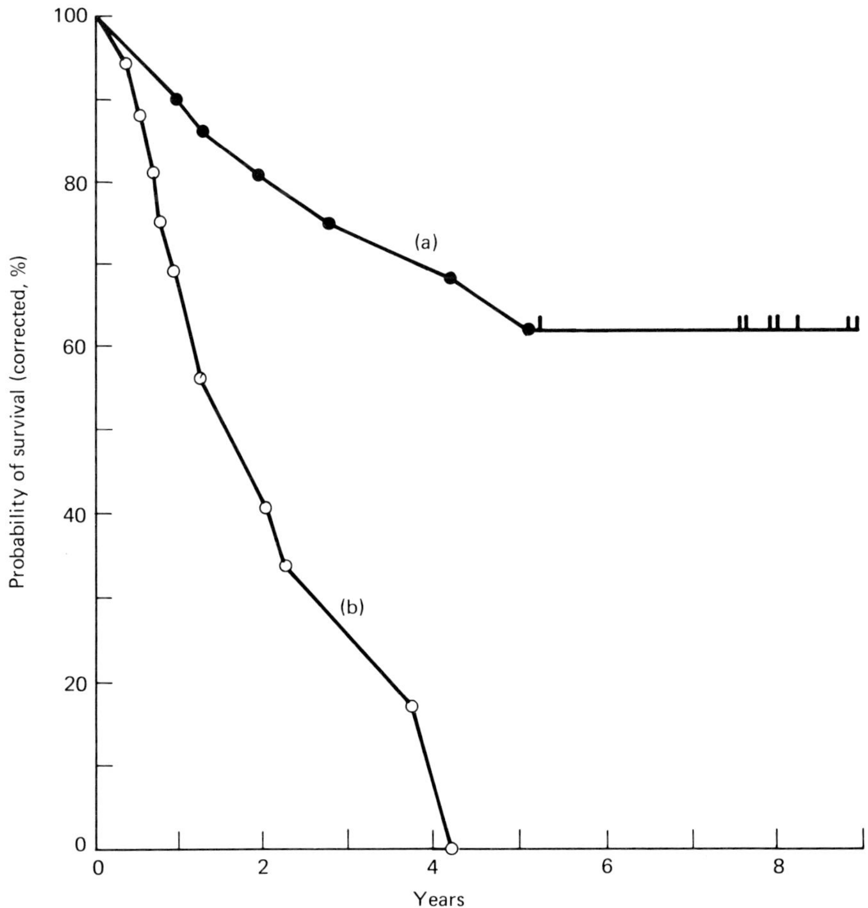

Fig. 8.8 Effect of histology on survival after full-dose irradiation. (a) Papillary histology, $N=21$; (b) solid or flat, $N=16$. $p=0.002$

ably these patients had the most advanced tumours and the electron energies used (3.5 and 7.0 MeV) may not have been adequate. Local recurrence rates in this series were quite low: 5.7 per cent in the group with solitary tumours and 23.1 per cent in the group with multiple tumours. Abe and Takahashi (1981) also reported intraoperative data from Japan. At the time of this report, 171 patients had been treated in a 10-institution trial, with 117 patients still alive. Intraoperative irradiation requires a high-energy therapy unit in the operating suite, or transportation of the patient under anaesthesia to the therapy unit with the attendant risks. More data will be generated as IORT gains widespread use. For invasive tumours, IORT of approximately 2000 cGy is likely to be optimally combined with 5000 cGy external-beam irradiation to the bladder and pelvic lymph nodes.

Radiation sensitizers

There have been two reports of studies combining radiation with misonidazole, a radiation sensitizer, in order to improve local control of bladder cancer. In the first study, a phase-I/II trial from the RTOG, 9 patients received oral misonidazole, 1.5 g/m^2 on Monday for 8 weeks followed in 4–6 hours by 400 cGy (Mohiuddin *et al.*, 1982). The remainder of the radiation was given in 200 cGy fractions on Wednesdays and Fridays for a total dose of 6800 cGy. Eight patients had T3 and T4 disease. Out of 9 patients treated, 7 achieved complete regression of their tumour. The trial was terminated when 3 patients developed small-bowel complications, presumably secondary to the unconventional fractionation schedule. A second trial, a phase-I/II study from South Africa, was reported by Abratt and colleagues in 1983. In the first pilot study, 11 patients received whole pelvic irradiation, then oral misonidazole during the boost (600 cGy×2) to the bladder. In the second pilot study, patients received intravesical misonidazole in addition to their oral dose. Sixteen of 22 patients achieved a complete response (73 per cent). This figure was significantly better than the 43 per cent complete response rate achieved by external-beam irradiation alone at the same institutions. Although these studies are small, the complete response rates are encouraging in that they may predict a favourably long-term survival with preservation of bladder function.

Chemotherapy and radiation (see also Chapters 15 and 17)

Just as local persistence and regrowth of bladder cancer has been a major problem in the treatment of this disease, the attempt to prevent distant metastases has been an equally difficult task. Up to 40 per cent of patients treated with full-dose irradiation will die of distant disease alone. In the last few years efforts to combine the most effective chemotherapy with external-beam irradiation have proven fruitful. Phase-II institutional trials of cisplatin (DDP) reported 30–50 per cent objective response rates when used alone or in combination with other chemotherapeutic agents in patients with measurable metastatic bladder cancer (Hahn, 1979). On this basis, Collaborative Group A of the National Bladder Cancer Project combined cisplatin (70 mg/m^2 every 3 weeks for up to 8 courses) with 6400 cGy of irradiation in patients considered unsuitable for a cystectomy (Shipley *et al.*, 1984). Twenty-seven patients have been reviewed with follow-up from 6 to 27 months. Of 17 evaluable patients, complete responses of the primary tumour were achieved in 11 of 13 clinical stage-T2 and T3 patients and in 2 of the 4 clinical T4 patients. Actuarial survival of the patients in this study is 63 per cent at 3 years (W.U. Shipley, unpublished data, 1985). Significant toxicity occurred in 3 of 27 patients and included 1 patient each with renal failure, sepsis and small-bowel obstruction. The University of Innsbruck, Austria, has undertaken a similar study using 1.6 mg/kg of cisplatin every 3 weeks for four cycles in combination with 6000 cGy (Jakse *et al.*, 1985). The rate of tumour-free bladders with a mean follow-up of 14 months was 17 of 22 patients, with an actuarial 3-year survival of 86 per cent. Finally, Raghavan and colleagues (1985) recently reported the results of an Australian collaborative trial using cisplatin, 100 mg/m^2 every 3 weeks times two, followed by standard definitive therapy, either radiation or cystectomy. This therapy was administered to 50 patients who were in a very poor prognostic group, with 82 per cent having T3–T4 tumours and 50 per cent having evidence of ureteral obstruction. At restaging after cisplatin, the objective response rate was 60 per cent which increased to 85 per cent after definitive therapy. The 3-year actuarial survival is 64 per cent. Clearly the combination of cisplatin and radiation is proving beneficial for patients with advanced, but localized, disease. The combination of cisplatin and radiation appears less toxic to normal tissues, if the drug is given before rather than simultaneously with the radiation (Shipley *et al.*, 1985; Pearson and Steel, 1984).

Summary

Radiation therapy can be curative treatment in up to 40 per cent of patients who present with invasive but otherwise operable bladder cancer. Careful attention to technique may result in a higher cure rate with a better functional result. Prospective randomized trials have yielded contradictory evidence for the superiority of surgery or radiation, perhaps secondary to small numbers of patients and failure to stratify results by stage and other prognostic variables. These factors which seem to be significant on the basis of retrospective reviews include radiation dose, radiation response, findings of excretory urogram, completeness of transurethral resection, and histopathology. Future considerations in attempting to improve the results of radiation therapy in bladder cancer may involve intraoperative irradiation, radiation sensitizing agents and, most promising, the combination of aggressive cisplatin therapy and full-dose irradiation.

References

Abe, M. and Takahashi, M. (1981). Intraoperative radiotherapy: the Japanese experience. *International Journal of Radiation Oncology* **7**: 863–8.

Abratt, R.P., Sealy, R., Tucker, R.D. *et al.* (1983). Radical irradiation and misonidazole in treatment of T2 grade III and T3 bladder cancer. *International Journal of Radiation Oncology* **9**: 629–32.

Batata, M.A., Chu, F.C.H., Hilaris, B.S. *et al.* (1981). Factors of prognostic and therapeutic significance in patients with bladder cancer. *International Journal of Radiation Oncology* **7**: 576–9.

Blandy, J.P., England, H.R., Evans, S.J.W. *et al.* (1980). T3 bladder cancer—the case for salvage cystectomy. *British Journal of Urology* **52**: 506–10.

Bloom, H.J.G., Hendry, W.F., Wallace, D.M. *et al.* (1982). Treatment of T3 bladder cancer: controlled trial of preoperative radiotherapy and radical cystectomy versus radical radiotherapy; second report and review. *British Journal of Urology* **54**: 136–51.

Fletcher, G.H. (1984). Radiation therapy in subclinical disease. *Cancer* **53**: 1274–84.

Goffinet, D.R., Schneider, N.J., Glastein, E.J. *et al.* (1975). Bladder cancer: results of radiation therapy in 384 patients. *Radiology* **117**:149–53.

Goodman, G.B., Hislop, T.G., Elwood, J.M. *et al.* (1981). Conservation of bladder function in patients with invasive bladder cancer treated by definitive irradiation and selective cystectomy. *International Journal of Radiation Oncology* **7**: 559–73.

Gospodarowicz, M., Rider, W.D., Hawkins, N.V. *et al.* (1984). Definitive radiation therapy in the management of bladder cancer. *International Journal of Radiation Oncology* **10**: 118.

Greiner, R., Skaleric, C. and Veraguth, P. (1977). The prognostic significance of ureteral obstruction in carcinoma of the bladder. *International Journal of Radiation Oncology* **2**: 1095–1100.

Hahn, R.G. (1979). Bladder cancer treatment considerations for metastatic disease. *Seminars in Oncology* **6**: 236–9.

Heney, N.M., Proppe, K., Prout, G.R. *et al.* (1983). Invasive bladder cancer: tumor configuration, lymphatic invasion and survival. *Journal of Urology* **130**: 895–7.

Hodson, N.J., Husband, J.E. and MacDonald, J.S. (1979). The role of computed tomography in the staging of bladder cancer. *Clinical Radiology* **30**: 389–95.

Jakse, G., Frommhold, H. and Nedden, D.Z. (1985). Combined radiation and chemotherapy for locally advanced transitional cell carcinoma of the urinary bladder. *Cancer* **55**: 1659–64.

Madsen, P.D., Hoyme, U.B. and Byar, D.B. (1980). No differences in 10-year survival rates in 3 bladder cancer groups. *Urology Times*: April.

Matsumoto, L., Kakizoe, T., Mikuriya, S. *et al.* (1981). Clinical evaluation of intraoperative radiotherapy for carcinoma of the urinary bladder. *Cancer* **47**: 509–13.

Miller, L.S. (1977). Bladder cancer: superiority of preoperative irradiation therapy and cystectomy in clinical stages B2 and C. *Cancer* **39**: 973–80.

Mohiuddin, M., Kramer, S., Phillips, T. *et al.* (1982). Preliminary results of RTOG phase I/II study of misonidazole and radiation for bladder cancer. *American Journal of Clinical Oncology* **5**: 551–4.

Morrison, R. (1975). The results of radiation treatment of cancer of the bladder—the clinical contribution of radiobiology. *Clinical Radiology* **76**: 67–75.

Nakamura, S. and Niijima, T. (1980). Staging of bladder cancer by ultrasonography: a new technique by transurethral intravesical scanning. *Journal of Urology* **124**: 341–4.

Parsons, J.T., Thar, T.L., Bova, F.S. *et al.* (1980). An evaluation of split-course irradiation for pelvic malignancies. *International Journal of Radiation Oncology* **6**: 175–81.

Pearson, A.E. and Steel, G.G. (1984). Chemotherapy in combination with pelvic irradiation: a time dependence study in mice. *Radiotherapy and Oncology* **2**: 49–55.

Prout, G.R. (1977). Bladder carcinoma and a TNM system of staging. *Journal of Urology* **117**: 583–90.

Prout, G.R. (1984). Radiation therapy and cystectomy. *Urology* **23** (Suppl. 4): 104–9.

Raghavan, D., Pearson, B., Duval, P. *et al.* (1985). Initial intravenous cisplatin therapy: improved management for invasive high risk bladder cancer? *Journal of Urology* **133**: 399–402.

Shipley, W.U., Coombs, L.J., Einstein, A.B. *et al.* (1984). Cisplatin and full-dose irradiation for patients with invasive bladder carcinoma: a preliminary report of tolerance and local response. *Journal of Urology* **132**: 899–903.

Shipley, W.U., Rose, M.A., Perrone, T. *et al.* (1985). Full-dose irradiation for patients with invasive bladder carcinoma: clinical and histologic factors prognostic of improved survival. *Journal of Urology* **134**: 679–83.

Soto, E.A., Freidell, G.H. and Tiltman, A.J. (1977). Bladder cancer as seen in giant histologic sections. *Cancer* **39**: 447–55.

Straus, K.L., Littman, P., Wein, A.J. *et al.* (1985). Interstitial iridium-192 treatment for invasive bladder carcinoma. *International Journal of Radiation Oncology* **11**: 188.

Tannock, I., Choo, B. and Buick, R. (1984). The radiation response of human bladder cancer assessed *in vitro* or as xenografts in immune deprived mice. *International Journal of Radiation Oncology* **10**: 1897–1902.

Van der Werf Messing, B., Star, W.M. and Memon, R.S. (1980). T1-3NXM0 bladder cancer treated by radium implant and external irradiation. *International Journal of Radiation Oncology* **6**: 1723–5.

Van der Werf Messing, B.H.P., Memon, R.S. and Hop, W.C.J. (1983). Cancer of the urinary bladder treated by interstitial radium implant: second report. *International Journal of Radiation Oncology* **9**: 481–5.

9

Cytotoxic chemotherapy in the elderly

D. Raghavan, R. Grundy and L.T. Malden

Introduction

In the past 50 years, the proportion of people older than 65–70 years in Western society has increased, and now approaches 15 per cent (Vestal, 1978; WHO, 1981). However, this group consumes nearly 30 per cent of health funds and uses a similar proportion of acute hospital beds (WHO, 1981). It is likely that this substantial requirement for health resources will continue to increase.

The prevalence of malignant disease increases with age, including cancers of the urothelium, in which the median age at presentation is approximately 65 years (see Chapters 1 and 15). An important clinical and philosophical concern has been to define the level of activity or aggression that should be employed in the management of these older patients: what are the guidelines that should be used in the clinical decision-making process? For example, should a different approach be used for an ailing 65-year-old with cancer and several intercurrent diseases from that employed for a fit and active 78-year-old with invasive non-metastatic bladder cancer? Should age *per se* preclude an active management policy?

Elderly patients have age-related changes in their physiology which may result in a reduced tolerance to the side effects of surgery or radiotherapy (Gunn, 1980; Cohen, 1985) or which may alter the pharmacological disposition of drugs, including cytotoxics (see Table 9.1). Many factors influence the dose–response relationships for drug use in the elderly (Triggs and Nation, 1975; Vestal, 1978; Greenblatt *et al.*, 1982; Ho and Triggs, 1984). Ageing is associated with a progressive alteration of many cellular and organic functions which produce changes in the pharmacokinetics and pharmacodynamics of many drugs (Cohen, 1986). In many cases, the pharmacokinetic changes are easier to define as they can be inferred from analysis of simple concentration–time data. The alterations in pharmacodynamic indices may be more complex, relating to altered binding, receptor or transport states.

Several factors make the interpretation of data more difficult in an elderly patient population (see Table 9.2). For example, it has been estimated that 80 per cent of these patients have one or more chronic disorders (WHO, 1981) for which they may receive between three and twelve medications simultaneously (Shaw, 1982). Thus the assessment of the disposition and effects of any drug may be complicated by potential interactions with other

Table 9.1 Factors affecting the pharmacology of cytotoxic drugs in the elderly

Physiological
Reduced cardiac output
Reduced perfusion of kidneys
Reduced hepatic perfusion
Reduced perfusion of GIT
Decreased gastric acid secretion
Increased gastric emptying time
Decreased intestinal motility
Reduced GI absorptive cells

Pharmacological
Variable absorption
Altered distribution—increased lipid–water partition ratio?
Third spaces
Altered plasma protein binding
Reduced metabolism—e.g. reduced hepatic microsomal enzyme function
Reduced excretion
Altered pharmacodynamics—receptor sensitivity?
Chronic diseases—impaired organ function?
Multiple medications—drug interactions?

Table 9.2 Factors influencing the outcome of cytotoxic chemotherapy in the elderly

The patient
General 'fitness'/activity
Age
Mental function—dementia?
Ocular/auditory function
Prior treatment experiences
Prior toxins—smoking, analgesics
Level of family/social support
Expectation of outcome/perceptions of aims of treatment
Financial constraints from disease and treatment
Reduced reporting of adverse drug reactions

The disease
Sites of involvement
Damage to normal tissues
Initial presentation/relapse?
Acute versus chronic
Expectation of outcome—cure versus palliation
Symptoms from the disease

The drugs
Side effects
Interactions with other medications
Complexity of schedule
Route of administration
Cost

medications in use. The prevalence of adverse drug reactions has been reported to rise with age and with the number of drugs administered, and may be as high as 27 per cent in elderly patients receiving six drugs (Williamson, 1979). These figures may represent an underestimate as elderly patients tend to report side effects less reliably (or perhaps they are recorded with less enthusiasm by their physicians). Psychotropic and cardiovascular drugs appear to be responsible for the most serious side effects in this group of patients (Ho and Triggs, 1984). Thus in elderly patients receiving cytotoxic chemotherapy, the antiemetics and sedatives used to ameliorate toxicity may, in fact, themselves cause dramatic side effects.

An additional problem is raised by poor compliance in adhering to schedules of medication, particularly when prescribed orally. In the elderly, factors that contribute to this include decreased memory or senile dementia, impaired eyesight and hearing, complex medication regimens, lack of family or social support, the direct or incidental effects of the medications themselves, and occasionally the financial constraints imposed from the costs of the drugs.

The physiology of ageing

One of the most important physiological changes to occur with ageing is a reduction in cardiac output, which alters by about 1 per cent per year between the ages of 25 and 80 years (Bender, 1965). As a result, there is a reduced perfusion of the kidneys, liver, gastrointestinal tract and skeletal muscles. Compensatory mechanisms retain the blood flow to the brain and heart. These vascular changes may reduce the absorption, distribution and elimination of some drugs. The renal blood flow is reduced to a greater extent than would be predicted solely on the basis of reduced cardiac output (Triggs and Nation, 1975). Furthermore, among the population of patients with urothelial cancer, renal function may be further compromised by a past history of analgesic abuse (see Chapters 1 and 16).

In the elderly, a substantial decrease in lean muscle mass results in reduced creatinine excretion. This reduction, and the decrease in creatinine clearance with ageing, may not necessarily be reflected by a fall of serum creatinine (Rowe *et al.*, 1976). Hence, serum creatinine may be misleading as the sole index of renal function in the aged, and may result in incorrect calculation of drug doses. The creatinine clearance should be used to estimate the renal function in the elderly and is more sensitive to the changes in renal blood flow that occur with ageing.

In this aged population, other changes in organ function may predispose to increased toxicity of treatment. For example, the peripheral neuropathies commonly associated with ageing may enhance the sensitivity to vinca alkaloids. Similar effects may occur as a result of peripheral vascular disease. Cigarette smoking, an aetiological factor in bladder cancer (see Chapter 1), causes chronic bronchitis and pulmonary interstitial damage, and may leave the lungs more sensitive to damage from bleomycin. Similarly, the cardiovascular disorders that are characteristic of ageing (e.g. myocardial ischaemia and infarction, congestive cardiac failure) may sensitize the heart to the effects of the anthracyclines, such as doxorubicin.

Pharmacological considerations

As cytotoxic drugs usually have a relatively narrow therapeutic index, any factors that potentially alter the pharmacokinetics in the elderly may be of great importance with regard to efficacy and toxicity of the chemotherapy regimens employed. Traditionally, many of the detailed phase I–II and pharmacological studies of new and conventional agents have been carried out in younger patients. As a result, less information is available regarding their use in the older population.

Absorption

Although most cytotoxic chemotherapy is delivered parenterally, some agents can be taken by mouth (e.g. methotrexate, cyclophosphamide, VP-16,213 and demethoxy-daunorubicin). To our knowledge, methotrexate is the only one of these drugs that may have a role in the management of bladder cancer when administered orally. Hall *et al.* (1981) reported a series of 17 patients with superficial TCCs who were treated with weekly doses of 50 mg methotrexate in syrup. Measurement of urinary methotrexate levels showed substantial variation, but in each instance the level was greater than 10^{-6} M for 24 hours after dosing. A total of 428 doses of weekly oral methotrexate were delivered; only three patients experienced myelosuppression that delayed treatment, two patients had mucositis and there were two reported episodes of conjunctivitis. One patient suffered severe toxicity owing to an error in taking medications. The variability in urinary methotrexate concentrations could have been due to variations in absorption, distribution or excretion, as discussed below.

In addition to these cytotoxic agents, a variety of ancillary medications are administered orally to this group of patients (for example, analgesics, antiemetics, laxatives, steroids, calcium leucovorin). It is thus appropriate to consider the factors that affect systemic bioavailability (the proportion of the dose that reaches the systemic circulation). The major factors that determine bioavailability include the absorption process *per se* and initial elimination (such as first-pass hepatic metabolism or degradation in the small intestine). Several changes in gastrointestinal function occur with increasing age and may affect absorption. Gastric acid secretion is reduced, as is gastrointestinal blood flow and the number of functional absorbing cells. The gastric emptying time rises, while intestinal motility is reduced. These changes may cause a reduction in the absorption of basic and poorly lipid soluble drugs. Furthermore, as noted above, hepatic blood flow decreases in the elderly, which may either increase or decrease bioavailability, depending on the drug under consideration. These factors may be compounded by changes in diet, excessive ingestion of antacids or laxatives, and the presence of intercurrent diseases, such as congestive cardiac failure or cirrhosis. The metabolic implications of metastases in the liver are variable and poorly characterized. In fact, the true impact of most of these factors with regard to absorption of cytotoxic agents is not clear, and further studies will be required to define more accurate indices of drug absorption, especially if the orally administered agents come into increasing use.

Drug distribution

Several factors can alter the patterns of distribution of drugs in the elderly. The distribution of a drug is a function of its relative lipid–water partition characteristics, the degree of binding to plasma proteins and other tissues, and overall blood flow. The lipid composition of the body doubles in men between the ages of 25 and 75 years (Forbes and Reina, 1970). At the same time, the total body water decreases, although the situation may be complicated in the presence of significant third spaces (e.g. ascites, pleural effusions). Highly lipid-soluble drugs (e.g. diazepam) have an increased volume of distribution in the elderly and hence may remain in their bodies for longer periods of time than is usual (Greenblatt *et al.*, 1980). This effect is not seen in its more water-soluble analogue, lorazepam (Greenblatt *et al.*, 1979), which we use routinely as part of an antiemetic regimen (see Chapter 15).

Plasma protein binding is altered in old patients. The serum albumin falls, which can cause a reduced drug binding with a concomitant rise in the level of free drug. Reduced protein binding can be caused by a reduced protein intake, uraemia or as a result of competition for binding sites when multiple drugs are in use.

It should be emphasized that the prediction of the effects of the changes associated with ageing can be very difficult: each of the age-related changes in physiology and pharmacology may have opposite effects on drug availability. For instance, in an elderly patient with bladder cancer, antecedent analgesic nephropathy and mild cardiac failure, the conflicting factors that affect bioavailability include reduced plasma protein binding, reduced hepatic and renal perfusion, altered lipid/water ratios, etc. The prediction of the pharmacology of cytotoxic drug use in such a patient will also depend on the physicochemical traits of the drug under consideration.

Metabolism

Drug metabolism is also a complex process, involving hepatic and extrahepatic enzyme systems. There have been extensive studies with respect to the effects of ageing on drug metabolism (summarized by Ho and Triggs, 1984; Cohen, 1986). The rate of drug metabolism is influenced by the state of nutrition, hepatic function, the use of other drugs, intercurrent diseases, smoking and serum albumin. However, no simple predictor or index of drug metabolism has been defined, regardless of the age of the patient. The conventional tests of liver function (enzyme levels, coagulation profiles, serum bilirubin) are usually not sufficiently reliable indices for routine use.

The 1 per cent annual decrease of hepatic blood flow (Vestal *et al.*, 1975) and of hepatic parenchymal mass (Wood *et al.*, 1979) may have opposite effects in drug metabolism, and it is difficult to predict which will have a greater impact in a specific patient. The situation is even more complex: some hepatic functions (e.g. acetylation, conjugation) usually do not change with age, whereas others (e.g. function of the microsomal oxidative enzymes) become reduced with increasing age.

Hepatic metabolism is of particular importance in the case of doxorubicin and the other anthracycline analogues (mitoxantrone, 4′-epiadriamycin, demethoxy-daunorubicin) which are excreted via the biliary route. It is well known that the haematological and gastrointestinal toxicity of doxorubicin is increased in patients with biliary obstruction (Chabner and Myers, 1985). However, after more than a decade of clinical use, a concordance of opinion with respect to dose modification in the presence of abnormal liver function tests (other than serum bilirubin) has not been achieved.

Many other drugs, including phenytoin, the tricyclic antidepressants, non-steroidal anti-inflammatory drugs and analgesics show marked variability of metabolism in clinical studies of older patients. Hence increased clinical monitoring is of particular importance in the elderly, especially if repeated or continuous treatment is planned. It may even be prudent, in some clinical settings, to consider a dosage reduction initially (on a trial basis) in order to define the level of toxicity for a particular patient. However, in that situation, caution should be exercised in the interpretation of the efficacy of treatment.

Excretion

The kidneys provide the major route of excretion for many anticancer drugs, including methotrexate, bleomycin and cisplatinum. Renal function decreases with age. The glomerular filtration rate falls by 35 per cent between the ages of 25 and 65 years (Bender, 1965). The ability of the kidneys to concentrate urine and to conserve sodium also decreases with age. There is also a reduction in renal mass and in the number of functioning nephrons (Hollenberg *et al.*, 1974).

If renal function is impaired, drugs that are predominantly excreted by the kidneys will have prolonged half-lives and increased plasma concentrations, a factor of particular importance if the therapeutic index is narrow. Dose modification can be carried out on the basis of creatinine clearance or through the monitoring of plasma levels (e.g. by high-pressure liquid chromatography).

However, another approach has been reported for the use of methotrexate in the elderly. A low test dose is first administered and the pharmacokinetic parameters for that patient are then calculated; based on these estimations, plasma methotrexate concentrations at higher doses can be predicted (Kerr *et al.*, 1983). Nevertheless, it should not be forgotten that delayed toxicity can occur in this situation in patients with large third spaces (e.g. pleural effusions, ascites) as methotrexate is predominantly water-soluble.

In patients with urothelial cancer, the impact of underlying disease can be of great importance. These patients may have chronic urinary tract infection, antecedent analgesic nephropathy, renal calculi or obstruction, or they may even have undergone surgery (nephrectomy, cystectomy). In the geriatric patient, the ability of a solitary kidney to compensate after nephrectomy is reduced. In younger patients, a 60–80 per cent increase in renal function in a solitary kidney is possible; whereas a compensatory increase of only about 30 per cent occurs in the elderly (Moussad, 1984).

Pharmacodynamics

Alterations in therapeutic response (e.g. dose–response relationships) are often seen in geriatric patients, and are most commonly due to changes in the pharmacokinetics of the drugs (see above). For example, the duration of analgesia after the administration of morphine is increased in the elderly (Kaiko, 1980). By contrast, no change has been shown in the peak level of pain relief. Differences in response to morphine in the aged may be due to a reduction in clearance of the drug (Kaiko *et al.*, 1982).

Alternatively, aberrant responses in the elderly may reflect changes in sensitivity of drug receptors or other undefined factors. For example, this population is particularly susceptible to the effects of some benzodiazepines, even in the absence of the pharmacokinetic changes outlined above. Castleden *et al.* (1979) reported a greater level of impairment of psychomotor function in elderly patients than in a young cohort after a dose of 10 mg of nitrazepam. However, in this study, no difference in pharmacokinetics was detected.

Cytotoxic chemotherapy in the elderly

Against a background of an increasing knowledge and understanding of the physiology and pharmacology of drug treatment in the elderly, it is only relatively recently that specific attention has been paid to the problems associated with cytotoxic treatment in this group. A general dictum, perhaps unsupported by firm evidence, has related increased toxicity of chemotherapy as a function of advanced age, irrespective of the general condition of the patient. The original data that were available referred to relatively small numbers of patients. For example, methotrexate was reported to cause increased haematological toxicity in the elderly (Hansen *et al.*, 1971), and bleomycin was noted to be associated with increased pulmonary damage in these patients (Haas *et al.*, 1976).

More recently, the Eastern Cooperative Oncology Group (ECOG) has specifically addressed the issue of toxicity, response and survival in the elderly receiving chemotherapy for cancer (Begg and Carbone, 1983). Data obtained from more than 5000 patients treated in 19 randomized studies concerning 8 types of cancer were reported. The tumours under consideration included lung, colorectal, gastric, sarcoma, epithelial cancer of head and neck, melanoma, kidney and ovary. A wide spectrum of cytotoxic drugs was used, including doxorubicin, cyclophosphamide, the vinca alkaloids, mitomycin C, bleomycin, methyl-CCNU, and VP-16,213. The extent and severity of toxicity was a function of the agents and doses employed. For example, the investigators showed that haematological toxicity with doxorubicin is independent of age in doses ranging from 50 to 75 mg/m^2, administered every 3 weeks, and even in weekly schedules of delivery of lower doses. By contrast, they reported that age-related toxicity occurred with methotrexate and methyl-CCNU. In the case of methotrexate, the side effects may have been a function of impaired renal function (outlined above). In the case of methyl-CCNU, the lipid solubility of the drug, accompanied by the higher fat/water ratio of the elderly, could explain the effect.

Of particular importance, Begg and Carbone were unable to detect a significant difference in the overall prevalence or severity of side effects between patients less than 70 years of age and those in the older age group. However, it should be noted that only 13 per cent of the patients assessed in the total group were aged 70 years or more, and this group may have been the product of a careful (inadvertent?) process of patient selection. Although the investigators attempted to ensure balance between the total population and the geriatric group, by comparing factors such as performance status, loss of weight and prior radiotherapy, it remains possible that a bias of referral was present (i.e. the selection of the 'fit 70 year old' for chemotherapy). However, this does not weaken their argument that fit geriatric patients can tolerate cytotoxic drugs as well as the younger age groups and may thus be entered into clinical trials without undue concern about the toxic consequences. Furthermore, Begg and Carbone demonstrated equivalent response rates and survival figures in the groups of older and younger patients.

This view, however, is not unchallenged. Another study from the ECOG, in this case referring to the treatment of breast cancer in the elderly, demonstrated a steady increase in toxicity (except nausea and vomiting) with increasing age if a standard regimen of cyclophosphamide, methotrexate and 5-fluorouracil (CMF) was used (Gelman and Taylor, 1984). In patients in whom the dose of CMF was modified on the basis of creatinine clearance, no trend of increased toxicity with advanced age was demonstrated. Some of the discrepancies with the data from Begg and Carbone (1983) may be explained by the variety of treatment regimens in the former study, compared with the uniform approach to CMF chemotherapy reported by Gelman and Taylor. Furthermore, the diseases under consideration were different.

Further support for a policy of dose-modification in the elderly has been provided by another study from ECOG. Kahn *et al.* (1984) randomly allocated geriatric patients with acute leukaemia to receive full- or attenuated-dose regimens of doxorubicin, cytosine arabinoside and 6-thioguanine. The patients who received the reduced-dose schedule suffered less toxicity, spent less time in hospital, and had a lower induction death rate, with a longer median survival.

Similarly, with regard to the management of diffuse histiocytic lymphoma, Armitage and Potter (1984) reported increased complications from aggressive treatment of elderly patients and speculated that a high early death rate was due to altered drug metabolism or increased sensitivity of normal tissues to the drugs used. However, Dixon *et al.* (1986) documented a worse prognosis in older patients treated on two Southwest Oncology Group protocols, but suggested that this could be a function of the dose-reduction schedule employed for elderly patients. This view was confirmed recently by O'Connell *et al.* (1986), who demonstrated a higher complete remission rate and median survival in elderly patients with diffuse lymphoma who received full-dose doxorubicin-containing combination regimens.

It is clear that the approach to chemotherapy in the elderly is not a simple issue, and several factors influence the outcome of these endeavours (see Table 9.2). Of particular importance are the performance status and general fitness of the patient, the nature and side effects of the drug(s) in use, and the aims of the chemotherapy regimen (cure versus palliation). These considerations have particular application in the management of invasive and metastatic bladder cancer, a disease that occurs predominantly in the elderly.

Chemotherapy of bladder cancer in the elderly

Extensive data have been reported with respect to the response rate and survival of patients with recurrent and metastatic bladder cancer treated with single-agent and combination chemotherapy (reviewed in Chapters 10–15). However, in the majority of reports, it has proved difficult to demonstrate whether the efficacy and toxicity of treatment differs in the elderly subgroup of patients. In most of the published series, the ages of the patients have been expressed in terms of mean values (with a range), thus making it almost impossible to define accurately the proportion of treated patients over the age of 70 years. Furthermore, no data are provided with regard to referral patterns or the criteria used to exclude elderly patients.

In several of the reports of aggressive combination regimens, relatively young median ages and upper age limits suggest that few older patients have undergone treatment. For example, in the first full report of the use of the MVAC regimen (see Chapter 12 for details), 25 patients with a median age of only 60 years (range 23 to 72 years) were treated; it is unlikely that more than two or three patients older than 70 years were treated in this initial programme (Sternberg *et al.*, 1985). In this report, no distinction was made with regard to the older patient in the reporting of toxicity, a feature common to most reported series. Similarly, Harker *et al.* (1985), in reporting the CMV regimen (see Chapter 12), described the response rate and toxicity in 50 evaluable patients with a median age of 61.5 years. No attempt was made to distinguish the extent and distribution of side effects in the younger (46–61 years) and older (62–77 years) patients. Durable complete remissions were obtained in four patients older than 70 years, but the extent of the side effects that they experienced was not specified.

We believe that the reporting of the results of chemotherapy for recurrent or metastatic bladder cancer should specify the factors summarized in Table 9.3. In this way, it may prove easier for the practising clinician to assess the applicability of the published results to his or her own clinical practice.

Practical application: assessment of acute and late toxicity with neoadjuvant cisplatin plus radiotherapy in elderly patients with invasive bladder cancer

As discussed in Chapter 15, we treated 70 patients with high-grade, invasive non-metastatic TCC of the bladder between August 1981 and November 1984 (Raghavan *et al.*, 1985; Pearson and Raghavan, 1985). This protocol involved the administration of cisplatinum $100\,\text{mg/m}^2$ intravenously every three weeks ($\times 2$), followed by check cystoscopy and subsequent definitive treatment (usually radiotherapy, 60 Gy to the bladder and 45–50 Gy to the pelvis). Fifteen of these patients (21 per cent) were aged 70 years or more. Five additional patients were rejected for entry into the protocol either

Table 9.3 Chemotherapy for bladder cancer in the elderly: requirements for optimal reporting of results

---

Patient population
Numbers of patients $\geqslant$70 years
Criteria of inclusion/exclusion
Intercurrent illnesses
Percentage of the population treated:
   number treated/number referred?
   number treated/number in community?
Prior treatment
'Special' baseline tests—e.g. ejection fraction, lung function tests, etc.

Treatment regimen
Drugs and doses
Dose modifications for the elderly
Added measures—modified antiemetic drugs/schedules, hydration
   regimens, sedatives
Other modalities of treatment

Outcome
Percentage of 'dropouts'/reasons
Toxicity profile—spectrum, duration and severity
Treatment-related deaths
Intercurrent diseases/complications
Treatment aims/outcome:
   cure?
   palliation?

---

because of advanced age (greater than 80 years) or intercurrent diseases (predominantly unstable congestive cardiac failure). As can be seen from Table 9.4, the acute toxicity was acceptable, with no episodes of grade-IV toxicity (WHO scale) and no toxic deaths. The mean age of this group was 73.1 years (median 71, range 70–79 years) and six patients were aged 75 or more. The median survival was 22 months, with five patients surviving three years or longer.

The issue of delayed toxicity was evaluated in an unconventional fashion. As part of a broader survey of the quality of life among long-term survivors, questionnaires were presented to 12 of these elderly patients; the other elderly patients had either died (2) or were unable to speak English. Nine patients responded. The questionnaires consisted of linear analogue self-assessment scales (see Chapters 11 and 15) and multiple-choice questions. They were designed to assess physical wellbeing, symptoms of disease, side effects of treatment, functional status, sexual function, social interactions and satisfaction with treatment (Raghavan *et al.*, in press). The major issue under consideration was whether the morbidity of the treatment programme was justified by the long-term quality of life.

As can be seen in Table 9.5, the majority of respondents in this elderly population sample suffered few major long-term complications of treatment and assessed themselves overall as having a satisfactory quality of life. Of some importance, however, was the fact that the quality of sexual function after this programme was not satisfactory (in old and young alike); this factor should be taken into consideration when allocating a preference

Table 9.4 Elderly patients with bladder cancer treated with neoadjuvant cisplatinum plus radiotherapy

Sex	Age	Grade	Stage	Other diseases	Acute toxicity	Late toxicity	Months of survival
F	71	III	T3	Fibroids	—	Subacute bowel obstruction ×1	35
M	76	III	T4a	—	N&V gd 2	? Necr. femoral head	60+
F	72	III	T3	Hypertension	N&V gd 3 Renal gd 2 High tone deafness	Not applicable	6
M	70	III	T3	Aortic aneurysm Diabetes mellitis	N&V gd 2 Diarrhoea gd 2	Occasional cystitis	50+
M	78	III	T3	—	N&V gd 2 Renal gd 2	Not applicable	8
M	70	III	T3	Hypertension Inguinal hernia	N&V gd 2 Renal gd 2	Radiation colitis	13
M	79	III	T4a	Atrial fibrillation Congestive cardiac failure (controlled)	N&V gd 2 Transient confusion		13
M	71	III	T2+	—	N&V gd 2		36
M	70	III	T2	COAD Inquinal hernia	N&V gd 2 Neutropenia gd 1		36+
M	71	III	T2	Duodenal ulcer Renal calculi Thrombasthenia	N&V gd 3 Neutropenia gd 2		22
M	75	III	T2+	—	N&V gd 2		28+
M	70	III	T3	COAD Renal calculi	N&V gd 3	Intermittent cystitis	17
F	76	II	T2+	Hypertension 'Palpitations'	N&V gd 3 Atrial fibrillation Femoral embolus	Unknown	14
M	77	III	T4a	Ischaemic heart disease	Neutropenia gd 1	Ototoxicity gd 2 Colitis gd 2	14
F	71	III	T3	Varicose veins	N&V gd 2–3	Colitis gd 1	24+

Table 9.5 Aspects of quality of life: assessment after neoadjuvant chemotherapy plus radiotherapy in nine elderly patients

Abbreviated questions	Responses	
As fit as before illness?	Yes	7
	No	2
Maintain hobbies/interests as desired?	Yes	8
	No	1
Do you spend most days?	Out	7
	At home	2
	In chair	0
	In bed	0
Should a friend with bladder cancer have this therapy?	Yes	9
	No	0
Hearing problems since therapy?	Yes	2
	No	6
	—	1
Episodes of nocturia per night	0	0
	1	1
	2	5
	3	3
	>3	0
Does nocturia bother you?	Yes	2
	No	7
Do you have diarrhoea?	No	1
	Sometimes	7
	Often	1

Sexual function since illness?

Much worse ^{XXXX} .... ^{XXX} .... Much better

Overall quality of life?

Excellent ^{XXXXXXX} .... ^{XX} .... Very poor

In LASA scales a cross denotes the approximate position of responses in a 10 cm linear analogue scale.

between the known side effects of cystectomy and radiotherapy for invasive bladder cancer.

Of the three non-respondents, two were shown subsequently to be dissatisfied with the long-term results of treatment (because of recurrent symptoms of cystitis in particular).

In this highly selected example, we have shown that it is possible to treat elderly patients in an active fashion (using intravenous cisplatinum) without unacceptable toxicity, and to achieve long-term survival in approximately one-third of cases. In a population group over the age of 70 years, a shift of the survival curve to the right, with a prolongation of good-quality life of two to five years, can be a very worthwhile achievement. However, it should be emphasized that this series has been highly selected in that the expectation of 5-year survival in this elderly group, treated by radiotherapy alone for invasive non-metastatic bladder cancer, is approximately 20 per cent; i.e. there is at least a reasonable chance of securing a sustained remission by active treatment.

However, it may well be that the use of cytotoxic chemotherapy for patients with recurrent or metastatic bladder cancer in this age group is not appropriate. In this context, variables such as the expected duration of survival, the quality of life and the likely toxicity of prolonged chemotherapy (as distinct from the short courses in the neoadjuvant programme) must be taken into account. Further data from the available trials, including formal evaluation of toxicity, survival and quality of life, will be required before a definitive statement can be made regarding the use of chemotherapy for metastatic bladder cancer in elderly patients.

It should also be emphasized that the role of first-line or neoadjuvant intravenous chemotherapy for invasive, non-metastatic TCC of the bladder has not yet been validated in the population as a whole. As discussed in Chapter 15, we are currently conducting a national, multicentre, randomized trial to test the true utility of this approach to management. It may ultimately be possible to compare the indices discussed above for the elderly patients randomized to each arm of this trial. Until that time, the use of first-line intravenous cytotoxics cannot be recommended as the 'state of the art' in the management of invasive bladder cancer in the elderly patient.

There is a particular responsibility in treating the aged patient to do no harm. To this end, it is important to define clearly the aims of treatment, emphasizing the balance between 'cure' and 'palliation'. The changes in pharmacology and physiology of the aged, accompanied by the likely use of multiple medications, problems with compliance, and the stresses imposed by intercurrent diseases, should not be forgotten when planning a regimen of treatment for such a patient. However, with these constraints in mind, the judicious use of single cytotoxic agents, such as methotrexate or cisplatinum, can effectively palliate the symptoms of invasive or metastatic bladder cancer and, in some cases, can achieve cure, allowing the elderly patient to live the full extent of his life without the symptoms or the complications of the disease.

References

Armitage, J.O. and Potter, J.F. (1984). Aggressive chemotherapy for diffuse histiocytic lymphoma in the elderly: increased complications with advancing age. *Journal of the American Geriatric Society* **32**: 269–73.

Begg, C. and Carbone, P.P. (1983). Clinical trials and drug toxicity in the elderly: the experience of Eastern Cooperative Oncology Group. *Cancer* **52**: 1986–92.

Bender, A.D. (1965). The effects of increasing age on the distribution of peripheral blood flow in man. *Journal of the American Geriatric Society* **13**: 192–8.

Castleden, C.M., George, C.F., Mercer, D. and Hallet, C. (1979). Increased sensitivity to nitrazepam in old age. *British Medical Journal* **i**: 10–12.

Chabner, B.A. and Myers, C.E. (1985). Clinical pharmacology of cancer chemotherapy. In *Cancer: Principles and Practice of Oncology*, pp. 156–97. Edited by DeVita, V.T., Hellman, S. and Rosenberg, S.A. Lippincott, Philadelphia.

Cohen, H.J. (1985). Clinical aspects of cancer in the elderly. In *Interrelationship among Aging, Cancer and Differentiation*, pp. 15–21. Edited by Pullman, B., Ts'o, P.O.P. and Schneider, E.L. Reidel Publishing Co., Dordrecht.

Cohen, J.L. (1986). Pharmacokinetic changes in aging. *American Journal of Medicine* **80** (Suppl. 5A): 31–8.

Dixon, D.O., Neilan, B., Jones, S.E., Lipschitz, D.A., Miller, T.P., Grozea, P.N. and Wilson, H.E. (1986). Effect of age on therapeutic outcome in advanced diffuse histiocytic lymphoma: the Southwest Oncology Group experience. *Journal of Clinical Oncology* **4**: 295–305.

Forbes, G.B. and Reina, J.C. (1970). Adult lean body mass declines with age: some longitudinal observations. *Metabolism* **19**: 653–63.

Gelman, R.S. and Taylor, S.G. (1984). CMF chemotherapy in women more than 65 years old with advanced breast cancer: the elimination of age trends in toxicity by using doses based on creatinine clearance. *Journal of Clinical Oncology* **2**: 1404–13.

Greenblatt, D.J., Allen, M.D., Harmatz, J.S. and Shader, R.I. (1980). Diazepam disposition determinations. *Clinical Pharmacology and Therapeutics* **27**: 301–12.

Greenblatt, D.J., Allen, M.D., Locnisker, A., Harmatz, J.S. and Shader R.I. (1979). Lorazepam kinetics in the elderly. *Clinical Pharmacology and Therapeutics* **26**: 103–13.

Greenblatt, D.J., Sellers, E.M. and Shader, R.I. (1982). Drug disposition in old age. *New England Journal of Medicine* **306**: 1081–8.

Gunn, W.G. (1980). Radiation therapy for the aging patient. *Ca–A Cancer Journal for Clinicians* **30**: 337–47.

Haas, C.D., Coltman, C.A., Gottlieb, A.J. *et al.* (1976). Phase II evaluation of bleomycin: a Southwest Oncology Group study. *Cancer* **38**: 8–12.

Hall, R.R., Herring, D.W., McGill, A.C. and Gibb, I. (1981). Oral methotrexate therapy for multiple superficial bladder carcinoma. *Cancer Treatment Reports* **65** (Suppl.): 175–8.

Hansen, H.H., Selawry, O.S., Holland, J.F. and McCall, C.B. (1971). The variability of individual tolerance to methotrexate in cancer patients. *British Journal of Cancer* **25**: 298–305.

Harker, W.G., Meyers, F.I., Freiha, F.R. *et al.* (1985). Cisplatin, methotrexate and vinblastine (CMV): an effective chemotherapy regimen for metastatic transitional cell carcinoma of the urinary tract. *Journal of Clinical Oncology* **3**: 1463–70.

Ho, P.C. and Triggs, E.J. (1984). Drug therapy in the elderly. *Australia and New Zealand Journal of Medicine* **14**: 179–90.

Hollenberg, N.K., Adams, D.F., Solomon, H.S., Rashid, A., Abrams, H.L. and Merrill, J.P. (1974). Senescence and the renal vasculature in normal man. *Circulation Research* **34**: 309–16.

Kahn, S.B., Begg, C.J., Mazza, J.J., Bennett, J.M., Bonner, H. and Glick, J.H. (1984). Full dose versus attenuated dose daunorubicin, cytosine arabinoside, and 6-thioguanine in the treatment of acute non-lymphocytic leukaemia in the elderly. *Journal of Clinical Oncology* **2**: 865–70.

Kaiko, R.F. (1980). Age and morphine analgesia in cancer patients with postoperative pain. *Clinical Pharmacology and Therapeutics* **28**: 823–6.

Kaiko, R.F., Wallenstein, S.L., Rogers, A.G., Grabinski, P.Y. and Honde, R.W. (1982). Narcotics in the elderly. *Medical Clinics of North America* **66**: 1079–89.

Kerr, I.G., Jolivet, J., Collins, J.M., Drake, J.C. and Chabner, B.A. (1983). Test dose for predicting high dose methotrexate infusions. *Clinical Pharmacology and Therapeutics* **33**: 44–51.

Moussad, N. (1984). Pharmacokinetic considerations in geriatric patients. In *Pharmacokinetic Bases for Drug Treatment*. Edited by Bennett, L.Z. Raven Press, New York.

O'Connell, M.J., Earle, J.D., Harrington, D.P., Johnson, G.J. and Blick, J.H.

(1986). Initial chemotherapy doses for elderly patients with malignant lymphoma. *Journal of Clinical Oncology* **4**:1418.

Ouslander, J.G. (1981). Drug therapy in the elderly. *Annals of Internal Medicine* **95**: 711–22.

Pearson, B.S. and Raghavan, D. (1985). First line intravenous cisplatin for deeply invasive bladder cancer: update on seventy cases. *British Journal of Urology* **57**: 690–3.

Raghavan, D., Grundy, R., Greenaway, T.M. *et al.* (in press). Pre-emptive intravenous cisplatin plus radical radiotherapy for fit septuagenarians with bladder cancer: Age itself is not a contra-indication. *British Journal of Urology* (in press).

Raghavan, D., Pearson, B., Duval, P., Rogers, J., Meagher, M., Wines, R., Mameghan, H., Boulas, J. and Green, D. (1985). Initial intravenous cis-platinum therapy: improved management for invasive high risk bladder cancer? *Journal of Urology* **133**: 399–402.

Rowe, J.W., Andres, R., Tobin, J.D., Norris, A.H. and Shock, N.H. (1976). The effect of age on creatinine clearance in man: a cross sectional and longitudinal study. *Journal of Gerontology* **31**: 155–63.

Shaw, P.G. (1982). Common pitfalls in geriatric drug prescribing. *Drugs* **23**: 324–8.

Sternberg, C.N., Yagoda, A. and Scher, H.I. *et al.* (1985). Preliminary results of MVAC (methotrexate, vinblastine, doxorubicin and cisplatin) for transition-al cell carcinoma of the urothelium. *Journal of Urology* **133**: 403–7.

Triggs, E.J. and Nation, R.L. (1975). Pharmacokinetics in the aged: a review. *Journal of Pharmacokinetics and Biopharmacology* **3**: 387–418.

Vestal, R.E. (1978). Drug use in the elderly: a review of problems and special considerations. *Drugs* **16**: 358–82.

Vestal, R.E., Norris, A.H., Tobin, J.D., Cohen, B.H., Shock, N.W. and Andres, R. (1975). Antipyrine metabolism in man: influence of age, alcohol, caffeine and smoking. *Clinical Pharmacology and Therapeutics* **18**: 425–32.

WHO (1981). Health care in the elderly: report of the technical group on use of medicaments by the elderly. *Drugs* **22**: 279–94.

Williamson, J. (1979). Adverse reactions to prescribed drugs in the elderly. In *Drugs and the Elderly: Perspectives in Geriatric Clinical Pharmacology*, pp. 239–57. Edited by Crooks, J. and Stevenson, I.H. Macmillan, London.

Wood, A.J., Vestal, R.E., Wilkinson, G.R., Branch, R.A. and Shard, D.G. (1979). Effect of aging and cigarette smoking on antipyrene and indocyanine green elimination. *Clinical Pharmacology and Therapeutics* **26**: 16–20.

10

New drugs and old toxicities

Stephen P. Ackland and Nicholas J. Vogelzang

Introduction

Over the last two decades a large number of agents have been studied for activity in metastatic bladder carcinoma. Early chemotherapy trials were frequently suboptimal, and assessment of results and comparison between studies has been hampered by a number of factors: lack of imaging techniques which allowed assessment of pelvic and retroperitoneal nodes, poor study design and lack of uniform criteria of reporting responses. In recent years these problems have been largely surmounted and clinical trials are mostly conducted in a reproducible manner which allows accurate analysis and comparison between studies. By such means a number of single agents and combinations have been recognized which have significant activity in advanced bladder carcinoma (see Tables 10.1–10.3).

Cisplatin is the most active single agent reported to date (Merrin, 1975; Price and Goldie, 1971; Rossof *et al.*, 1979; Soloway *et al.*, 1981b; Yagoda, 1979; Soloway *et al.*, 1981a; Khandekar *et al.*, 1985; Hillcoat and Raghavan, 1986). The combined response rate in this series is 30 per cent; however the response rate has been reported to approach 50 per cent in previously untreated patients. Other active agents include cyclophosphamide, doxorubicin, methotrexate, vinblastine and 5-fluorouracil. Initial claims that VM-26 and neocarzinostatin are also active (Sakamoto *et al.*, 1980a; Mechl *et al.*, 1977) have not been substantiated (Natale *et al.*, 1980; Qazi *et al.*, 1982). The trials involving single-agent 5-FU were mostly conducted in the early 1970s and suffered from the problems alluded to above. A recent study of 46 patients with advanced, pretreated transitional cell carcinoma of the bladder demonstrated a response rate of 15 per cent (Knight *et al.*, 1983). Whether this agent has significant activity in minimally treated disease remains to be explored.

Until recently, no combination of these active drugs had shown clear superiority over single-agent cisplatin (Tables 10.2 and 10.3). Recent reports of cisplatin–methotrexate combinations have described high response rates in small unselected numbers of patients (see Table 10.3) (Sternberg *et al.*, 1985; Carmichael *et al.*, 1985; Hillcoat and Raghavan, 1986; Harker *et al.*, 1985). Although confirmation of these results will require larger studies with longer periods of follow-up, these results are gratifying, especially in regard to unprecedented complete response rates—48 per cent with the MVAC

Table 10.1 Single agents with demonstrable activity in advanced bladder carcinoma

Drug	Number of patients	Average response (%)	References
Cisplatin	288	30	Merrin (1975); Price and Goldie (1971); Rossof *et al.* (1979); Soloway *et al.* (1981a,b); Yagoda (1979); Khandekar *et al.* (1985); Hillcoat and Raghavan (1986)
Cyclophosphamide	98	31	Fox (1965); Merrin *et al.* (1975); Yagoda (1980); de Kernion (1977)
Doxorubicin	280+	21	de Kernion (1977); Carter and Wasserman (1975); Tan *et al.* (1973); Knight *et al.* (1983)
Methotrexate	140	29	Altman *et al.* (1972); Andrews and Wilson (1976); Burfield (1972); Natale *et al.* (1981); Pavone-Macaluso (1971); Turner *et al.* (1977)
5-fluorouracil	120	27	Carter and Wasserman (1975); Knight *et al.* (1983)
Mitomycin C	48	21	Pavone-Macaluso (1971); Early *et al.* (1973)
Hexamethyl-melamine	50	26	Blum *et al.* (1973); Wilson *et al.* (1969); Gagliano *et al.* (1984)
Vinblastine	35	17	Pavone-Macaluso (1971); Blumenreich *et al.* (1982)

regimen and 29 per cent with cisplatin–methotrexate (Sternberg *et al.*, 1985; Carmichael *et al.*, 1985; Hillcoat and Raghavan, 1986). However, an Australian study failed to show a significant advantage for cisplatin–methotrexate (response rate 45 per cent) compared with cisplatin alone (response rate 33 per cent), although the trend favoured the combination (Hillcoat and Raghavan, 1986; see also Chapter 15). The recent study reported by Harker *et al.* (1985), where the combination of cisplatin, methotrexate and vinblastine produced a 56 per cent overall response rate with 28 per cent complete responses in 50 patients, is also of interest. These recent studies suggest that progress is being made in the management of this disease.

Despite these apparent advances, such factors as performance status, cardiac disease and renal insufficiency mandate limitations to the use of these drugs in this predominantly elderly group of patients. In bladder carcinoma, as in other malignancies, these limitations have prompted investigators to search for methods or agents which are more effective and/or less toxic.

This quest has been conducted in several directions: (1) new chemotherapeutic agents, primarily synthesized analogues of existing drugs; (2) new

Table 10.2 Combinations not containing cisplatin but with significant activity against advanced bladder carcinoma

Drug	Number of patients	Average response (%)	References
DOX + CTX	35	34	Merrin *et al.* (1975); Yagoda *et al.* (1977)
DOX + 5-FU	85	41	Cross *et al.* (1976); EORTC (1977); Martino *et al.* (1980)
DOX + CTX + MTX	38	39	Tannock *et al.* (1983)
VLB + MTX	47	19	Ahmed *et al.* (1985)

Legend: CTX = cyclophosphamide; DOX = doxorubicin; 5-FU = 5-fluorouracil; MTX = methotrexate; VLB = vinblastine.

methods of administering existing drugs, to increase antitumour activity or reduce toxicity; (3) rationally designed multimodality therapy, such as combination chemotherapy and radiotherapy, and pre-operative chemotherapy and/or radiotherapy.

This chapter will focus on new agents, and the attempts to modify existing agents to improve their therapeutic index, and on the potential or demonstrated benefit that these drugs may have in bladder carcinoma. Comparison with the parent drug will be made in each case and the differences in pharmacology, toxicity and antitumour activity will be highlighted.

Table 10.3 Cisplatin-containing combination regimens for advanced bladder carcinoma

Drug	Number of patients	Average response (%)	References
Cisplatin + CTX	91	24	Yagoda (1979); Soloway *et al.* (1981a)
Cisplatin + DOX	64	42	Yagoda (1979); Gagliano (1980); Vogl *et al.* (1976); Mills *et al.* (1977)
Cisplatin + CTX + DOX	385	46	Khandekar (1985); Samuels *et al.* (1980); Kedia *et al.* (1981); Kedia (1983); Campbell *et al.* (1981); Al-Sarraf *et al.* (1985); Troner and Hemstreet (1981); Troner (1985); Sternberg *et al.* (1977); Mulder *et al.* (1982); Schwartz *et al.* (1983)
Cisplatin + DOX + 5-FU	39	46	Williams *et al.* (1979)
MTX + VLB + DOX + Cisplatin (MVAC)	25	68	Sternberg *et al.* (1985)
MTX + cisplatin	19	68	Carmichael *et al.* (1985)
Cisplatin + MTX + VLB	50	56	Harker *et al.* (1985)

Legend: CTX = cyclophosphamide; DOX = doxorubicin; 5-FU = 5-fluorouracil; MTX = methotrexate; VLB = vinblastine.

Cisplatin and platinum analogues

The biological activity of platinum (Pt) coordination complexes was first observed in 1965 when Rosenberg and colleagues fortuitously observed inhibition of *E. coli* growth in a medium subjected to electrolysis with Pt electrodes (Rosenberg *et al.*, 1965). The similarity of this inhibition to that produced by radiation and alkylating agents ultimately led to the discovery of the active antineoplastic agent cis-dichloro-diammine platinum II (cisplatin, c-DDP) (Rosenberg *et al.*, 1969).

C-DDP was almost discarded in the early 1970s when trials showed marked gastrointestinal effects and nephrotoxicity. Interest was rejuvenated when responses were seen in testicular malignancies, and nephrotoxicity was reduced by hydration (Higby *et al.*, 1973; Higby *et al.*, 1974; Rossof *et al.*, 1972; Talley *et al.*, 1973). Over the last decade there has been a proliferation of information regarding the pharmacology, toxicity and clinical applications of c-DDP (Loehrer and Einhorn, 1984).

However, like many antineoplastic drugs, c-DDP has a low therapeutic index when given by these schedules. Thus, a variety of modifications have ensued, including variations on the method of drug delivery, and synthetic analogues of the parent compound have been developed.

Mechanism of action and pharmacology

The mechanism of action of c-DDP begins with displacement of the chloride ions in a low-chloride environment (such as intracellular fluid) to yield a number of positively charged aquated complexes. These reactive intermediates then interact with nucleophilic sites on DNA, RNA or protein. Particularly susceptible is the N-7 position of guanine in DNA resulting in formation of bifunctional covalent links analogous to alkylating reactions (Zwelling and Kohn, 1979; Rosenberg, 1979; Drobnick and Horacek, 1973). Interstrand and intrastrand cross-links are thought to be the major cytotoxic lesions as cytotoxicity is most closely related to extent of DNA binding (Zwelling *et al.*, 1979). The formation of cross-links is a slow process, taking several hours, and is opposed by excision repair mechanisms (Zwelling *et al.*, 1979; Fraval and Roberts, 1979; Plooy *et al.*, 1985). Cross-links result in conformational DNA changes and inhibition of DNA synthesis.

C-DDP concentrations in biological fluids can be determined by a number of analytical techniques, including atomic absorption spectrophotometry and high-pressure liquid chromatography (LeRoy *et al.*, 1977; Bannister *et al.*, 1977; Bannister *et al.*, 1978). Recent applications of high-pressure liquid chromatography techniques have allowed measurement of both protein-bound and free Pt species as well as partial analysis of the various c-DDP transformation products (see Fig. 10.1) (Daley-Yates and McBrien, 1984, 1983; Andrews *et al.*, 1984). Of considerable pharmacokinetic importance is the binding of c-DDP to plasma protein (gamma globulin and transferrin as well as albumin (Gullo *et al.*, 1980)), which is felt to be covalent and irreversible and renders the drug no longer cytotoxic to cells (Litterst *et al.*, 1976; LeRoy 1979; Gormley *et al.*, 1979; Vermorken *et al.*, 1984). This occurs with a half-life of 2.7 hours (Litterst *et al.*, 1976). However, owing to tissue distribution and renal clearance of unbound Pt species, greater than

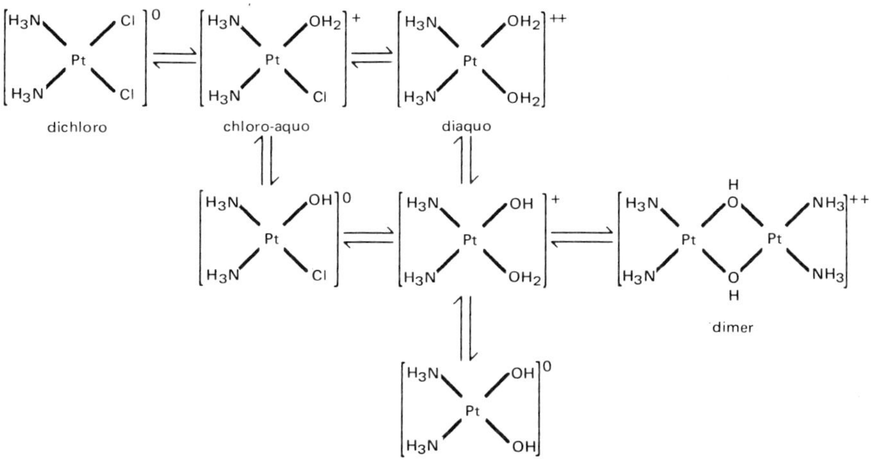

Fig. 10.1 Reactions of cisplatin with water

90 per cent of total plasma Pt is protein-bound 2 hours after administration (Daley-Yates and McBrien 1984; Gullo *et al.*, 1980; DeConti *et al.*, 1973; Himmelstein *et al.*, 1981). Unbound c-DDP undergoes a number of chemical transformations in aqueous media or plasma (Fig. 10.1). The chloride concentration of plasma tends to retard the aquation reactions and maintains the drug in the 'dichloro' form. However, recent investigators have indicated that the active unchanged c-DDP may be almost completely eliminated from plasma within 3 hours of dosing, and that the predominant forms are hydrolysis products, presumably 'chloro-aquo' and 'diaquo' species (Daley-Yates and McBrien, 1984). As well, a significant amount of Pt appears to be converted to methionine complexes (Daley-Yates and McBrien, 1984).

After bolus injection of c-DDP, a triphasic plasma disappearance curve for total platinum is demonstrated, consisting of an initial rapid distribution phase, a secondary phase with t1/2 of 17–54 minutes, caused predominantly by renal excretion of unbound Pt, and a tertiary phase with t1/2 of 1.2–8.5 days owing to slow disappearance of protein-bound Pt (Gullo *et al.*, 1980; Gormley *et al.*, 1979; Vermorken *et al.*, 1984; Himmelstein *et al.*, 1981; Patton *et al.*, 1978; Belt *et al.*, 1979 C.J. Williams *et al.*, 1979; Vermorken *et al.*, 1982; Sasaki *et al.*, 1985).

Neither mannitol, hypertonic saline nor forced diuresis affect either peak plasma levels or terminal half-life of total or filterable Pt (Himmelstein *et al.*, 1981; Bajorin *et al.*, 1985).

Very little is known about the transport of Pt species into cells. On physicochemical grounds, it is generally believed that the uncharged species can enter the cell by passive diffusion and that charged species are excluded.

During the first few hours after bolus dosing, elimination of Pt species from the body is mainly by renal excretion. The rate of renal excretion is inversely proportional to the extent of plasma protein binding (Gormley *et al.*, 1979), which would be expected if only non-protein bound species were excretable. In humans, 15–27 per cent can be excreted in 3–6 hours, and 27–45 per cent by 5 days (Gormley *et al.*, 1979; DeConti *et al.*, 1973; Sasaki *et al.*, 1985). Excretion occurs by filtration and probably also by active tubular secretion (Nelson *et al.*, 1984; Daley-Yates and McBrien, 1982). Some minimal bilary excretion also occurs (LeRoy *et al.*, 1979; Casper *et al.*, 1979; DiSimone *et al.*, 1979). C-DDP species rapidly enter tissues after intravenous administration and a fraction is retained in tissue for long periods (Litterst *et al.*, 1976; Himmelstein *et al.*, 1981; LeRoy *et al.*, 1979).

Toxicity

Nephrotoxicity remains incompletely understood, but until recently was the predominant dose-limiting toxicity. In humans distal tubular and collecting duct abnormalities predominate (Leonard *et al.*, 1971; Ward and Fauvie, 1976; Kociba and Sleight, 1971; Dentino *et al.*, 1978; Gonzalez-Vitale *et al.*, 1977). Hypomagnesemia associated with renal tubular magnesium wasting has been observed frequently (Schilsky and Anderson, 1979; Volgelzang *et al.*, 1985). Nephrotoxicity may be reduced effectively by diuresis or mannitol (Cvitkovic *et al.*, 1977; Carey *et al.*, 1977; Hayes *et al.*, 1977; Merrin, 1976), without apparently altering pharmacokinetic parameters or antineoplastic activity (Himmelstein *et al.*, 1981; Belt *et al.*, 1979; Kociba and Sleight, 1971; Pera and Harder, 1979). The Pt species responsible for nephrotoxicity is not known; one or more c-DDP metabolites have been incriminated (Daley-Yates and McBrien, 1984). Reduction of nephrotoxicity by concomitant administration of sodium thiosulphate or diethyldithiocarbamate (DDTC) derivatives lends further support to the impression that reactive species formed in plasma are the likely causes (Poore *et al.*, 1984; Iwatmoto *et al.*, 1984; Dedon and Borch, 1984; Pfeifle *et al.*, 1985; Juckett *et al.*, 1984; Glover *et al.*, 1984; Roemeling *et al.*, 1985). One group of investigators have demonstrated a circadian influence on renal toxicity, with the least toxicity occurring if the drug is given when the normal circadian maximum in urinary volume occurs (Levi *et al.*, 1982; Hrushesky, 1984). The significance of this finding to scheduling of drugs is yet to be fully determined.

Nausea and vomiting is a severe toxicity often causing poor patient compliance (VonHoff *et al.*, 1979). Numerous trials have shown partial alleviation of these side effects using various antiemetic drugs and combinations (Gagen *et al.*, 1984). Subclinical ototoxicity is common, but tinnitus and deafness are infrequently seen; this effect appears to be age- and dose-related (Reddel *et al.*, 1982). Myelosuppression and peripheral neuropathy are infrequently seen but can be cumulative (VonHoff, 1979; Thompson *et al.*, 1984; Mollman *et al.*, 1985; Hadley and Herr, 1979).

In summary, the low therapeutic index for c-DDP is due to a compilation of several factors: (1) rapid metabolism of a large percentage of the drug in plasma to inactive species, including protein-bound drug; (2) rapid excretion of unbound drug by the kidney; and (3) significant toxicity, especially nephrotoxicity and emesis. These factors tend to limit the utility of c-DDP in all tumours, including bladder carcinoma which tends to affect an elderly population and has a modest incidence of associated renal dysfunction (see also Chapter 9).

In an attempt to overcome these problems, variations on the method of drug delivery have been utilized. These include continuous intravenous infusions, and intra-arterial infusion.

Continuous infusion of c-DDP

The rationale for continuous infusion (c.i.) c-DDP is based on cytokinetic, pharmacological and preclinical studies. Cytokinetically, various investigators have observed that c-DDP preferentially kills cells following exposure in the G1 phase, although the drug is active in all phases (Drewinko *et al.*, 1973; Sigdestad *et al.*, 1979). Continuous infusion theoretically allows more cells to be exposed during the most sensitive phase of their cycle.

In preclinical studies using cultured human lymphoma cells, Drewinko *et al.* showed that a longer-term exposure to low doses of c-DDP was more cytotoxic (Drewinko *et al.*, 1973), but this did not occur with colon carcinoma cells (Bergerat, 1979). No preclinical data for exposure longer than 24 hours are currently available.

There is very little pharmacological data to support the use of c.i. c-DDP. The levels of total and filterable Pt after infusion are 10–20 per cent of those after intravenous bolus, although other pharmacokinetic parameters are not significantly different (Himmelstein *et al.*, 1981; Patton *et al.*, 1978; C.J. Williams *et al.*, 1979; Vermorken *et al.*, 1982; Posner *et al.*, 1985). Posner *et al.* compared 30-minute c-DDP infusion with a 5-day continuous infusion and found that, although peak free plasma Pt levels were only 10 per cent of those of rapid infusion, the half-life (40–206 versus 25–36 minutes) and 'concentration times time' ($C \times T$) factor (6.4–15 versus 0.4–1.7 µg/ml-h) favoured improved efficacy for longer-term infusion c-DDP. If the area under the plasma $C \times T$ curve is the important parameter in determining cytotoxicity, rather than the peak dose, then long-term infusions may be more effective (Posner *et al.*, 1985). Whether a sufficient extracellular fluid concentration of Pt species capable of crossing the cell membrane can be obtained to allow cytotoxic intracellular levels is not known.

The few clinical studies of c.i. c-DDP performed to date have mostly involved 24–120 hour venous c-DDP infusions. Studies in a variety of tumours have shown that nausea and vomiting is reduced in proportion to the rate of infusion. Nephrotoxicity is inconsistent; some studies have shown little or no nephrotoxicity (Posner *et al.*, 1985; Bozzino *et al.*, 1981; Richardson *et al.*, 1985; Tisman *et al.*, 1984), whereas in other studies the incidence of this complication has been similar to that for intravenous bolus administration (C.J. Williams *et al.*, 1979; Jacobs *et al.*, 1978; Amrein and Weitzman, 1985; Salem *et al.*, 1978; Salem *et al.*, 1984; Lokich, 1980; Lokich and Zipoli, 1984). Gratifying responses have been seen in head and neck cancer (Jacobs *et al.*, 1978; Amrein and Weitzman, 1985), ovarian cancer (Bozzino *et al.*, 1981), non-small cell carcinoma of lung (Salem *et al.*, 1978; Loh *et al.*, 1985) and testicular cancer (Richardson *et al.*, 1985) and sporadic responses in other tumours (Salem *et al.*, 1978; Lokich, 1980; Lokich and Zipoli, 1984; Loh *et al.*, 1985; Sand *et al.*, 1984). Few patients with bladder carcinoma have been studied in this manner, and no responses were observed (Salem *et al.*, 1984; Lokich and Zipoli, 1984; Sand *et al.*, 1984).

In summary, although there is little preclinical data to support or refute a hypothesis that continuous infusion may improve the therapeutic index for c-DDP, clinical studies using infusions up to 5 days have demonstrated that this schedule allows larger total doses of c-DDP to be given safely and effectively, provided adequate hydration and diuresis are maintained.

Lokich *et al.* (1984) studied long-term, continuous, low-dose infusions of c-DDP for up to 30 days in 14 patients. Nausea and vomiting was dose-limiting and, despite absence of hydration, clinical nephrotoxicity was rare. The cumulative dose of cisplatin delivered by this schedule was comparable to intermittent high-dose treatment but with less toxicity. A response was seen in one patient with thyroid carcinoma, and a single patient with bladder cancer did not respond. Further studies of this nature are needed to define the value of this form of therapy in the antineoplastic armamentarium. However, catheter complications may limit the usefulness of this technique (Lokich and Becker, 1983).

Intra-arterial cisplatin
Another means of theoretically improving the therapeutic index for c-DDP is by regional arterial perfusion for locally confined malignancies. This offers the potential advantage of greater total drug exposure for the tumour, and possibly a reduction in systemic toxicity. Theoretical principles dictate that a proportional increase in local drug concentration is conditional upon a low blood flow rate through the infusing artery and a high systemic drug elimination rate (Chen and Gross, 1980; Collins, 1984). Furthermore, reduction in systemic drug delivery depends on the ability of the infused region to eliminate the drug (Chen and Gross, 1980; Collins, 1984; Campbell *et al.*, 1983), or the ability to give an antidote of the drug 'downstream' from the infused region (Iwatmoto *et al.*, 1984).

Comparisons of the pharmacokinetics of intravenous and intra-arterial (i.a.) c-DDP have demonstrated minimal differences in the various parameters with the exception of hepatic arterial infusion, where some first-pass extraction of total Pt by the liver is apparent (Stewart *et al.*, 1983). An elegant study by Campbell *et al.* (1983) made direct comparisons of steady-state reactive (non-protein bound) Pt concentrations during i.a. and i.v. infusions in the same subject. No significant difference was found for either intrahepatic or femoral artery infusions at several different dose rates: the plasma clearance associated with i.a. infusion averaged only an insignificant 19 per cent greater than that associated with i.v. infusion. By contrast, D.J. Stewart *et al.* (1985), in analysing tissues collected at autopsy, found that Pt concentrations tended to be higher in areas of i.a. c-DDP infusion. Despite a lack of preclinical data to support the concept, several phase I–II studies have been conducted to analyse the clinical value of i.a. c-DDP (see Table 10.4). In primary and metastatic brain tumours, intracarotid infusions over a 1-hour period have resulted in remarkable response rates but some severe neurological toxicities (Lehane *et al.*, 1983; Feun *et al.*, 1984; Khan *et al.*, 1982; Kapp and Vance, 1984; Vance and Kapp, 1985).

Recent studies of regional perfusion for head and neck squamous cell carcinomas, regionally confined sarcomas, and a variety of other malignancies, have shown some useful responses (Frustaci *et al.*, 1984; Mortimer *et al.*, 1985; Calvo *et al.*, 1980; Jaffe *et al.*, 1984; Benjamin *et al.*, 1984). One of these patients had bladder cancer, and had stable disease for at least 8 months after two courses of c-DDP given via the internal iliac artery (Calvo *et al.*, 1980). At the M.D. Anderson Hospital, Logothetis and colleagues treated 38 patients with locally advanced bladder carcinoma using cisplatin, cyclophosphamide and doxorubicin given by both i.a. and i.v. routes (Logothetis *et al.*, 1985). Of 10 patients who had i.a. treatment only, 4

Table 10.4 Regional intra-arterial cisplatin

Tumour	Dose (route)	Response rate	Toxicity	References
Brain (1° and 2°)	100 mg (carotid)	8/10	Deafness Visual/CNS-10%	Lehane *et al.* (1983)
Brain—1° —2°	60–120 mg/m^2 (carotid)	6/20 5/10	Seizures; agitation; transient hemiparesis; retinal; encephalopathy	Feun *et al.* (1984)
Glioma	150–200 mg (supraophthalmic)	83%	No neurologic deficit; lower doses—lower response rate	Kapp and Vance (1984); Vance and Kapp (1985)
Head and neck	100 mg/m^2/5 days (regional)	50%	As per i.v. administration	Frustaci *et al.* (1984)
Head and neck	100 mg/m^2 (carotid)	14/20	Unilateral alopecia; transient facial palsy; blurred vision; tongue infarction; others as per i.v.	Mortimer *et al.* (1985)
Various	120 mg/m^2	Overall 45% (5/19 melanoma, 4/10 sarcoma, 2/9 breast, 3/11 others)	As per i.v.; local pain; erythema; oedema	Calvo *et al.* (1980)
Osteosarcoma	150 mg/m^2	12/18	Local erythema and induration Others as per i.v.	Jaffe *et al.* (1984)

responses (one complete) were observed, which is not significantly different from the small number of patients who responded to i.v. treatment only.

Whether these responses are due to delivery of low but effective concentrations of drug to poorly perfused areas of tumour, or achievement of higher peak concentrations of active c-DDP species at the tumour cell membrane than can be attained by i.v. c-DDP, is unclear. Nonetheless, intra-arterial infusion of c-DDP may be a useful preoperative technique in patients with bulky primary bladder carcinoma, or in localized tumours relatively resistant to c-DDP given intravenously where the higher doses achievable by i.a. infusion may be efficacious. Carefully designed studies are needed.

Platinum analogues

Clinical success with c-DDP and awareness of its narrow therapeutic index has led to the development of several analogues, with less nephrotoxicity and emetic potential and equal or greater antitumour effect. A number of these compounds have been evaluated in clinical trials (Lee *et al.*, 1983). Two in particular appear to have some advantages over c-DDP in these respects: CBDCA (JM-8, carboplatin, cis-diammine 1,1-cyclobutane dicarboxlato Pt II) and CHIP (JM-9, iproplatin, cis-dichloro-trans dihydroxyl-bis-isopropylamine Pt IV) (see Fig. 10.2).

CBDCA (carboplatin) has demonstrated activity comparable to c-DDP against many *in vitro* tumour systems, but superior activity in others (Lee *et al.*, 1983). The mode of antitumour action of CBDCA is not known, but is expected to be similar to c-DDP (Micetich *et al.*, 1985). Similarly, comparisons of the efficacy of c-DDP, CBDCA and CHIP against xenograft models of bladder carcinoma have demonstrated comparable results (Russell *et al.*, 1986; see also Chapter 1).

In animal and human toxicity studies, CBDCA has demonstrated comparable haematological toxicity to c-DDP, manifest primarily as thrombocytopenia. It has little or no nephrotoxicity, ototoxicity or neurotoxicity, even in the absence of diuresis, and is also less emetogenic than c-DDP (Lee *et al.*, 1983; Calvert *et al.*, 1982; Curt *et al.*, 1983; Egorin *et al.*, 1983; Leyvraz *et al.*, 1985; Koeller *et al.*, 1983; Evans *et al.*, 1983; Kaplan *et al.*, 1983; Kelsen *et al.*, 1984; Ten Bokkel Huinink *et al.*, 1984; Rosencweig *et al.*, 1983; Ohnuma *et al.*, 1984; Creekmore *et al.*, 1985; Siddik *et al.*, 1982; Priego *et al.*, 1983; Tauer *et al.*, 1985; Ozols *et al.*, 1985; Creekmore *et al.*, 1986; Wiltshaw *et al.*, 1985; Smith *et al.*, 1985; Egorin *et al.*, 1984).

Pharmacokinetic studies have demonstrated a much lower rate of plasma protein binding of CBDCA compared with c-DDP. In one study, 20–40 per cent of total plasma Pt was present as ultrafiltrable (UF) Pt after 1 hour (Priego *et al.*, 1983), and in other studies, 35–45 per cent at 4–6 hours (Egorin *et al.*, 1983; Harland *et al.*, 1984). Most of the ultrafilterable Pt present within the first 4 hours or more after administration is unchanged CBDCA (Harland *et al.*, 1984). As a consequence the rate of renal excretion of elemental Pt is much higher, accounting for the relatively higher molar dose required for the same biological activity. Rates of disappearance of UF Pt from plasma have been reported to be triphasic with half-lives of 1–7

Cisplatin

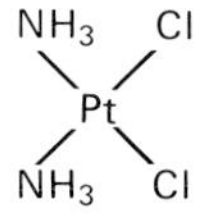

JM-8
(CBDCA,
carboplatin)

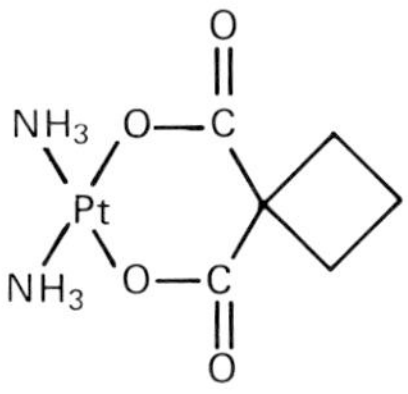

JM-9
(chip)

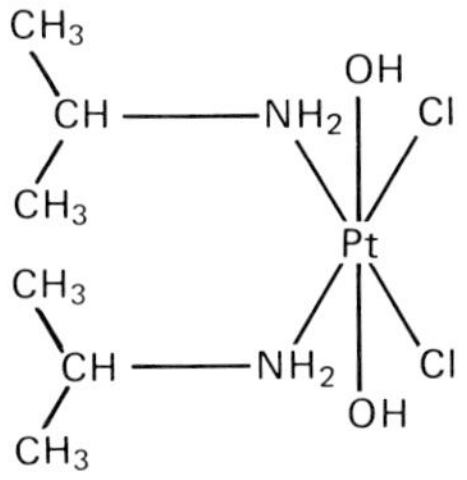

Fig. 10.2 Structures of cisplatin and its analogues

minutes, 25–87 minutes, and 100–345 minutes respectively (Calvert *et al.*, 1982; Curt *et al.*, 1983; Egorin *et al.*, 1983; Siddik *et al.*, 1982; Priego *et al.*, 1983; Harland *et al.*, 1984). Considerable interpatient variability is apparent with respect to half-lives, protein binding and renal excretion rates, some of which is accounted for by variations in baseline glomerular filtration rate.

In clinical phase I and II studies, the *in vivo* antitumour spectrum of CBDCA seems similar to c-DDP, with activity shown against ovarian cancer (Curt *et al.*, 1983; Evans *et al.*, 1983; Ten Bokkel Huinink *et al.*, 1984; Creekmore *et al.*, 1985; Tauer *et al.*, 1985), squamous cell carcinoma of the head and neck (Ohnuma *et al.*, 1984; Creekmore *et al.*, 1985), and small- and non-small-cell lung carcinoma (Creekmore *et al.*, 1985; Smith *et al.*, 1985; Harland *et al.*, 1984). However, responses have been seen in some c-DDP-resistant tumours (Curt *et al.*, 1983; Egorin *et al.*, 1983; Leyvraz *et al.*, 1985; Koeller *et al.*, 1983; Evans *et al.*, 1983; Tauer *et al.*, 1985). Its true response rate in bladder carcinoma has not been defined. No significant nephrotoxicity has been demonstrated in any of these studies.

To date, little or no data are available in regard to continuous i.v. CBDCA. One preliminary report comparing 24-hour infusion to i.v. bolus administration did not demonstrate a difference in toxicity between these two schedules, but the numbers of patients were extremely small (Leyvraz *et al.*, 1985). In another study a 48-hour continuous infusion of 800 mg/m^2

produced responses in 2 of 8 patients with c-DDP-resistant ovarian carcinoma; the only toxicities observed with this schedule were nausea, vomiting and myelosuppression (Ozols *et al.*, 1985). A 24-hour infusion of CBDCA given to patients with bladder carcinoma induced objective responses in 4 of 19 patients, with one complete remission (Creekmore *et al.*, 1986). Although the activity of CBDCA in this study was similar to c-DDP, the drug was well-tolerated, with thrombocytopenia being the only significant toxicity.

CHIP (iproplatin) is a quadrivalent Pt complex with an octahedral rather than a planar configuration. As such it may have a different antitumour spectrum from c-DDP and other divalent platinum analogues. It has demonstrated activity against a large variety of experimental tumour systems although, unlike CBDCA, sensitivity in c-DDP-resistant tumours has been demonstrated (Lee *et al.*, 1983).

The spectrum of clinical toxicity of CHIP when given by i.v. bolus was predicted from rat and dog toxicity data. Myelosuppression is dose-limiting, with thrombocytopenia being more severe than neutropenia. Nausea and vomiting are mild to moderate and, in contrast to c-DDP, there is little or no nephrotoxicity, ototoxicity, neurotoxicity or alopecia (B.S. Yap *et al.*, 1983; Ginsberg *et al.*, 1983; Creaven *et al.*, 1983; Sessa *et al.*, 1985).

Pharmacokinetic studies in dogs suggested a biphasic decay with a $t1/2\alpha$ of 0.6 hours, which is similar to that of c-DDP (Pendyala *et al.*, 1982). However, the $t1/2\beta$ was only 39.4 hours, which is much shorter than that reported following c-DDP administration in the dog (Litterst *et al.*, 1976). Similar results have been observed in the rat (Pendyala *et al.*, 1982). CHIP does not bind to plasma protein *in vitro*, in contrast to c-DDP (Pendyala *et al.*, 1982). These data, coupled with the finding that most unchanged CHIP is excreted by the kidneys early after administration, leads to the supposition that the long half-life is due to retention of non-protein-bound metabolites (Pendyala *et al.*, 1982). In humans, the pharmacokinetic parameters of CHIP have been described as being remarkably similar to c-DDP (Creaven *et al.*, 1983; Pendyala *et al.*, 1982). However, further study is required to confirm these impressions.

Clinical trials to date have suggested superior activity to c-DDP in non-small-cell lung cancer (Kriesman *et al.*, 1985), and responses have been seen in some c-DDP-resistant tumours (Sessa *et al.*, 1985). Only a handful of patients with bladder carcinoma have been reported in phase-I trials of CHIP to date. Phase-II trials of this compound in bladder carcinoma are currently in progress.

New anthraquinones

Doxorubicin (Adriamycin) has been in widespread and routine clinical use for more than a decade. It has significant activity in a wide spectrum of malignancies. Although it is not the most active drug in bladder carcinoma, it has activity such as to warrant its inclusion in combinations against this disease (see Tables 10.1 and 10.2). The primary toxicities of doxorubicin are myelosuppression, nausea and vomiting, mucositis and alopecia. Myelosuppression limits the individual dose given, but the toxicity of greatest concern in the responding patient is cumulative cardiac toxicity, which reaches significance at 450–550 mg/m^2 total dose. These toxicities seriously limit the use of this drug, especially in elderly patients and those with pre-existing cardiac disease, such as is common in the population with bladder carcinoma.

The rational development of new anthraquinones is one way of circumventing these toxicities. A large number of analogues have been synthesized; one of these has entered clinical trial in bladder carcinoma, and several others are suitable candidates for study in this disease.

Mitoxantrone (dihydroxyanthracenedione) was one of many compounds synthesized by the American Cyanamid Co. laboratories after antitumour activity was found to be associated with a polycyclic aromatic structure that had been selected for its ability to intercalate with DNA. Studies in mouse tumour models resulted in selection of mitoxantrone as the most effective derivative synthesized. It differs from doxorubicin in that it is a 3-ring planar anthraquinone rather than a 4-ring anthracycline, and does not have a sugar moiety attached (see Fig. 10.4). Mitoxantrone intercalates DNA in a manner analogous to doxorubicin, but in addition causes inter- and intra-strand cross-linking possibly associated with its charged side-arms. It induces single-strand and double-strand breaks in DNA and is a strong inhibitor of DNA and RNA synthesis (Durr *et al.*, 1983). Mitoxantrone was predicted to have minimal or no cardiotoxicity since it does not induce free-radical formation or lipid peroxidation; these mechanisms have been incriminated

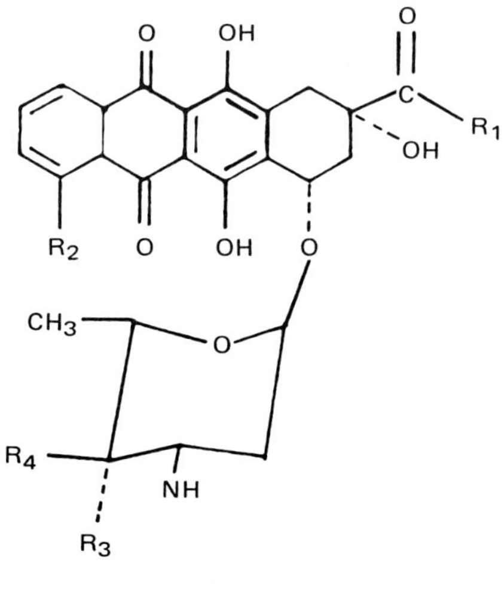

	R_1	R_2	R_3	R_4
doxorubicin	CH_2OH	OCH_3	OH	H
daunorubicin	CH_3	OCH_3	OH	H
4'-deoxydoxorubicin	CH_2OH	OCH_3	H	H
4-demethoxy daunorubicin	CH_3	H	OH	H
4'-epidoxorubicin	CH_2OH	OCH_3	H	OH

Fig. 10.3 Structure of anthracyclines

in doxorubicin cardiotoxicity (Doroshow, 1983; Kharasch and Novak, 1982). It is active in a variety of murine tumour systems and human tumour cell lines transplanted into mice (Schabel *et al.*, 1983). In humans, predictable neutropenia is the dose-limiting toxicity, although anaemia or thrombocytopenia are uncommon (Crossley, 1984). The commonest toxicities are nausea and vomiting, stomatitis and alopecia, although in most patients these adverse reactions are mild or non-existent, in contrast to the experience with doxorubicin. Congestive cardiac failure has been noted in occasional patients treated with mitoxantrone, but the risk appears to be reduced in patients not previously treated with chest irradiation or other anthracyclines (Crossley, 1984). Thus, the preclinical prediction of reduced cardiotoxicity has been confirmed.

Phase-I clinical studies suggested activity in breast cancer, lymphoma and leukaemia, which has been confirmed in phase-II and III studies (Smyth *et al.*, 1984; Levin *et al.*, 1984; Gams *et al.*, 1985; Arlin *et al.*, 1985). Preliminary data in these tumours suggested activity comparable to doxorubicin but fewer adverse effects for mitoxanthrone (Vogel *et al.*, 1985; Case *et al.*, 1985). In phase-I studies, although activity was seen in bladder carcinoma, too few patients were studied for independent analysis (Smith, 1983; VonHoff *et al.*, 1980). A single phase-II study in bladder carcinoma, utilizing a dose of 12 mg/m^2 intravenously every 3 weeks, failed to produce a response in 28 patients (Van Oosterom *et al.*, 1985). However, 13 of these patients had received prior chemotherapy, and all but 2 had received other treatment modalities, tending to bias the results towards failure. In spite of this discouraging result, and since in other tumours mitoxantrone has similar activity to doxorubicin, further studies of mitoxantrone both singly and in combinations may be worth while.

Bisantrene (9,10-anthracenedicarboxaldehyde bis [4,5-dihydro-1-H-imidazol-2-yl] hydrazone dihydrochloride) is an antitumour agent selected for clinical trial on the basis of its novel chemical structure and its significant activity against a wide variety of animal tumour models (Giuliani and Kaplan, 1980; Citarella *et al.*, 1980). Its chemical structure and molecular mechanism of action are similar to mitoxantrone (see Fig. 10.4) (Bowden *et al.*, 1985). In phase-I studies using a variety of schedules, neutropenia was the dose-limiting toxicity (VonHoff *et al.*, 1981; Spiegel *et al.*, 1982; Alberts *et al.*, 1982). Phlebitis and drug-induced hypotension, which related to the concentration and rate of infusion, were sometimes seen; but nausea and vomiting were uncommon. Unusual local cutaneous reactions including local erythema and a delayed oedema and erythema of the infused limb were seen in about one-third of patients. Responses have been seen in hypernephroma, hepatoma, bladder carcinoma, adenocarcinoma of lung, melanoma and myeloma in these studies. Phase-II studies have shown significant activity in breast carcinoma (Osborne *et al.*, 1984; H.Y. Yap *et al.*, 1983), but not in melanoma (Papadopoulos *et al.*, 1985). Phase-II studies in bladder carcinoma are awaited. However, in view of the structural similarity of this agent to mitoxantrone, and the additional toxicities described, the ultimate value of this drug as an anticancer agent may be limited.

4'epi-doxorubicin (epirubicin) is an anthracycline antibiotic differing from doxorubicin in the epimerization of the OH-group in position 4' of the

MITOXANTRONE

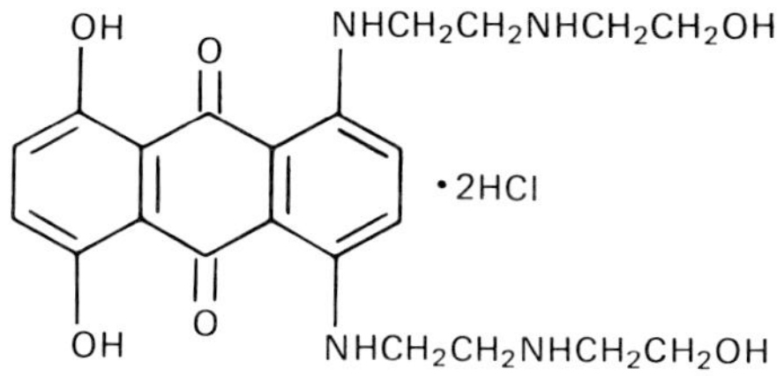

OH   O   NHCH₂CH₂NHCH₂CH₂OH

$\cdot$ 2HCl

OH   O   NHCH₂CH₂NHCH₂CH₂OH

BISANTRENE

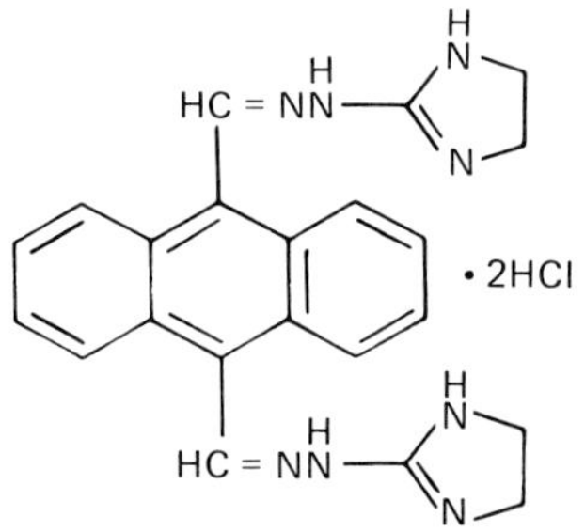

HC = NN

$\cdot$ 2HCl

HC = NN

Fig. 10.4 Structures of substituted anthraquinones

amino sugar moiety (see Fig. 10.3). It binds to DNA in a manner analogous to doxorubicin (Plumridge and Brown, 1978). In several experimental tumour models, antitumour activity similar to doxorubicin was demonstrated (Casazza *et al.*, 1978). However, in Lewis lung carcinoma, MS-2 sarcoma lung metastases and human melanoma heterotransplanted into mice, greater activity than doxorubicin was shown (Casazza *et al.*, 1978; Giuliani *et al.*, 1981).

In phase-I studies, epirubicin has demonstrated a pattern of toxicity qualitatively similar to doxorubicin at identical doses but quantitatively less severe, particularly for leukopenia and gastrointestinal toxicity (Bonfanti *et al.*, 1982; Young, 1984; Bonnadonna *et al.*, 1984). Chronic toxicity studies in animals revealed the same pattern of cardiac toxicity for both doxorubicin and epirubicin, but it was less marked with epirubicin (Villani *et al.*, 1980). In human studies a limited number of patients have developed cardiotoxicity at relatively high doses (Young, 1984; Bonnadonna *et al.*, 1984). The overall impression is that epirubicin may be slightly less cardiotoxic than doxorubicin but specific and comparative studies await completion.

Clinical studies have shown significant antitumour activity against breast carcinoma, ovarian carcinoma, soft-tissue sarcomas, non-Hodgkin's lymphonas, leukaemias and gastric cancer (Clinical brochure, 1985). In bladder carcinoma, 15 evaluable patients have been studied, with responses observed in 3 (response rate 20 per cent) (Clinical Brochure, 1985). Although these results are not encouraging, responses in heavily pretreated patients with advanced disease have been observed, and further studies are needed to define accurately the single-agent response rate. Furthermore, as with the other new anthracyclines, the lower toxicity compared to doxorubicin may make it suitable for up-front comparison with doxorubicin or inclusion in combination chemotherapy programmes.

4'deoxydoxorubicin (esorubicin, DxDx) is another analogue which structurally differs from doxorubicin by the lack of an oxygen atom at the 4' position of the amino sugar moiety. DxDx demonstrated equal or greater antitumour activity than doxorubicin against a spectrum of murine tumours and human xenografts, including doxorubicin-resistant tumours (Casazza, 1979; Cagnassa, 1982; Henry, 1979; Giuliani and Kaplan, 1980). Toxicity in animals appeared comparable to doxorubicin, with the exception that no significant cardiotoxicity occurred with DxDx (Casazza, 1979; Cagnasso, 1982). In phase-I studies myelosuppression, predominantly neutropenia, was dose-limiting, with only mild nausea and vomiting and occasional alopecia being reported (Ferrari *et al.*, 1984; Stanton *et al.*, 1985). Insufficient data has accumulated to date to assess the cardiotoxicity of this drug, although 3 cases of possible cardiac damage by DxDx have been reported to the NCI (NCI Memorandum, 1985). Responses have been seen in breast, head and neck, colon, pancreatic and endometrial carcinomas, and non-Hodgkin's lymphomas (Ferrari *et al.*, 1984; Stanton *et al.*, 1985). Disease-oriented phase-II studies are currently under way, but preliminary results are not yet available. No data have been forthcoming on actual or predicted effects in bladder carcinoma.

4-demethoxydaunorubicin (Idarubicin, DMDR) is a new analogue of daunorubicin which differs from its parent compound by the absence of a methoxy group in position 4 in the Ring D of the aglycone moiety (see Fig. 10.3). This change renders DMDR more lipophilic than daunorubicin (Plumridge and Brown, 1979). Preclinical studies demonstrated activity against a variety of tumours, including L1210, P388 leukaemia, sarcomas MS-2 and 180 (Arcamone *et al.*, 1976). Against some tumours the drug was much more active than daunorubicin or doxorubicin. Furthermore, unlike the parent compound, the major hydroxy metabolite DMDR-ol retains significant cytotoxic activity, and has prolonged retention in tissues, indicating that hydroxylation of DMDR is an important step in the metabolism of this compound (Italia *et al.*, 1983; Casazza *et al.*, 1983). Tumour tissue appears capable of selective retention of the drug. Also, elimination of DMDR-ol is mainly urinary, in contrast to the hydroxy metabolite of daunorubicin, which is mainly excreted in bile (Tamassia *et al.*, 1983).

Myelosuppression, predominantly neutropenia, is the dose-limiting toxicity. Non-haematological toxicities at equivalent myelosuppressive doses appear to be less than that reported with doxorubicin or daunorubicin (Berman *et al.*, 1983; Kaplan *et al.*, 1984a,b; Bonfante *et al.*, 1983). Mild to moderate nausea and vomiting have been reported, and are less frequent and less severe with intravenous than with oral administration. Mild to moderate alopecia occurs, and occasional transient elevation of liver enzymes has been reported (Berman *et al.*, 1983; Kaplan *et al.*, 1984a,b; Bonfante *et al.*, 1983). Cardiotoxicity occurs but appears to be much less common than with doxorubicin. Preliminary data suggest that it is additive to that produced by previous anthracycline therapy. Animal data, however, suggest that the cardiotoxic–therapeutic ratio is better than for either daunorubicin or doxorubicin.

Phase I–II studies of i.v. idarubicin indicate that it is effective against all lymphomas (Hodgkin's and non-Hodgkin's), carcinoma of the breast and leukaemias (Berman *et al.*, 1983; Kaplan *et al.*, 1984a,b; Bonfante *et al.*, 1983; Bastholt *et al.*, 1985; Bacha *et al.*, 1985). To date, little or no activity against a variety of other solid tumours has been seen. The possibility of oral administration of this drug make it a preferred anthracycline in some circumstances (Berman *et al.*, 1983; Kaplan *et al.*, 1984a,b; Bonfante *et al.*, 1983).

In summary, a large number of analogues of doxorubicin and daunorubicin have been synthesized. These compounds are the products of attempts to reduce the toxicity of these drugs to normal tissues, particularly the myocardium, while at the same time maintaining or enhancing the anti-tumour activity. Several of these compounds appear to have partly achieved this aim and have entered clinical trial. Although the clinical spectrum of activity of these analogues generally appears similar to the parent drugs, the toxicities (especially cardiotoxicity) appear to be less. For these reasons, and since the discovery of a less toxic analogue which is active in bladder carcinoma may be of significant benefit in this population, continuation of studies of anthracycline analogues in bladder carcinoma may be productive.

Other agents

Etoposide and teniposide

The root of the mandrake (Popophyllum peltatum) is the source of podophyllotoxins. Two derivatives have been developed and used clinically: etoposide (VP-16,213) and teniposide (VM-26). In adult solid tumours, etoposide has seen more widespread usage, although this was fortuitous and had no rational basis.

In preclinical studies encouraging activity was seen. Etoposide is one of the most active plant products ever tested against L1210 leukaemia (Dombernowsky and Nissen, 1976). Significant activity was seen against a variety of solid tumours in animals (Rozencweig *et al.*, 1977; Stahelin, 1973). Synergism with cisplatin, cyclophosphamide and cytarabine has also been demonstrated in several animal tumours.

Unlike the vinca alkaloids and the parent compound podophyllum, etoposide does not bind to tubulin or inhibit microtubule assembly (Loike *et al.*, 1978). Both VP-16 and VM-26 induce dose-dependent single-strand DNA breaks *in vivo* and in isolated nuclei; however, this effect does not occur when the drugs are incubated with purified DNA *in vitro* (Loike and Horwitz, 1976; Roberts *et al.*, 1980; Long *et al.*, 1985; Ross *et al.*, 1984). This suggests that the target for etoposide activity is a nuclear component other than DNA and that strand breaks are a secondary phenomenon. A novel explanation for this apparently unique mechanism by which VP-16 and VM-26 introduce DNA breaks is by inhibition of type-II topoisomerase, an enzyme with DNA ligase activity (Long *et al.*, 1985; Ross *et al.*, 1984). However, to date, this proposed mechanism has not been unequivocally confirmed.

The development of a variety of high-pressure liquid chromatography assays has allowed accurate delineation of the pharmacokinetics of these drugs. After a short intravenous infusion, plasma levels of etoposide and teniposide follow a biexponential decay curve, with a terminal half-life of 6–8 hours in most studies (Arnold *et al.*, 1980; Scalzo *et al.*, 1982; D'Incalci *et al.*, 1982; Hande *et al.*, 1984; Evans *et al.*, 1982). Renal clearance accounts for 30–40 per cent of plasma clearance of etoposide (Scalzo *et al.*, 1982; D'Incalci *et al.*, 1982; Hande *et al.*, 1984). The fate of the remaining 60 per cent is still unclear. For teniposide, the individual components of systemic clearance are also not well known; one study showed a renal clearance of about 45 per cent of administered drug (Creaven and Allen, 1975).

Etoposide and teniposide are unusual among the known anticancer agents in that, at standard doses, the only frequent toxicities encountered are alopecia and myelosuppression. Nausea and vomiting are mild even with high doses, and mucositis and diarrhoea are common but rarely severe (Rozencweig *et al.*, 1977; Aisner *et al.*, 1982). Once haematological toxicity is overcome by autologous bone marrow rescue, mucositis or hepatotoxicity become dose-limiting at greater than 8 times the dose which causes modest myelosuppression (Wolff *et al.*, 1982; Postmus *et al.*, 1984).

For etoposide, significant responses have been demonstrated in a variety of cancers, most importantly germ cell tumours, small-cell lung carcinoma, lymphoma, leukaemia, uterine carcinoma, and a variety of sarcomas (Nissen *et al.*, 1980; Fitzharris *et al.*, 1980; S.D. Williams *et al.*, 1980; Cecil *et al.*, 1978; Mathe *et al.*, 1974; Taylor *et al.*, 1982; Smith *et al.*, 1976; Chard *et al.*, 1979; Hayes *et al.*, 1983). Etoposide has been incorporated into first- and second-line combination chemotherapy regimens for these tumours, but to date there have been few definitive randomized trials to establish the contribution of etoposide to these combinations. However, some trials have demonstrated significant enhancement of response rate or survival by the addition of etoposide (Zekan *et al.*, 1983; Osterlind *et al.*, 1982).

Little information is available about the value of etoposide in the treatment of bladder cancer. Nissen *et al.* (1980) included 13 patients with bladder carcinoma in their broad phase-II study, and found no responses. However, the dosage was relatively low and all had received prior treatment. Ponder and Oliver (1984) treated 15 patients with adequate doses of VP-16 without seeing any responses. All had failed previous therapy, which included chemotherapy in 9 patients. These studies, however, may underestimate the activity of the drug because of the opportunity for the tumour to develop drug resistance following prior exposure to chemotherapy. Furthermore, in other tumours with relatively low response rates to etoposide alone (such as small-cell lung cancer and leukaemias), augmented response rates have been seen when etoposide has been given in combination with cisplatin, anthracyclines and cytarabine (Zekan *et al.*, 1983; Hurd *et al.*, 1981; Look *et al.*, 1981; Sauter *et al.*, 1982). It is possible that similar synergy would be seen in bladder carcinoma, but this possibility has not yet been explored. Etoposide is a drug worthy of further exploration because of its apparently novel mechanism of action, relatively low toxicity apart from myelosuppression, and its ability to operate synergistically with other drugs useful in bladder carcinoma, such as cisplatin.

Teniposide has a place in the management of patients with leukaemia, pediatric and adult lymphomas and some brain tumours, although its true efficacy is still incompletely defined (O'Dwyer *et al.*, 1984). Responses have been seen in relapsed small-cell lung cancer and non-small-cell lung cancer, so its spectrum of activity appears similar to etoposide. The single-agent activity in bladder cancer is low (Qazi *et al.*, 1982; Garcia-Giralt *et al.*, 1981); however, the same reservations with regard to these preliminary data apply as were expressed for etoposide. Furthermore, activity of the drug has been demonstrated against superficial bladder cancer in studies performed by the EORTC (see Chapter 14).

Dihydrofolate reductase inhibitors

These agents are all structural analogues of folic acid and all inhibit DNA and RNA synthesis by binding tightly to dihydrofolate reductase DHFR, preventing maintenance of the tetrahydrofolate pools necessary for thymidine and purine synthesis (Chabner, 1982). Many DHFR inhibitors are unusual in that intracellular formation of polyglutamates provides a pool from which the active drug can be released slowly to cause prolonged effects or toxicity (Schilsky *et al.*, 1980).

Methotrexate (MTX) is the most commonly used DHFR inhibitor in clinical practice. In bladder cancer, it has a single-agent response rate of around 30 per cent (see above), and forms part of most front-line combination chemotherapy protocols. The toxicity of methotrexate in relatively low doses (less than 250 mg/m^2) is generally acceptable, with bone marrow suppression and oral mucositis predominating. Since MTX is both filtered at the glomerulus and secreted by renal tubules, adequate renal function is an essential prerequisite to drug administration. The concurrent use of nephrotoxic agents, including cisplatin, may abruptly reduce MTX clearance and lead to prolonged duration of exposure with unexpected toxicity. These factors provide a high risk of methotrexate toxicity in patients with bladder carcinoma. The rational development of new MTX analogues to circumvent these problems may lead to a safer dihydrofolate reductase inhibitor without compromising activity. A number of analogues have been developed and tested, but none has yet shown an advantage over methotrexate to the point where it can be a replacement in clinical practice.

Trimetrexate (TMQ), a recently developed 'non-classical' quinazoline antifolate, may have an advantage over methotrexate (see Fig. 10.5) (Elslager *et al.*, 1983). It is a potent growth inhibitor of cultured human neoplastic cells and is concentrated in leukaemic cells to a greater extent than MTX (Bertino and Sawicki, 1977; Bertino *et al.*, 1979; Bertino *et al.*, 1985). Furthermore, efficacy has been demonstrated in cell lines resistant to MTX on the basis of decreased membrane transport and increased DHFR (Kamen *et al.*, 1984; Scanlon *et al.*, 1982). The fact that, unlike MTX, TMQ is not polyglutamated does not seem adversely to affect its cytotoxicity; a sustained inhibition of DNA synthesis is still possible owing to initial high levels of accumulation (Legha *et al.*, 1985). However, in clinical studies, the toxicities of the drug are not dissimilar to MTX (Legha *et al.*, 1985; Donehower *et al.*, 1985; Lin *et al.*, 1985; Fanucchi *et al.*, 1985; J.A. Stewart *et al.*, 1985). In addition, the method of excretion is still predominantly renal, with up to 70 per cent of

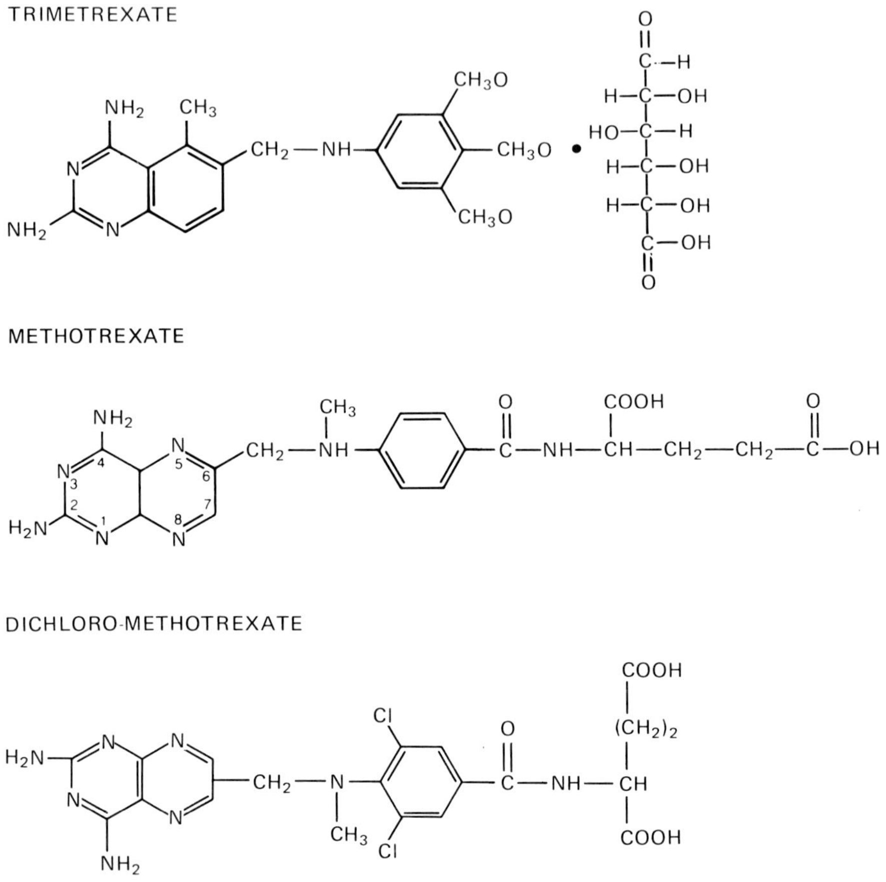

TRIMETREXATE

METHOTREXATE

DICHLORO-METHOTREXATE

Fig. 10.5 Structures of dihydrofolate reductase inhibitors

the administered dose being excreted in 48–72 hours (Legha *et al.*, 1985; Donehower *et al.*, 1985).

TMQ has demonstrated antitumour activity against a variety of murine tumours, including B-16 melanoma, CD8F1 mammary tumours, colon 26 and 38 tumours, Lewis lung carcinoma, and L1210 and P388 leukaemia (Bertino *et al.*, 1979; Kamen *et al.*, 1984).

To date, there is insufficient data concerning the clinical antitumour efficacy of TMQ. In phase-I studies toxicity was similar to MTX, and a small number of responses were seen in heavily pretreated patients with a variety of tumours (Legha *et al.*, 1985; Donehower *et al.*, 1985; Lin *et al.*, 1985; Fanucchi *et al.*, 1985; J.A. Stewart *et al.*, 1985). Phase-II studies in potentially sensitive tumours are continuing. Whether any advantage over MTX in bladder carcinoma will ultimately be shown remains to be seen.

Dichloromethotrexate (DCMTX) is a dihalogenated analogue of MTX originally synthesized in the 1950s, which has undergone a recent rejuvenation (see Fig. 10.5). DCMTX is unique among antimetabolites in that it is curative in mice with L1210 leukaemia, even in those with advanced infiltrative disease (Goldin *et al.*, 1959). Early clinical trials, however, did not support a theoretical advantage over methotrexate (Frei *et al.*, 1965). The resurgence of interest is based on its potential application in combination chemotherapy, and in particular its intra-arterial administration.

The mechanism of action is identical to MTX, but it may be a better substrate for the active transport mechanism at the cell membrane, accounting for the increased intracellular antifolate levels achieved (Kessel and Hall, 1967). Although intracellular polyglutamate formation is presumed to occur, this has not yet been clearly shown. DCMTX has a shorter plasma half-life than MTX (10 minutes versus 25 minutes) with more rapid conversion to the 7-hydroxy metabolite (Tong *et al.*, 1980). In addition, up to 60 per cent of administered DCMTX is excreted via bile and faeces, one-third as the inactive 7-hydroxy metabolite, accounting for the negligible nephrotoxicity seen with this agent. This may indicate a significant advantage of DCMTX over MTX in patients with bladder carcinoma where questionable renal function is common, or if concomitant administration of other nephrotoxic antineoplastic agents is contemplated (e.g. cisplatin).

In solid tumours, DCMTX has shown activity against colon carcinoma, breast carcinoma, hepatoma, chordoma and adenocarcinoma of unknown primary (Fernbach *et al.*, 1979; Tester *et al.*, 1982).

Natale and colleagues have reported encouraging results using DCMTX in conjunction with cisplatin in head and neck, bladder and cervical carcinomas (Natale *et al.*, 1983; Wheeler *et al.*, 1984). They demonstrated that with this combination both drugs can be used at doses very close to their individual maximally tolerated doses and that renal toxicity is minimal. Furthermore, good response rates were seen in all three tumour types studied, with a 62 per cent overall response rate in 13 patients with bladder carcinoma. These response rates are in the same range as for cisplatin–MTX combinations, so that if comparative studies demonstrate reduced toxicity and confirm similar efficacy for cisplatin–DCMTX, then DCMTX may ultimately supersede MTX as the DHFR inhibitor of choice in bladder carcinoma.

Immunotherapy in advanced bladder carcinoma

BCG (bacillus Calmette–Guerin) has enjoyed considerable success in recent years in the management of superficial bladder carcinoma. It is assumed to act locally by stimulating a host response to antigens on superficial bladder tumour cells. Several studies documenting control of recurrent or residual local tumour using intravesical BCG, with or without concurrent intradermal injections, have been summarized in a recent review (Torti and Lum, 1984), and more recent studies continue to support the use of BCG in this condition (Pinsky *et al.*, 1985; Lamm, 1985) (see also Chapters 4 and 6). Systemic BCG has not been studied in patients with advanced bladder carcinoma.

Interferons have been shown to induce responses in malignant papilloma-tosis of the bladder (Ikic *et al.*, 1981; Scorticatti *et al.*, 1982), with complete responses observed in a number of patients. Although being extensively studied for antitumour effects in a variety of malignant diseases (Kirkwood and Enstoff, 1984), with the exception of hairy cell leukaemia (Golomb *et al.*, 1986), interferon has not so far been shown to significantly benefit patients with advanced cancer.

Summary

In conclusion, a large number of new agents have become available to the oncologist for assessment in various cancers, including bladder carcinoma. Many of these drugs are rationally synthesized analogues of known antineoplastic agents, and have been developed with the intention of avoiding toxicity to normal host tissues, without compromising and perhaps augmenting antitumour effects. Several of these compounds have at least partially achieved these aims, particularly anthracycline and cisplatin analogues. Whether or not these agents have a different spectrum of clinical activity is not yet fully known, but several appear at least as potent as the parent drug and may have a role in the management of bladder carcinoma. Since the patients with bladder carcinoma are often in poor health and frequently unable to tolerate more than mild toxicity, proper evaluation of these compounds is particularly important in this disease. The inclusion of all eligible patients in studies to evaluate these agents would hasten the development of these potentially useful compounds and should ultimately bring about advances in the management of advanced bladder carcinoma.

References

Ahmed, T., Yagoda, A., Needles, B. *et al.* Vinblastine and methotrexate for advanced bladder cancer. *Journal of Urology* **133**: 602–4.

Aisner, J., Van Echo, D.A., Whitacre, M. and Wiernick, P.H. (1982). A phase I trial of continuous infusion VP-16-213 (etoposide). *Cancer Chemotherapy and Pharmacology* **7**: 157–60.

Alberts, D.S., Mackel, C., Pocelinko, R. and Salmon, S.E. (1982). Phase I clinical investigation of 9,10-anthracenedicarboxyaldehyde bis[4,5-dihydro-lH-imidazol-2-yl)-hydrazone] dihydrochloride with correlative *in vitro* human tumor clonogenic assay. *Cancer Research* **42**: 1170–75.

Al-Sarraf, M., Frank, J., Smith, J.A., O'Bryan, R.M., Constanzi, J.J., Stephans, R.L., Caraveo, J. and Crawford, E.D. (1985). Phase II trial of cyclophosphamide, doxorubicin, and cisplatin (CAP) versus amsacrine in patients with transitional cell carcinoma of the urinary bladder: a Southwest Oncology Group study. *Cancer Treatment Reports* **69**: 189–94.

Altman, C.C., McCague, N.J., Ripepi, A.C. and Cardoza, M. (1972). The use of methotrexate in advanced carcinoma of the bladder. *Journal of Urology* **198**: 271–3.

Amrein, P. and Weitzman, S. (1985). Treatment of squamous cell carcinoma of the head and neck with cisplatin and 5-fluorouracil. *Journal of Clinical Oncology* **3**: 1632–9.

Andrews, M.C. and Wilson, W.L. (1976). Phase II study of methotrexate (NSC 740) in solid tumors. *Cancer Chemotherapy Reports* **51**: 471–4.

Andrews, P.A., Wung, W.E. and Howell, S.B. (1984). An HPLC analysis of active cisplatin in plasma ultrafiltrate. *Proceedings of the American Association for Cancer Research* **25**: 647.

Arcamone, F., Bernard, L., Giardino, P. *et al.* (1976). Synthesis and antitumour activity of 4' demethoxydaunorubicin, 4-demethoxy-7,9-diepidaunorubicin and their beta-anomers. *Cancer Treatment Reports* **60**: 829–34.

Arlin, Z.A., Silver, R.T., Cassileth, P. *et al.* (1985). Further evaluation of mitoxantrone in acute leukemia. In *The Current Status of Novantrone*, pp. 91–4. John Wiley, New York.

Arnold, A.M., Dodson, M., Renwick, A. and Whitehouse, J.M.A. (1980). Pharmacokinetics of VP-16-213 using a new HPLC assay. *Cancer Chemotherapy and Pharmacology* **5** (Suppl.): 2 (Abstract).

Bacha, D., Steinherz, L., Dantis, E. *et al.* (1985). Phase I study of oral idarubicin (4DMDR) in children with cancer. *Proceedings of the American Association for Cancer Research* **26**: 186.

Bajorin, D., Bosl, G.J., Alcock, N. *et al.* (1986). Pharmacokinetics of cis-Diamminedichloroplatinum (II) after administration in hypertonic saline. *Cancer Research* **46**: 5969–72.

Bannister, S.J., Chang, Y., Sternson, L.A. *et al.* (1978). Atomic absorption spectro-photometry of free circulating platinum species in plasma derived from cis-dichlorodiammineplatinum (II). *Clinical Chemistry* **24**: 877–80.

Bannister, S.J., Sternson, L.A. and Repta, A.J. (1977). Measurement of free-circulating cis-dichlorodiammineplatinum (II) in plasma. *Clinical Chemistry* **23**: 2258–62.

Bastholt, L., Ejlertsen, B. and Dalmark, M. (1985). A phase II trial of oral 4-dimethoxydaunorubicin (DMDR) in patients with measurable advanced carcinoma of the breast. *Proceedings of the American Association for Cancer Research* **26**: 164.

Belt, R.J., Himmelstein, K.J., Patton, T.F. *et al.* (1979). Pharmacokinetics of non-protein-bound platinum species following administration of cis-dichlorodiammineplatinum (II). *Cancer Treatment Reports* **63**: 1515–1521.

Benjamin, R.S., Murray, J.A. and Wallace, S. (1984). Intra-arterial preoperative chemotherapy for osteosarcoma—a judicious approach to limb salvage. *Cancer Bulletin* **36**: 32–6.

Bergerat, J.P., Barlogie, B. and Drewinko, B. (1979). Effects of cis-dichlorodiammine-platinum (II) on human colon carcinoma cells *in vitro*. *Cancer Research* **39**: 1334–8.

Berman, E., Wittes, R.E., Leyland-Jones, B. *et al.* (1983). Phase I and clinical pharmacology studies of intravenous and oral administration of 4-demethoxydaunorubicin in patients with advanced cancer. *Cancer Research* **43**: 6096–101.

Bertino, J.R., Mini, E., Sawicki, W.L. *et al.* (1985). Effects of trimetrexate on human leukemia cells from patients sensitive and resistant to methotrexate (MTX). *Proceedings of the American Society of Clinical Oncology* **4**: 44.

Bertino, J.R. and Sawicki, W.L. (1977). Potent inhibitory activity of trimethoxyquine (TMQ), a 'non-classical' 2,4-diaminoquinazoline, on mammalian DNA synthesis. *Proceedings of the American Association for Cancer Research* **18**: 168.

Bertino, J.R., Sawicki, W.L., Moroson, B.A. *et al.* (1979). 2,4-diamino-5-methyl-6-[(3,4,5-trimethoxyanilino) methyl] quinazoline (TMQ), a potent non-classical folate antagonist. I: Effects on dihydrofolate reductase and growth of rodent tumors *in vitro* and *in vivo*. *Biochemical Pharmacology* **28**: 1983–7.

Bloom, H.J.G., Hendry, W.F., Wallace, D.M. and Skeet, R.G. (1982). Treatment of T3 bladder cancer: controlled trial of preoperative radiotherapy and radical cystectomy versus radical radiotherapy. *British Journal of Urology* **54**: 136–51.

Blum, R.H., Livingston, R.B. and Carter, S.K. (1973). Hexamethylmelamine—a new drug with activity in solid tumours. *European Journal of Cancer* **9**: 195–202.

Blumenreich, M.S., Yagoda, A., Natale, R.B., Watson, R.C. *et al.* (1982). Phase II trial of vinblastine sulfate for metastatic urothelial tract tumors. *Cancer* **50**: 435–8.

Bonfanti, V., Ferrari, L., Villani, F. *et al.* (1983). Phase I study of 4-demethoxydaunorubicin. *Investigational New Drugs* **1**: 161–8.

Bonfanti, V., Villani, F. and Bonnadonna, G. (1982). Toxic and therapeutic activity of 4'-epidoxorubicin. *Tumori* **68**: 105–11.

Bonnadonna, G., Brambilla, C. and Rossi, A. (1984). Epirubicin in advanced breast cancer: the experience of the Milan Cancer Institute. In *Advances in Anthracycline Chemotherapy*, p. 63. Edited by Bonnadonna, G. Masson, Milan.

Bowden, G.T., Roberts, R., Alberts, D.S. *et al.* (1985). Comparative molecular pharmacology in leukemic L1210 cells of the anthracene anticancer drugs mitoxantrone and bisantrene. *Cancer Research* **45**: 4915–20.

Bozzino, J.M., Prasad, V. and Koriech, O.M. (1981). Avoidance of renal toxicity by 24-hour infusion of cisplatin. *Cancer Treatment Reports* **65**: 351–2.

Burfield, G.D. (1972). Intravenous methotrexate in the treatment of advanced bladder cancer. *British Journal of Urology* **44**: 121–4.

Cagnasso, M. (Ed.) (1982). Summary of pre-clinical studies in IMI-58 (4'-deoxyrubicin) up to April 1981. Milan, Farmitalia Carlo Erba.

Calvert, A.H., Harland, S.J., Newell, D.R. *et al.* (1982). Early clinical studies with cis-diammine-1,1-cyclobutane dicarboxylate platinum (II). *Cancer Chemotherapy and Pharmacology* **9**: 140–7.

Calvo, D.B., Patt, Y.Z., Wallace, S. *et al.* (1980). Phase I–II trial of percutaneous intra-arterial cis-diamminedichloroplatinum (II) for regionally confined malignancy. *Cancer* **45**: 1278–83.

Campbell, M., Baker, L.H., Opipari, M. and Al-Sarraf, M. (1981). Phase II trial with cisplatin, doxorubicin, and cyclophosphamide (CAP) in the treatment of urothelial transitional cell carcinoma. *Cancer Treatment Reports* **65**: 897–9.

Campbell, T.N., Howell, S.B., Pfeifle, C.E. *et al.* (1983). Clinical pharmacokinetics of intra-arterial cisplatin in humans. *Journal of Clinical Oncology* **1**: 755–61.

Carmichael, J., Cornbleet, M.A., MacDougall, R.H. *et al.* (1985). Cis-platin and methotrexate in the treatment of transitional cell carcinoma of the urinary tract. *British Journal of Urology* **57**: 299–302.

Carter, S.K. and Wasserman, T.H. (1975). The chemotherapy of urologic cancer. *Cancer* **36**: 729–47.

Casazza, A.M. (1979). Experimental evaluation of anthracycline analogs. *Cancer Treatment Reports* **63**: 835–44.

Casazza, A.M. *et al.* (1985). Biologic activity of 4-demethoxy-13-dihydrodaunorubicin (4-dm-33-OH-DNR). *Proceedings of the American Association for Cancer Research* **24**: 251.

Casazza, A.M., DiManco, A., Bertazzoli, C. and Formelli, F. (1978). Antitumor activity, toxicity and pharmacological properties of 4'-epi-adriamycin. In *Current Chemotherapy*, pp. 1257–60. American Society for Microbiology, International Society of Chemotherapy.

Case, D.C., Wolff, S., Arlin, Z.A. *et al.* (1985). Phase III comparative trial of Adriamycin versus Novantrone in combination chemotherapy for the treatment of stages II to IV lymphomas. In *The Current Status of Novantrone*, pp. 79–84. John Wiley, New York.

Casper, E.S., Kelson, D.P., Alcock, N.W. *et al.* (1979). Platinum concentrations in bile and plasma following rapid and six-hour infusion of cis-dichlorodiammenplatinum (II). *Cancer Treatment Reports* **63**: 2023–5.

Cecil, J.W., Quagliana, J.M., Coltman, C.A. *et al.* (1978). Evaluation of VP-16-213 in malignant lymphoma and melanoma. *Cancer Treatment Reports* **62**: 801–3.

Chabner, B.A. (1982). Methotrexate. In *Pharmacologic Principles of Cancer Treatment*, pp. 229–55. Edited by Chabner, B.A. W.B. Saunders, Philadelphia.

Chard, R.L., Krivit, W., Bleyer, W.A. and Hammond, D. (1979). Phase II study of VP-16-213 in childhood malignant disease: a Children's Cancer Study Group report. *Cancer Treatment Reports* **63**: 1755–9.

Chary, K.K., Higby, D.J., Henderson, E.S. *et al.* (1977). Phase I study of high dose cis-dichlorodiammineplatinum (II) with forced diuresis. *Cancer Treatment Reports* **61**: 367–70.

Chen, H.S.G. and Gross, J.F. (1980). Intra-arterial infusion of anticancer drugs: theoretic aspects of drug delivery and review of responses. *Cancer Treatment Reports* **64**: 31–40.

Citarella, R.V., Wallace, R.E., Murdock, K.C. *et al.* (1980). Antitumor activity of CL 216,942: 9,10-anthracenedicarboxaldehyde bis[(4,5-dihydro-IH-imidazol-2-yl)-hydrazone] dihydrochloride. In *Abstracts of the 20th Interscience Conference on Antimicrobial Agents and Chemotherapy, Bethesda, MD*. American Society of Microbiology.

Clinical brochure (1985). Epirubicin (4'-epidoxorubicin). Adria Laboratories.

Collins, J.E. (1984). Pharmacologic rationale for regional drug delivery. *Journal of Clinical Oncology* **2**: 498–504.

Creaven, J.P. and Allen, L.M. (1975). PTG, a new antineoplastic epipodophyllotoxin. *Clinical Pharmacology and Therapeutics* **18**: 221–6.

Creaven, P.J., Madajewicz, S., Pendyala, L. *et al.* (1983). Phase I clinical trial of cis-dichloro-trans-dihydroxy-bis-isopropylamine platinum IV (CHIP). *Cancer Treatment Reports* **67**: 795–800.

Creekmore, S.P., Micetich, K.C., Vogelzang, N.J. *et al.* (1985). Low toxicity and significant tumor responses in phase II trials of carboplatin (CBDCA) in head and neck, non small cell lung, urothelial and ovarian cancers. *Proceedings of the American Society of Clinical Oncology* **4**: C562.

Creekmore, S.P., Waters, W.B., Vogelzang, N.J., Micetich, V.C. and Fisher, R.I. (1986). Antitumor activity of 24-hour CBDCA infusions in metastatic TCC *Proceedings of the American Society of Clinical Oncology* **5**: 101.

Cross, R.J., Glashan, R.W., Humphrey, C.S., Robinson, M.R.G., Smith, P.H. and Williams, R.E. (1976). Treatment of advanced bladder cancer with Adriamycin and 5-flurouracil. *British Journal of Urology* **48**: 609–615.

Crossley, R.J. (1984). Clinical safety and tolerance of mitoxantrone. *Seminars in Oncology* **11** (Suppl. 1): 54–8.

Curt, G.A., Grygiel, J.J., Corden, B.J. *et al.* (1983). A phase I and pharmacokinetic study of diamminecyclobutane dicarboxylato platinum (NSC 241,240). *Cancer Research* **43**: 4470–3.

Cvitkovic, E., Spaulding, J., Bethune, V. *et al.* (1977). Improvement of cis-dichlorodiammineplatinum (NSC-119875) therapeutic index in an animal mode. *Cancer* **39**: 1357–61.

Daley-Yates, P.T. and McBrien, D.C.H. (1982). The mechanism of renal clearance of cis-platin (cis-dichlorodiammineplatinum (II) and its modification by furosemide and probenecid. *Biochemical Pharmacology* **31**: 2243–6.

Daley-Yates, P.T. and McBrien, D.C.H. (1983). Cisplatin metabolites: a method for their separation and for measurement of their renal clearance *in vivo*. *Biochemical Pharmacology* **32**: 181–4.

Daley-Yates, P.T. and McBrien, D.C.H. (1984). Cisplatin metabolites in plasma: a study of their pharmacokinetics and importance in the nephrotoxic and antitumor activity of cisplatin. *Biochemical Pharmacology* **33**: 3063–70.

DeConti, R.C., Toftness, B.R., Lange, R.C. *et al.* (1973). Clinical and pharmacological studies with cis-diamminedichloroplatinum (II). *Cancer Research* **33**: 1310–15.

Dedon, P.C. and Borch, R.F. (1984). Diethyldithiocarbamate (DDTC) reversal of cisplatin (DDP) nephrotoxicity. *Proceedings of the American Association for Cancer Research* **25**: 1470.

de Kernion, J.B. (1977). The chemotherapy of advanced bladder carcinoma. *Cancer Research* **37**: 2771–4.

Dentino, M., Luft, F.L., Yum, M.N. *et al.* (1978). Long-term effect of cis-diammine-dichloro platinum (CDDP) on renal function and structure in man. *Cancer* **41**: 2174–81.

D'Incalci, M., Farina, P., Sessa, C. *et al.* (1982). Pharmacokinetics of VP-16-213 given by different administration methods. *Cancer Chemotherapy and Pharmacology* **7**: 141–5.

DiSimone, P.A., Yancey, R.S., Coupal, J.J. *et al.* (1979). Effect of a forced diuresis on distribution and excretion (via urine and bile of ^{195m}platinum when given as ^{195m}platinum cis-dichlorodiammine platinum. *Cancer Treatment Reports* **63**: 951–60.

Dombernowsky, P. and Nissen, N.I. (1976). Combination chemotherapy with 4'-demethylepipodophyllotoxin   9-(4,6-0-ethylene-B-D-glucopyranoside), VP-16-213 (NSC 141540) in L-1210 leukemia. *European Journal of Cancer* **12**: 181–8.

Donehower, R.C., Graham, M.L., Thompson, G.E. *et al.* (1985). Phase I and pharmacokinetic study of trimetrexate (TMTX) in patients with advanced cancer. *Proceedings of the American Society of Clinical Oncology* **4**: 32.

Doroshow, J.H. (1983). Comparative cardiac oxygen radical production by anthracycline antibiotics, mitoxantrone, bisantrene, m-AM5A and neocarzinostatin. *Clinical Research* **31**: 67 (abstract).

Drewinko, B., Brown, B.W. and Gottlieb, J.A. (1973). The effect of cis-diammine-dichloroplatinum (II) on cultured human lymphoma cells and its therapeutic implications. *Cancer Research* **33**: 3091–5.

Drobnick, J. and Horacek, P. (1973). Specific biological activity of platinum complexes. Contribution to the theory of molecular mechanism. *Chemical and Biological Interactions* **7**: 223–9.

Durr, F.E., Wallace, R.E. and Citarella, R.V. (1983). Molecular and biochemical pharmacology of mitoxantrone. *Cancer Treatment Reviews* **10** (Suppl. B): 3–11.

Early, K., Elias, E.G., Mittelson, A., Albert, A. and Murphy, G.P. (1973). Mitomycin C in the treatment of metastatic transitional cell carcinoma of the bladder. *Cancer* **31**: 1150–3.

Egorin, M.J., Van Echo, D.A., Tipping, S.J. *et al.* (1984). Pharmacokinetics and dosage reduction of cis-diammine-1,1-cyclobutane-dicharboxylatoplatinum in patients with impaired renal function. *Cancer Research* **44**: 5432–8.

Egorin, M.J., Van Echo, D.A., Whitacre, M.Y. *et al.* (1983). Phase I study and clinical pharmacokinetics of carboplatin (CBDCA) (NSC 241 240). *Proceedings of the American Society of Clinical Oncology* **2**: C109.

Elslager, E.F., Johnson, J.L. and Werbel, L.M. (1983). Folate antagonists 20: synthesis, antitumor and antimalarial properties of trimetrexate and related 6-[[(phenyl) amino]-methyl]-2,4-quinazolinediamines. *Journal of Medicinal Chemistry* **26**: 1753–60.

EORTC (1977). The treatment of advanced carcinoma of the bladder with a combination of Adriamycin and 5-FU. *European Urology* **3**: 276–8.

Evans, B.D., Raju, K.S., Calvert, A.H. *et al.* (1983). Phase II study of JM-8, a new platinum analog, in advanced carcinoma. *Cancer Treatment Reports* **67**: 997–1000.

Evans, W.E., Sinkule, J.A., Crom, W.R. *et al.* (1982). Pharmacokinetics of teniposide (VM-26) and etoposide (VP-16-213) in children with cancer. *Cancer Chemotherapy and Pharmacology* **7**: 147–50.

Fanucchi, M., Fleischer, M., Vidal, P. *et al.* (1985). Phase I and pharmacologic study of trimetrexate (TMTX). *Proceedings of the American Association for Cancer Research* **26**: 179.

Fernbach, B., Takahashi, I., Ohmuma, T. *et al.* (1979). Clinical and laboratory reevaluation of dichloromethotrexate. *Recent Results in Cancer Research* **74**: 56–64.

Ferrari, L., Rossi, A., Brambilla, C. *et al.* (1984). Phase I study with 4′ deoxydoxorubicin. *Investigational New Drugs* **2**: 287–95.

Feun, L.G., Wallace, S., Steward, D.J. *et al.* (1984). Intercarotid infusion of cis-diamminedichloroplatinum in the treatment of recurrent malignant brain tumors. *Cancer* **54**: 794–9.

Fitzharris, B.M., Kaye, S.B., Saverymuttu, S. *et al.* (1980). VP-16-213 as a single agent in advanced testicular tumors. *European Journal of Cancer* **16**: 1193–7.

Fox, M. (1965). The effect of cyclophosphamide on some urinary tract tumors. *British Journal of Urology* **37**: 399–403.

Fraval, H.N.A. and Roberts, J.J. (1979). Excision repair of cis-diammine dichloroplatinum(II)-induced damage to DNA of chinese hamster cells. *Cancer Research* **39**: 1793–7.

Frei, E., Spurr, C.L., Brindley, C.O. *et al.* (1965). Clinical studies of dichloromethotrexate (NSC 29630). *Clinical Pharmacology and Therapeutics* **6**: 160–71.

Frustaci, S., Tumolo, S., Veronesi, A. *et al.* (1984). Intra-arterial cisplatin (IA-CDDP) in head and neck cancer. *Proceedings of the American Society of Clinical Oncology* **3**: C697.

Gagen, M., Gochnour, D., Young, D. *et al.* (1984). A randomized trial of metoclopramide and a combination of dexamethasone and lorazepam for prevention of chemotherapy-induced vomiting. *Journal of Clinical Oncology* **2**: 696–701.

Gagliano, R. (1980). Adriamycin versus Adriamycin plus cisplatin in transitional cell bladder carcinoma: a SWOG study. *Proceedings of the American Society of Clinical Oncology* **21**: 347.

Gagliano, R.G., Stephens, R.L., Costanzi, J.J., Oishi, N., Stuckey, W.J., Grozea, P.N., Frank, J. and Crawford, E.D. (1984). Randomized trial of hexamethylmelamine versus 5-FU, doxorubicin, and cyclophosphamide (FAC) in advanced transitional cell bladder carcinoma: a Southwest Oncology Group study. *Cancer Treatment Reports* **68**: 1025–6.

Gams, R.A., Keller, J., Case, D.J. *et al.* (1985). Novantrone in malignant lymphoma. In *The Current Status of Novantrone*, pp. 75–8. John Wiley, New York.

Garcia-Giralt, E., Auvert, J., Lachand, A.T. *et al.* (1981). Combined chemotherapy in the management of metastatic bladder cancer. *British Journal of Urology* **53**: 318–19.

Ginsberg, S.J., Lee, F., Issell, B. *et al.* (1983). A phase I study of cis-dichloro-trans-dihydroxy-bis (isopropylamine)-platinum IV (CHIP) administered by intravenous bolus daily for 5 days. *Proceedings of the American Society for Clinical Oncology* **2**: C139.

Giuliani, F.C., Coirin, A.K., Rene Rice, M. and Kaplan, N.O. (1981) The effect of 4'-epi-doxorubicin analogues on heterotransplantation of human tumors in congenitally athymic mice. *Cancer Treatment Reports* **65**: 1063–75.

Giuliani, F.C. and Kaplan, N.O. (1980). New doxorubisin analogs active against doxorubicin-resistant colon tumor xenografts in the nude mouse. *Cancer Research* **40**: 4682–7.

Glover, D., Glick, J.H., Weiler, C. *et al.* (1984). Phase I trials of WR-2721 and cis-platinum. *Proceedings of the American Association for Cancer Research* **25**: 720.

Goldin, A., Humphreys, S.R., Venditti, J.M. *et al.* (1959). Prolongation of the lifespan of mice with advanced leukemia (L1210) by treatment with halogenated derivatives of amethopterin. *Journal of National Cancer Institute* **22**: 811–23.

Golomb, H.M., Ratain, M.J. and Vardiman, J.W. (1986). Sequential treatment of hairy cell leukemia: a new role for interferon. In *Important Advances in Oncology 1986*, pp. 311–21. Edited by DeVita, V.T. Lippincott, Philadelphia.

Gonzalez-Vitale, J.C., Hayes, D.M., Cvitkovic, E. *et al.* (1977). The renal pathology in clinical trials of cis-platinum (II) diamminedichloride. *Cancer* **39**: 1362–71.

Gormley, P.E., Bull, J.M., LeRoy, A.F. *et al.* (1979). Kinetics of cis-dichlorodiammine-platinum. *Clinical Pharmacology and Therapeutics* **25**: 351–7.

Gullo, J.J., Litterst, C.L., Maguire, P.J. *et al.* (1980). Pharmacokinetics and protein binding of cis-dichlorodiammine platinum (II) administered as a one hour or as a twenty hour infusion. *Cancer Chemotherapy and Pharmacology* **5**: 21–6.

Hadley, D. and Herr, H.W. (1979). Peripheral neuropathy associated with cis-dichlorodiammineplatinum (II) treatment. *Cancer* **44**: 2026–8.

Hande, K.R., Wedlund, P.J., Noone, R.M. *et al.* (1984). Pharmacokinetics of high-dose etoposide (VP-16-213) administered to cancer patients. *Cancer Research* **44**: 379–82.

Harker, W.G., Meyers, F.J., Freiha, F.S. *et al.* (1985). Cisplatin, methotrexate, and vinblastine (CMV): an effective chemotherapy regimen for metastatic transitional cell carcinoma of the urinary tract: a Northern California Oncology Group study. *Journal of Clinical Oncology* **3**: 1463–70.

Harland, S.J., Newell, D.R., Siddik, Z.H. *et al.* (1984). Pharmacokinetics of cis-diammine-1,1-cyclobutane dicarboxylate platinum (II) in patients with normal and impaired renal function. *Cancer Research* **44**: 1693–7.

Hayes, D.M., Cvitkovic, E., Golbey, R.B. *et al.* (1977). High dose cisplatinum diamminedichloride: amelioration of renal toxicity by mannitol diuresis. *Cancer* **39**: 1372–81.

Hayes, F.A., Green, A., Thompson, E. *et al.* (1983). Phase II trial of VP-16-213 in pediatric solid tumors. *Proceedings of the American Association for Cancer Research* **2**: 66.

Henry, D.W. (1979). Structure activity relationships among daunorubicin and Adriamycin analogs. *Cancer Treatment Reports* **63**: 845–54.

Higby, D.J., Wallace, H.J., Albert, D.J. *et al.* (1974). Diammine dichloroplatinum: a phase I study showing responses in testicular and other tumors. *Cancer* **33**: 1219–25.

Higby, D.J., Wallace, H.J. and Holland, J.F. (1973). Cis-diammine dichloroplatinum (NSC-119875): a phase I study. *Cancer Chemotherapy Reports* **57**: 459–63.

Hillcoat, B.L. and Raghavan, D. (1986). A randomised comparison of cisplatinum (C) versus cisplatinum and methotrexate (C+M) in advanced bladder cancer. *Proceedings of the American Society of Clinical Oncology* **5**: 110.

Himmelstein, K.J., Patton, T.F., Belt, R.J. *et al.* (1981). Clinical kinetics of intact cisplatin and some related species. *Clinical Pharmacology and Therapeutics* **29**: 658–64.

Hrushesky, W.J.M. (1984). Circadian chromopharmacokinetics and chronotoxicology of doxorubicin and cisplatin in human beings with cancer. In *Annual Review of Chronopharmacology.* Edited by Reinberg, A., Smolensky, M. and Labreque, G. Pergamon Press, Oxford.

Hurd, D.D., Peterson, B.A., McKenna, R.W., Bloomfield, C.D. (1981). VP 16-213 and cyclophosphamide in the treatment of refractory acute nonlymphocytic leukemia with monocytic features. *Medical and Pediatric Oncology* **9**: 251–5.

Ikic, D., Maricic, Z., Dresic, V. *et al.* (1981). Application of leukocyte interferon in patients with urinary bladder papiliomatosis, breast cancer and melanoma. *Lancet* **1**: 1022–4.

Italia, C., Broginni, M., Colombo, T. *et al.* (1983). Comparative studies of the metabolism of 4-demethocydaunorubicin and daunoribicin and its contribution to the determination of cytotoxicity. In *Fourth NCI-EORTC Symposium on New Drugs in Cancer Therapy*, 14–17 December, p. 105 (abstract).

Iwatmoto, Y., Kawano, T. and Uozumi, J. (1984). 'Two-route chemotherapy' using high-dose i.p. cisplatin and i.v. sodium thiosulfate, it's antidote, for peritoneally disseminated cancer in mice. *Cancer Treatment Reports* **68**: 1367–73.

Jacobs, C., Bertino, J.R. and Goffinet, D.R. (1978). 24-hour infusion of cisplatin in head and neck cancers. *Cancer* **42**: 2135–40.

Jaffe, N., Bowman, R., Wang, Y. *et al.* (1984). Chemotherapy for primary osteosarcoma by intra-arterial infusion. *Cancer Bulletin* **36**: 37–42.

Juckett, D.A., Parham, D.M., Schonbaum, G.R. *et al.* (1984). A new treatment for prevention of cisplatin nephrotoxicity: adjunct therapy using polar dithiocarbamates. *Proceedings of the American Association for Cancer Research* **25**: 1274.

Kamen, B.A., Eibl, B., Cashmore, A. and Bertino, J. (1984). Uptake and efficacy of trimetrexate (TMQ, 2,4-diamino-5-methyl-6-[(3,4,5 trimethoxyanilino)methyl] quinazoline) a non-classical antifolate in methotrexate-resistant leukemia cells *in vitro. Biochemical Pharmacology* **33**: 1697–9.

Kaplan, S., Joss, R., Sessa, C. *et al.* (1983). Phase I trials of cis-diammine-1,1-cyclobutanedicarboxylate platinum (II) (CBDCA) in solid tumors. *Proceedings of the American Association for Cancer Research* **24**: 520.

Kaplan, S., Martini, A., Varini, M. *et al.* (1984a). Phase I trial of 4-demethoxydaunorubicin with single i.v. doses. *European Journal of Cancer and Clinical Oncology* **18**: 1303–6.

Kaplan, S., Sessa, C., Willens, Y. *et al.* (1984b). Phase I trial of 4-demethoxydaunorubicin (idarubicin) with single oral doses. *Investigational New Drugs* **2**: 281–6.

Kapp, J.P. and Vance, R.B. (1984). Supraophthalmic arterial infusion of cisplatinum and BCNU for recurrent malignant glioma. *Proceedings of the American Society of Clinical Oncology* **3**: C710.

Kedia, K.R. (1983). Role of systemic therapy in metastatic bladder carcinoma. In *78th Annual American Urology Association Meeting 1983*, p. 179. American Urological Association Inc.

Kedia, K.R., Gibbons, C. and Persky, L. (1981). The management of advanced bladder carcinoma. *Journal of Urology* **125**: 655–8.

Kelsen, D., Sternberg, C., Einzig, A. *et al.* (1984). Phase II study of carboplatin

(CBDCA) in advanced upper gastrointestinal tract (UGIT) malignancy. *Proceedings of the American Society of Clinical Oncology* **3**: C552.

Kessel, D. and Hall, T.C. (1967). Amethopterin transport in Ehrlich ascites carcinoma dn L1210 cells. *Cancer Research* **27**: 1539–43.

Khan, A.B., D'Souza, B.J., Wharam, M.D. *et al.* (1982). Cisplatin therapy in recurrent childhood brain tumors. *Cancer Treatment Reports* **66**: 2013–20.

Khandekar, J.D., Elson, P.J., DeWys, W.D., Slayton, R.E. and Harris, D.T. (1985). Comparative activity and toxicity of cis-diamminedichloroplatinum (DDP) and a combination of doxorubicin cyclophosphamide and DDP in disseminated transitional cell carcinoma of the urinary tract. *Journal of Clinical Oncology* **3**: 539–45.

Kharasch, E.D. and Novak, R.F. (1982). Inhibition of Adriamycin stimulated microsomal lipid peroxidation by mitoxantrone and ametantrone, two new anthracenedion antineoplastic agents. *Biochemica Biophys Research Committee* **108**: 1346–52.

Kirkwood, J.M. and Ernstoff, M.S. (1984). Interferons in the treatment of human cancers. *Journal of Clinical Oncology* **2**: 336–52.

Knight, E.W., Pagand, M., Hahn, R.G. and Horton, J. (1983). Comparison of 5-FU and doxorubicin in the treatment of carcinoma of the bladder. *Cancer Treatment Reports* **67**: 514–15.

Kociba, R.J. and Sleight, S.D. (1971). Acute toxicologic and pathologic effects of cis-diamminedichloroplatinum (NSC-119875) in the male rat. *Cancer Chemotherapy Reports* **55**: 1–8.

Koeller, J.M., Earhart, R.H., Davis, T.E. *et al.* (1983). Phase I trial of carboplatin (NSC 241 240) by bolus intravenous injection. *Proceedings of the American Association for Cancer Research* **24**: 643.

Kriesman, H., Ginsberg, S., Feldstein, M. *et al.* (1985). Iproplatin (CHIP) or carboplatin (CBDCA) in extensive non-small cell lung cancer. *Proceedings of the American Society of Clinical Oncology* **4**: C725.

Lamm, D.L. (1985). BCG versus adriamycin in bladder cancer: a Southern Oncology Group study. *Proceedings of the American Society of Clinical Oncology* **4**: 109.

Lee, F.H., Canetta, R., Issell, B.F. *et al.* (1983). New platinum complexes in clinical trials. *Cancer Treatment Reviews* **10**: 39–51.

Legha, S., Tenney, D., Ho, D.H. and Krakoff, I. (1985). Phase I clinical and pharmacology study of trimetrexate (TMQ). *Proceedings of the American Society of Clinical Oncology* **4**: 48.

Lehane, D.E., Bryan, R.N., Horowitz, B. *et al.* (1983). Intra-arterial displatinum chemotherapy for patients with primary and metastatic brain tumors. *Cancer Drug Delivery* **1**: 69–77.

Leonard, B.J., Eccleston, E. *et al.* (1971). Antileukemic and nephrotoxic properties of platinum compounds. *Nature* **234**: 43–5.

LeRoy, A.F. (1979). Some quantitative data on cis-dichlorodiammineplatinum (II) species in solution. *Cancer Treatment Reports* **63**: 231–3.

LeRoy, A.F., Lutz, R.J., Dedrick, R.L. *et al.* (1979). Pharmacokinetic study of cis-dichlorodiammineplatinum (II) (DDP) in the beagle dog: thermodynamic and kinetic behavior of DDP in a biologic milieu. *Cancer Treatment Reports* **63**: 59–71.

LeRoy, A.F., Wehling, M.L., Sponseller, H.L. *et al.* (1977). Analysis of platinum in biological materials by flameless atomic absorption spectrophotometry. *Biochemical Medicine* **18**: 184–91.

Levi, F., Hrushesky, W.J.M., Borch, R.F. *et al.* (1982). Cisplatin urinary pharmacokinetics and nephrotoxicity: a common circadian mechanism. *Cancer Treatment Reports* **66**: 1933–8.

Levin, M., Pandya, K.J., Khandekar, J.D. *et al.* (1984). Phase II study of mitoxantrone in advanced breast cancer: an Eastern Cooperative Oncology Group pilot study. *Cancer Treatment Reports* **68**: 1511–14.

Leyvraz, S., Ohnuma, T., Lassus, M. and Holland, J.F. (1985). Phase I study of carboplatin in patients with advanced cancer, intermittent intravenous bolus and 24-hour infusion. *Journal of Clinical Oncology* **3**: 1385–92.

Lin, J., Ernstoff, M., Cashmore, A. *et al.* (1985). A phase I study of trimetrexate. *Proceedings of the American Society of Clinical Oncology* **4**: 31.

Litterst, C.L., Gram, T.E., Dedrick, R.L. *et al.* (1976). Distribution and disposition of platinum following intravenous administration of cis-diamminedichloroplatinum II (NSC-119875) to dogs. *Cancer Research* **36**: 2340–4.

Loehrer, P.J. and Einhorn, L.H. (1984). Cisplatin. *Annals of Internal Medicine* **100**: 704–13.

Logothetis, C.J., Samuels, M.L., Ogden, S. *et al.* (1985). Cyclophosphamide, doxorubicin and cisplatin chemotherapy for patients with locally advanced urothelial tumors with or without nodal metastases. *Journal of Urology* **134**: 460–4.

Loh, S.H., Choi, K., Aziz, H. *et al.* (1985). Cis-platinum by continuous infusion with concomitant radiation effective in the therapy of primary advanced squamous cell carcinoma of the lung. *Proceedings of the American Society of Clinical Oncology* **4**: C741.

Loike, J.D., Brewer, C.F., Sternlicht, H. *et al.* (1978). Structure–activity study of the inhibition of microtubule assembly *in vitro* by podophyllotoxin and its congeners. *Cancer Research* **38**: 2688–93.

Loike, J.D. and Horwitz, S.B. (1976). Effect of VP-16-213 on the intracellular degradation of DNA in HeLa cells. *Biochemistry* **15**: 5443–8.

Lokich, J.J. (1980). Phase I study of cis-diamminedichloroplatinum (II) administered as a constant 5-day infusion. *Cancer Treatment Reports* **64**: 905–8.

Lokich, J.J. and Becker, B. (1983). Subclavian vein thrombosis in patients treated with infusion chemotherapy for advanced malignancy. *Cancer* **52**: 1586–9.

Lokich, J.J. and Zipoli, T.E. (1984). Phase I study of protracted infusion of cisplatin. *Cancer Drug Delivery* **1**: 247–50.

Long, B.H., Musial, S.T. and Brattain, M.G. (1985). Single- and double-strand DNA breakage and repair in human lung adenocarcinoma cells exposed to etoposide and teniposide. *Cancer Research* **45**: 3106–12.

Look, A.T., Dahl, G.C., Kalwinsky, D. *et al.* (1981). Effective remission induction of refractory childhood acute nonlymphocytic leukemia by VP-16-213 plus azacytidine. *Cancer Treatment Reports* **65**: 995–9.

Martino, S., Samal, B. and Al-Sarraf, M. (1980). Phase II study of 5-fluorouracil and Adriamycin in transitional cell carcinoma of the urinary tract. *Cancer Treatment Reports* **64**: 161–3.

Mathé, G., Schwarzenberg, L., Pouillart, P. *et al.* (1974). Epipodophyllotoxin derivatives, VM 26 and VP 16213, in the treatment of leukemias, hematosarcomas and lymphomas. *Cancer* **34**: 985.

Mechl, Z., Rovny, F. and Sopkova, B. (1977). VM-26 (4 demethyl-epipodophyllotoxin-B-d-thenylidine glucoside) in the treatment of urinary bladder tumors. *Neoplasma* **24**: 411–14.

Merrin, C. (1975). Treatment of advanced bladder cancer with cisdiammine dichloro platinum (II) (NSC 119875): a pilot study. *Journal of Urology* **114**: 884–7.

Merrin, C. (1976). A new method to prevent toxicity with high doses of cis-diammine platinum (therapeutic efficacy in previously treated widespread and recurrent testicular tumors). *Proceedings of the American Society of Clinical Oncology* **7**: 243.

Merrin, C., Cartegena, R., Wajsman, Z., Baumgartner, C. and Murphy, G.P. (1975). Chemotherapy of bladder cancer with cytoxan and Adriamycin. *Journal of Urology* **114**: 884–7.

Micetich, K.C., Barnes, D. and Erickson, L.C. (1985). A comparative study of cytotoxicity and DNA damaging effects of cis-(diammine) (1,1-cyclobutane dicarboxylato)platinum II and cis-diammainedichloro platinum II on L1210 cells. *Cancer Research* **45**: 4043–7.

Mills, R.C., Maurer, L.H., Forcier, R.J., Grace, W.R., Burke, G.P., Karp, D.O., Smith, R.L., McIntyre, O.R. and Bean, C. (1977). Clinical trial of combined therapy with Adriamycin and cis-dichlorodiammineplatinum (II). *Cancer Treatment Reports* **61**: 477–9.

Mollman, J.E., Glover, D.J., Hogan, W.M. *et al.* (1985). Cis-platin neuropathy: a possible protective agent. *Proceedings of the American Society of Clinical Oncology* **4**: C127.

Mortimer, J., Cummings, C., Laramore, G. *et al.* (1985). Selective intra-arterial (IA) cisplatin for localized (Stage 3 and 4) unresectable head and neck cancer. *Proceedings of the American Society of Clinical Oncology* **4**: C577.

Mulder, J.H., Fossa, S.D., DePauw, M. and Van Oosterom, A.T. (1982). Cyclophosphamide, Adriamycin and cisplatin combination chemotherapy in advanced bladder carcinoma: an EORTC phase II study. *European Journal of Cancer and Clinical Oncology* **18**: 111–12.

Natale, R.B., Wheeler, R.N., Ensminger, W. and Miller, D. (1983). Cisplatin and dichloromethotrexate (DCM): a pharmacologically rational combination with high activity. *Proceedings of the American Association for Cancer Research* **24**: 166.

Natale, R.B., Yagoda, A., Watson, R.C. *et al.* (1980). Phase II trial of neocarcinostatin in patients with bladder and prostatic cancer: toxicity of a 5-day i.v. bolus schedule. *Cancer* **45**: 2836–42.

Natale, R.B., Yagoda, A., Watson, R.C., Whitmore, W.F., Blumenreich, M. and Brain, D.W. (1981). Methotrexate: an active drug in bladder cancer. *Cancer* **47**: 1246–50.

NCI memorandum, 8 November 1985.

Nelson, J.A., Santos, G. and Herbert, B.H. (1984). Mechanisms for the renal excretion of cisplatin. *Cancer Treatment Reports* **68**: 849–53.

Nissen, N.I., Pajak, T.F., Leone, L.A. *et al.* (1980). Clinical trial of VP-16 (NSC 141540) i.v. twice weekly in advanced neoplastic disease. *Cancer* **45**: 232–5.

O'Dwyer, P.J., Alonso, M.T., Leyland-Jones, B. and Marsoni, S. (1984). Teniposide: a review of 12 years of experience. *Cancer Treatment Reports* **68**: 1455–66.

Ohnuma, T., Leyvraz, S., Coffey, C. *et al.* (1984). Carboplatin: activity in patients with head and neck (H&N), renal cell (RC) and ovarian carcinomas. *Proceedings of the American Association for Cancer Research* **25**: 710.

Osborne, C.K., VonHoff, D.D., Cowan, J.D. and Sandbach, J. (1984). Bisantrene, an active drug in patients with advanced breast cancer. *Cancer Treatment Reports* **68**: 357–60.

Osterlind, K., Hansen, H.H., Dombernowsky, P. *et al.* (1982). Combination chemotherapy of small cell lung cancer (SCC) based on *in vivo* cell cycle analysis. *Proceedings of the American Association for Cancer Research* **23**: 154 (abstract).

Ozols, R.F., Ostchega, Y., Curt, G. *et al.* (1985). High dose cisplatin and high dose carboplatinum in refractory ovarian cancer: salvage drugs with different toxicities. *Proceedings of the American Society of Clinical Oncology* **4**: C462.

Papadopoulos, N.E.J., Tenney, D.M., Chawla, S. *et al.* (1985). Phase II study of bisantrene in malignant melanoma. *Proceedings of the American Association for Cancer Research* **26**: 174.

Patton, T.F., Himmelstein, K.J., Belt, R. *et al.* (1978). Plasma levels and urinary excretion of filterable platinum species following bolus injection and i.v. infusion of cis-dichlorodiammineplatinum (II) in man. *Cancer Treatment Reports* **62**: 1359–62.

Pavone-Macaluso, M. (1971). Chemotherapy of vesical and prostatic tumors. *British Journal of Urology* **43**: 701–8.

Pendyala, L., Cowens, J.W., Creaven, P.J. *et al.* (1982a). Studies on the pharmacokinetics and metabolism of cis-dichloro-trans-dihydroxy-bis-isopropylamine platinum i.v. in the dog. *Cancer Treatment Reports* **66**: 509–16.

Pendyala, L., Cowens, J.W., Mittelman, A. *et al.* (1982b). Clinical pharmacokinetics of cis-dichloro-trans-dihydroxy-bis-isopropylamine platinum i.v. (CHIP): a new platinum drug in phase I trial. *Proceedings of the American Association for Cancer Research* **23**: 497.

Pera, M.F. and Harder, M.C. (1979). Effects of mannitol and furosemide diuresis on cis-dichlorodiammine platinum (II) antitumor activity and toxicity to host renewing cell populations in rats. *Cancer Research* **39**: 1279–86.

Pfeifle, E.C., Howell, S.B., Felthouse, R.D. *et al.* (1985). High-dose cisplatin with sodium thiosulfate protection. *Journal of Clinical Oncology* **3**: 237–44.

Pfister, M., Pavelic, Z., Bullard, G.A. *et al.* (1978). Dichloro-dihydroxy-bis-isopropylamine platinum i.v., a new antitumor platinum complex. Pharmacokinetics in the rat, relation to renal toxicity. *Biochimie* **60**: 1057–8.

Pinsky, C.M., Comacho, F.J., Kerr, D. *et al.* (1985). Intravesical administration of bacillus Calmette–Guerin in patients with recurrent superficial carcinoma of the urinary bladder: report of a prospective randomized trial. *Cancer Treatment Reports* **69**: 47–53.

Plooy, A.C.M., Van Dijk, M., Berends, F. and Lohman, P.H.M. (1985). Formation and repair of DNA interstrand cross-links in relation to cytotoxicity and unscheduled DNA synthesis induced in control and mutant human cells treated with cis-diamminedichloroplatinum (II). *Cancer Research* **45**: 4178–84.

Plumridge, T.W. and Brown J.R. (1978). Studies on the mode of interaction of 4'-epi-doxorubicin and 4-demethoxydaunomycin with DNA. *Biochemical Pharmacology* **27**: 1881–2.

Plumridge, T. and Brown, T.R. (1979). The interaction of Adriamycin and Adriamycin analogues with nucleic acids in the B and A conformations. *Biochimica Biophysica Acta* **563**: 181–92.

Ponder, B.A.J. and Oliver, R.T.D. (1984). Phase II study of VP 16-213 (etoposide) in metastatic transitional cell urothelial cancer. *Cancer Chemotherapy and Pharmacology* **12**: 64–5.

Poore, G.A., Todd, G.C. and Grindey, G.B. (1984). Effect of sodium thiosulfate (S_2O_3) on intravenous cisplatin (DDP) toxicity and antitumor activity. *Proceedings of the American Association for Cancer Research* **25**: 1466.

Posner, M.R., Bellieveau, J.F., Ferrari, L. *et al.* (1985). Clinical and pharmacokinetic study of 5-day continuous infusion cis-platinum. *Proceedings of the American Society of Clinical Oncology* **4**: C145.

Postmus, P.E., Mulder, N.H., Sleijfer, D.T. *et al.* (1984). High-dose etoposide for refractory malignancies: a phase I study. *Cancer Treatment Reports* **68**: 1471–4.

Price, L.A. and Goldie, J.H. (1971). Multiple drug therapy for disseminated malignant tumors. *British Medical Journal* **4**: 336–9.

Priego, V., Luc, V., Bonnem, E. *et al.* (1983). A phase I study and pharmacology of diammine (1,1) cyclobutane dicarboxylato (2-1-0) platinum (CDBCA) administered on a weekly schedule. *Proceedings of the American Society of Clinical Oncology* **2**: C117.

Qazi, R., Elson, P. and Khandekar, J.D. (1982). Phase II evaluation of VM-26 in patients with metastatic transitional cell carcinoma of the urinary tract: an Eastern Cooperative Oncology Group study. *Cancer Treatment Reports* **66**: 405–6.

Reddel, R.R., Kefford, R.F., Grant, J.M. *et al.* (1982). Ototoxicity in patients receiving cisplatin: importance of dose and method of drug administration. *Cancer Treatment Reports* **66**: 19–23.

Richardson, R.L., Hahn, R.G., Kvols, L.K. *et al.* (1985). Bleomycin, etoposide and continuous-infusion cisplatin in metastatic testicular cancer. *Proceedings of the American Association for Cancer Research* **4**: C410.

Roberts, D., Hilliard, S. and Peck, C. (1980). Sedimentation of DNA from L1210 cells after treatment with 4'-demethylepidophyllotoxin 9-(4,6-0-ethylidene-B-D-glucopyranoside) or 1-B-D-arabinofuranosylcytosine or both drugs. *Cancer Research* **40**: 4225–31.

Roemeling, R., Wick, M., Berestka, J. *et al.* (1985). Disulfiram and cisplatin chronotherapy allows safe and effective megadose therapy. *Proceedings of the American Association for Cancer Research* **26**: 1038.

Rosenberg, B. (1979). Anticancer activity of cis-dichlorodiammine platinum-(II) and some relevant chemistry. *Cancer Treatment Reports* **63**: 1433–8.

Rosenberg, B., Van Camp, L. and Krigas, T. (1965). Inhibition of cell division in *E. coli* by electrolysis products from a platinum electrode. *Nature* **205**: 698–9.

Rosenberg, B., Van Camp, L., Trosko, J.E. *et al.* (1969). Platinum compounds: a new class of potent antitumor agents. *Nature* **222**: 385–6.

Rosencweig, M., Nicaise, C., Beer, M. *et al.* (1983). Phase I study of carboplatin given on a five-day intravenous schedule. *Journal of Clinical Oncology* **1**: 621–6.

Rosencweig, M., VonHoff, D.D., Henney, J.E. and Muggia, F.M. (1977). VM26 and VP-16-213: a comparative analysis. *Cancer* **40**: 334–42.

Ross, W., Rowe, T., Glisson, B. *et al.* (1984). Role of topoisomerose II in mediating epipodophyllotoxin-induced DNA cleavage. *Cancer Research* **44**: 5857–60.

Rossof, A.H., Slayton, R.E. and Perlia, C.P. (1972). Preliminary clinical experience with cis-diamminedichloroplatinum(II) (NSC-119875), (CAP). *Cancer* **30**: 1451–6.

Rossof, A.H., Talley, R.W., Stephens, R., Thigpen, T., Samson, M.K., Groppe, C., Eyre, H.J. and Fisher, R. (1979). Phase II evaluation of cis-dichlorodiammineplatinum II in advanced malignancies of the genitourinary and gynecologic organs: a Southwest Oncology Group study. *Cancer Treatment Reports* **63**: 1557–64.

Russell, P.J., Raghavan, D., Gregory, P. *et al.* (1986). Bladder cancer xenografts: a model of tumor cell heterogeneity. *Cancer Research* **46**: 2035–40.

Sakamoto, S., Ogata, J., Ikegami, K. *et al.* (1980). Chemotherapy for bladder cancer with neocarzinostatin: evaluation of systemic administration. *European Journal of Cancer* **16**: 103–4.

Salem, P., Hall, S.W., Benjamin, R.S. *et al.* (1978). Clinical phase I–II study of cis-dichlorodiammine platinum II given by continuous i.v. infusion. *Cancer Treatment Reports* **62**: 1553–5.

Salem, P., Khalyl, M., Jabboury, K. *et al.* (1984). Cis-diammine-dichloroplatinum (II) by 5-day continuous infusion: a new dose schedule with minimal toxicity. *Cancer* **53**: 837–40.

Samuels, M.L., Logothetis, C., Trindade, A. and Johnson, P.E. (1980). Cytoxan, Adriamycin and cisplatinum (CISCA) in metastatic bladder cancer. *Proceedings of the American Association for Cancer Research* **21**: 137.

Sand, J., Rosenthal, C.J., Rotman, M. *et al.* (1984). Lack of toxicity of cisplatin administered as a radiosensitizer by long term continuous infusion. *Proceedings of the American Society of Clinical Oncology* **3**: C172.

Sasaki, K., Murakami, T. and Fujimoto, T. (1985). Clinical pharmacokinetics of cis-platinum in children. *Proceedings of the American Association for Cancer Research* **26**: 641.

Sauter, C., Fehr, J., Frick, P. *et al.* (1982). Acute myelogenous leukemia successful treatment of relapse with cytosine arabinoside, VP 16-213, vincristine and vinblastine (A-Triple-V. *European Journal of Cancer and Clinical Oncology* **18**: 733–7.

Scalzo, A.J., Comis, R., Fitzpatrick, A. *et al.* (1982). VP-16 pharmacokinetics in adults with cancer as determined by a new high-pressure liquid chromatography (HPLC) assay. *Proceedings of the American Society of Clinical Oncology* **1**: 129.

Scanlon, K., Ohnuma, T., Lo, R.J. *et al.* (1982). Effects of 2,4-diamino-6-(2,5-dimethoxybenzyl)-5-methylpyrido (2,3-D) pyrimidine (BW 301U) on methotrexate (MTX)-resistant human acute lymphoblastic leukemia (ALL) cell lines. *Proceedings of the American Society of Clinical Oncology* **23**: 12.

Schabel, F.M., Corbett, T.H., Griswold, D.P. *et al.* (1983). Therapeutic activity of mitoxantrone and ametantrone against murine tumors. *Cancer Treatment Reviews* **10** (Suppl. B): 12–21.

Schilsky, R.L. and Anderson, T. (1979). Hypomagnesemia and renal magnesium wasting in patients receiving cisplatin. *Annals of Internal Medicine* **90**: 929–31.

Schilsky, R.L., Bailey, B.D. and Chabner, B.A. (1980). Methotrexate polyglutamate synthesis by cultured human breast cancer cells. *Proceedings of the National Academy of Sciences* (USA) **77**: 2919–22.

Schwartz, S., Yagoda, A., Natale, R.B. *et al.* (1983). Phase II trial of sequentially administered cisplatin cyclophosphamide and doxorubicin for urothelial tract tumors. *Journal of Urology* **130**: 681–4.

Scorticatti, C.N., LaPena, N.C., Bellora, O.G. *et al.* (1982). Systemic IFN-alpha treatment of multiple bladder papilloma grade I or II patients: pilot study. *Journal of Interferon Research* **2**: 339–43.

Sessa, C., Cavalli, F., Kaye, S. *et al.* (1985). Phase II study of cis-dichloro-trans-dihydroxy-bis-isopropylamine platinum IV (CHIP) in advanced ovarian carcinoma. *Proceedings of the American Society of Clinical Oncology* **4**: C452.

Siddik, Z.H., Newell, D.R., Jones, M. *et al.* (1982). Pharmacokinetics of cis-diammine-1,1-cyclobutanedicarboxylato platinum (II) (CBDCA, JM 8) in mice and rats. *Proceedings of the American Association for Cancer Research* **23**: 659.

Sigdestad, C.P., Gardina, D.J., Peters, L.F. *et al.* (1979). Cell cycle phase preferential killing of fibrosarcoma tumor cells by cis-DDP or Adriamycin. *Proceedings of the American Association for Cancer Research* **20**: 1278.

Silverberg, E. (1985). Cancer statistics, 1985. *CA* **35**: 19–35.

Skinner, D.G. (1980). Current perspectives in the management of high grade invasive bladder cancer. *Cancer* **45**: 1866–74.

Smith, I.E. (1983). Mitoxantrone (novantrone): a review of experimental and early clinical studies. *Cancer Treatment Reviews* **10**: 103–15.

Smith, I.E., Evans, B.D. and Weston, C. (1985). Carboplatin (JM8) as a single agent and in combination in the treatment of small cell lung carcinoma. *Cancer Treatment Reviews* **12** (Suppl. A): 73–5.

Smith, I.E., Gerken, M.E., Clink, H.M. and McElwain, T.J. (1976). VP-16-213 in acute myelogenous leukemia. *Postgraduate Medical Journal* **52**: 66–70.

Smyth, J.F., Cornbleet, M.A., Stuart-Harris, R.C. *et al.* (1984). Mitoxantrone as first-line-chemotherapy for advanced breast cancer: results of a European collaborative study. *Seminars in Oncology* **11**: 15–18.

Soloway, M.S., Einstein, A., Corder, M.P., Bonney, W., Prout, G.R. and Coombs, J. (1981a). A comparison of cisplatin and the combination of cisplatin and cyclophosphamide in advanced urothelial cancer: a National Bladder Cancer Collaborative Group A study. *Cancer* **52**: 767–72.

Soloway, M.S., Jicard, M. and Ford, K. (1981b). Cis-diammine-dichloroplatinum II in locally advanced and metastatic cancer. *Cancer* **47**: 476–80.

Spiegel, R.J., Blum, R.H., Levin, M. *et al.* (1982). Phase I study of 9,10-anthracene dicarboxaldehyde (Bisantrene) administered on a five-day schedule. *Cancer Research* **42**: 354–8.

Stahelin, H. (1973). Activity of a new glycosidic lignan derivative (VP-16-213) related to podophyllotoxin in experimental tumors. *European Journal of Cancer* **9**: 213–21.

Stanton, G.F., Raymond, V. Wittes, R.E. *et al.* (1985). Phase I and clinical pharmacological evaluation of 4'-deoxydoxorubicin in patients with advanced cancer. *Cancer Research* **45**: 1862–8.

Sternberg, C.N., Yagoda, A., Scher, H.I., Watson, R.C. *et al.* (1985). Preliminary results of M-VAC (methotrexate, vinblastine, doxorubicin and cisplatin) for transitional cell carcinoma of the urothelium. *Journal of Urology* **133**: 403–7.

Sternberg, J., Bracken, R., Hundel, P. *et al.* (1977). Combination chemotherapy (CISCA) for advanced urinary tract carcinoma: a preliminary report. *JAMA* **238**: 2282–7.

Stewart, D.J., Benjamin, R.S., Zimmerman, S. *et al.* (1983). Clinical pharmacology of intra-arterial cis-diammendichloroplatinum (II). *Cancer Research* **43**: 917–20.

Stewart, D.J., Mikhael, N., Nanji, S. *et al.* (1985). Human tissue cisplatin pharmacology: clinical implications. *Proceedings of the American Association for Cancer Research* **26**: 608.

Stewart, J.A., McCormack, J.J., Tong, W. *et al.* (1985). A phase I study of trimetrexate. *Proceedings of the American Association for Cancer Research* **26**: 159.

Talley, R.W., O'Bryan, R.M., Gutterman, J.U. *et al.* (1973). Clinical evaluation of toxic effects of cis-diammine dichloroplatinum (NSC-119875): a phase I clinical study. *Cancer Chemotherapy Reports* **57**: 465–71.

Tamassia, V., Goldaniga, E., Moro, M.A. *et al.* (1985). Human pharmacokinetic studies on three new anthracyclines: epirubicin, idarubicin, esorubicin. In *Fourth NCI-EORTC Symposium on New Drugs in Cancer Therapy*, 14–17 December 1983: 16 (abstract).

Tan, C., Etcubanas, E., Wollner, N., Rosen, G., Gilladoga, A., Showel, J., Murphy, M.L. and Krakoff, I.H. (1973). Adriamycin—an antitumor antibiotic in the treatment of neoplastic disease. *Cancer* **32**: 9–17.

Tannock, I.F., Gospodarowicz, M. and Evans, W.K. (1983). Chemotherapy for metastatic transitional carcinoma of the urinary tract: a prospective trial of methotrexate, Adriamycin and cyclophosphamide (MAC) with cis-platinum for failure. *Cancer* **51**: 216–19.

Tauer, K., Bosl, G.J., Golbey, R.B. *et al.* (1985). A phase II trial of cis-diammine-1,1-cyclobutane dicarboxylate platinum II in patients with cis-platin-resistant germ cell tumors. *Proceedings of the American Society of Clinical Oncology* **4**: C406.

Taylor, R.E., McElwain, T.J., Barrett, A. and Peckham, M.J. (1982). Etoposide as a single agent in relapsed advanced lymphomas: a phase II study. *Cancer Chemotherapy and Pharmacology* **7**: 175–7.

Ten Bokkel Huinink, W.W., van der Burg, M.E.L., Vermorken, J.B. *et al.* (1984). Carboplatin in combination chemotherapy for ovarian cancer: a feasibility study. *Proceedings of the American Society of Clinical Oncology* **3**: C690.

Tester, W.J., Donehower, R.C., Eddy, J.L. *et al.* (1982). Evaluation of weekly escalating doses of dichloromethotrexate in patients with hepatocellular carcinoma and other solid tumors. *Cancer Chemotherapy and Pharmacology* **8**: 305–10.

Thompson, S.W., Davis, L.E., Kornfeld, M. *et al.* (1984). Cisplatin neuropathy: clinical, electrophysiologic, morphologic and toxicologic studies. *Cancer* **54**: 1269–75.

Tisman, G., Flener, V., Hsu, M.Y.K. *et al.* (1984). Outpatient high-dose cis-platinum continuous infusion chemotherapy. *Proceedings of the American Society of Clinical Oncology* **3**: C104.

Tong, W.P., Wisnicki, J.L., Horton, J. *et al.* (1980). A direct analysis of methotrexate, dichloromethotrexate and their 7-hydroxy metabolites in plasma by high pressure liquid chromatography. *Clinica Chimica Acta* **107**: 67–72.

Torti, F.M. and Lum, B.L. (1984). The biology and treatment of superficial bladder cancer. *Journal of Clinical Oncology* **2**: 505–31.

Troner, M. (1985). Cyclophosphamide (C), Adriamycin (A) and platinol (P) in the treatment of urothelial malignancy. *Proceedings of the American Society of Clinical Oncology* **4**: 106.

Troner, M. and Hemstreet, G. (1981). Cyclophosphamide, doxorubicin and cisplatin (CAP) chemotherapy in the treatment of urothelial malignancy: a pilot study of the Southeast Cancer Study Group. *Cancer Treatment Reports* **65**: 29–32.

Turner, A.G., Hendry, W.F., Williams, G.B. and Bloom, H.J.G. (1977). The treatment of advanced bladder carcinoma with methotrexate. *British Journal of Urology* **49**: 673–8.

Vance, R.B. and Kapp, J.P. (1985). Supraophthalmic arterial infusion of low dose cisplatin and BCNU for malignant glioma. *Proceedings of the American Society of Clinical Oncology* **4**: C125.

van der Werf-Messing, B. (1979). Preoperative irradiation followed by cystectomy to treat carcinoma of the urinary bladder category T3 Nx 0–4 M0. *International Journal of Radiation Oncology, Biology, Physics* **5**: 395–401.

Van Oosterom, A.T., Fossa, S.D., Mulder, J.H. *et al.* (1985). Mitoxantrone in advanced bladder carcinoma: a phase II study of the EORTC Genito-urinary Tract Cancer Cooperative Group. *European Journal of Cancer and Clinical Oncology* **21**: 1013–14.

Vermorken, J.B., Vander Vijgh, W.J.F., Klein, I. *et al.* (1982). Pharmacokinetics of free platinum species following rapid, 3-hr, and 24-hr infusions of cis-diamminedichloroplatinum (II) and its therapeutic implications. *European Journal of Cancer and Clinical Oncology* **18**: 1069–74.

Vermorken, J.B., Vander Vijgh, W.J.F., Klein, I. *et al.* (1984). Pharmacokinetics of free and total platinum species after short-term infusion of cisplatin. *Cancer Treatment Reports* **68**: 505–13.

Villani, F.P., Favalli, L. and Piccinini, F. (1980). Relationship between the effect on calcium turnover and early cardiotoxicity of doxorubicin and 4′-epidoxorubicin in guinea pig heart muscle. *Tumori* **66**: 689–97.

Vogel, C.L., Bennett, J.M., Byrne, P. *et al.* (1985). A randomized multicenter trial of Novantrone versus Adriamycin in combination chemotherapy for metastatic breast cancer. In *The Current Status of Novantrone*, pp. 59–64. John Wiley, New York.

Vogelzang, N.J., Torkelson, J.L. and Kennedy, B.J. (1985). Hypomagnesemia renal dysfunction and Raynaud's phenomenon in patients treated with cisplatin, vinblastine and bleomycin. *Cancer* **56**: 2765–70.

Vogl, S., Ohnuma, T., Perloff, M. and Holland, J.F. (1976). Combination chemotherapy with Adriamycin and cis-diamminedichloroplatinum II in patients with metastatic diseases. *Cancer* **38**: 21–6.

VonHoff, D.D., Myers, J.W., Kuhn, J. *et al.* (1981). Phase I clinical investigation of 9,10-anthracenedicarboxaldehyde bis[4,5-(dihydro-IH-imidazol-2-yl)-hydrazone] dihydrochloride (CL216,942). *Cancer Research* **41**: 3118–21.

VonHoff, D.D., Pollard, E., Kuhn, J. *et al.* (1980). Phase I clinical investigation of 1,4-dihydroxy-5,8-bis(2)(2-hydroxyethyl) amino-ethyl-amino (-9,10-anthracenedione dihydrochloride) (NSC 301739), a new anthracenedione. *Cancer Research* **40**: 1516–18.

VonHoff, D.D., Schilsky, R., Reichert, C.M. *et al.* (1979). Toxic effects of cis-dichlorodiammineplatinum (II) in man. *Cancer Treatment Reports* **63**: 1527–31.

Ward, J.M. and Fauvie, K.A. (1976). The nephrotoxic effects of cis-dichloroplatinum (II) (NSC-119875) in male F344 rats. *Toxicology and Applied Pharmacology* **38**: 535–47.

Wheeler, R.N., Natale, R.B., Roshon, S.G. and Baker, S.R. (1984). A phase I–II trial of cisplatin and dichloromethotrexate in squamous cell cancer of the head and neck. *Journal of Clinical Oncology* **2**: 831–5.

Whitmore, W.F. (1980). Integrated irradiation and cystectomy for bladder cancer. *British Journal of Urology* **52**: 1–9.

Williams, C.J., Stevenson, K.E., Buchanan, R.B. *et al.* (1979). Advanced ovarian carcinoma: a pilot study of cis-dichloro-diammine-platinum (II) in combination with Adriamycin and cyclophosphamide in previously treated patients. *Cancer Treatment Reports* **63**: 1745–53.

Williams, S.D., Einhorn, L.H. and Donohue, J.P. (1979). Cisplatinum combination chemotherapy of bladder cancer: an update. *Cancer Clinical Trials* **2**: 335–8.

Williams, S.D., Einhorn, L.H., Greco, F.A. *et al.* (1980). VP-16-213 salvage therapy for refractory germinal neoplasms. *Cancer* **46**: 2154–8.

Wilson, W.L., Schroeder, J.N., Bissel, H.F., Mrazek, R. and Hummel, R.P. (1969). Phase II study of hexamethylmelamine (NSC-13875). *Cancer* **23**: 132–6.

Wiltshaw, E., Evans, B. and Harland, S. (1985). Phase III randomized trial cisplatin versus JM8 (carboplatin) in 112 ovarian cancer patients, stages III & IV. *Proceedings of the American Society of Clinical Oncology* **4**: C471.

Wolff, S.N., Fer, M.F., McKay, C. *et al.* (1982). High dose VP-16 and autologous bone marrow transplantation (ABMTX) for advanced malignancies: a phase I study. *Proceedings of the American Association for Cancer Research* **23**: 134.

Yagoda, A. (1979). Phase II trials with cis-diamminedichloride platinum II in the treatment of urothelial tract tumors. *Cancer Treatment Reports* **63**: 1565–72.

Yagoda, A. (1980). Chemotherapy of metastatic bladder cancer. *Cancer* **45**: 1879–88.

Yagoda, A., Watson, R.C., Grabstald, H., Barzell, W.E. and Whitmore, W.F. (1977). Adriamycin and cyclophosphamide in advanced bladder cancer. *Cancer Treatment Reports* **61**: 97–9.

Yap, B.S., Tenney, D.M., Yap, H.Y. *et al.* (1983). Phase I clinical evaluation of cis-dichloro-trans-dihydroxy-bis-isopropylamine platinum IV (CHIP, JM9). *Proceedings of the American Association for Cancer Research* **24**: 658.

Yap, H.Y., Yap, B.S., Blumenschein, G.R. *et al.* (1983). Bisantrene, an active new drug in the treatment of metastatic breast cancer. *Cancer Research* **43**: 1402–4.

Young, C.W. (1984). Evaluation of epirubicin in patients with advanced breast cancer. In *Advances in Anthracycline Chemotherapy: Epirubicin*, p. 71. Edited by Bonnadonna, G. Masson, Milan.

Zekan, P., Jackson, D., Muss, H. *et al.* (1983). Cyclophosphamide, Adriamycin and vincristine (CAV) versus VP-16-213+CAV (VCAV) in the treatment of small cell carcinoma of the lung (SCC). *Proceedings of the American Society of Clinical Oncology* **2**: 193 (abstract).

Zwelling, L.A., Anderson, T. and Kohn, K.W. (1979). DNA-protein and DNA interstrand crosslinking by cis- and trans-platinum(II) diamminedichloride in L1210 mouse leukemia cells and relation to cytotoxicity. *Cancer Research* **39**: 365–9.

Zwelling, L.A. and Kohn, K.W. (1979). Mechanism of action of cis-dichlorodiammine platinum(II). *Cancer Treatment Reports* **63**: 1439–44.

11

Evaluation of response and morbidity following treatment of bladder cancer

Katia Tonkin and Ian Tannock

Introduction

The management of bladder cancer is controversial in many of its modes of presentation. In the treatment of recurrent multifocal superficial disease, for example, the choice lies between repeated transurethral resections, intravesical chemotherapy or cystectomy, while for locally invasive disease a clinician could recommend either radiation therapy, surgery, or a combination of both modalities. In the treatment of metastatic disease not only is supportive care important, but chemotherapy and/or radiation treatment may be employed for symptomatic control.

Thus far a multitude of clinical trials seems to indicate large variations in response to any one treatment modality. One example is shown in Table 11.1, which lists reported rates of response of patients with advanced bladder cancer who were treated with a three-drug regimen of chemotherapy. Reported rates of response vary from 13 to 81 per cent. This variability in results allows widely different interpretations of the available data.

Table 11.1 Variation in reported rate of response in patients with transitional cell carcinoma treated with cyclophosphamide, doxorubicin and cisplatin

Reference	Number of patients	Complete response (%)	Partial response (%)	Total (%)
Kedia *et al.* (1981)	23	22	61	81
Samuels *et al.* (1980)	50	18	34	52
Schwartz *et al.* (1983)	28	7	39	46
Al-Sarraf *et al.* (1985) (SWOG)	23	13	30	43
Smith *et al.* (1983) (EORTC)	42	12	28	40
Troner *et al.* (1981) (SECSG)	34	9	29	38
Khandekar *et al.* (1981) (ECOG)	45	22	11	33
Troner *et al.* (1985) (SECSG)	46	4	15	20
Campbell *et al.* (1981)	15	0	13	13

In this chapter we discuss parameters which may have a profound influence on the outcome of clinical trials and on the interpretation of their results. We suggest guidelines for the design and reporting of clinical trials, and the use of more stringent criteria of tumour response which would reduce the effect of errors in tumour measurement in phase-III trials of cancer chemotherapy. Finally, we review ways in which more global measures of patient benefit could be incorporated into future trial design.

Defining the goals of a clinical trial

Ethical considerations in clinical trials

The principle that patients must give informed consent before taking part in a clinical trial has received universal acceptance. Even in the absence of a formal clinical trial, it should be obligatory to discuss with the patient all reasonable options for treatment, and to allow the patient a greater part in the decision-making process. A number of problems may arise when treatment options are discussed with patients: the patient may not recall the information provided; the physician is liable to introduce personal bias in explaining the risks and benefits of various options; and the patient may have preconceived ideas about the merits of a particular treatment. In practice, informed consent is rarely achieved: studies of patients who have agreed to take part in clinical trials reveal that they have little insight about what they have consented to (Cassileth *et al.*, 1980). Many patients give consent either because of trust in their physician or because they suspect that a refusal might prejudice their care. In spite of these problems, the clinical trial remains the only route to improvements in therapy. What then constitutes an ethical trial? One major requirement is that the trial sets appropriate and attainable goals, and if randomization is involved, that it compares acceptable options for treatment.

One possible method for judging whether a clinical trial or a proposed treatment is appropriate is to ask physicians who treat bladder cancer to imagine that they have the disease and are faced with decisions about their own treatment: thus, they act as patient surrogates in simulated clinical scenarios. If a majority of specialist physicians accepted a particular treatment, or agreed to take part in a clinical trial for which the scenario made them eligible, then that treatment or trial could be regarded as ethically acceptable. This method has been applied to clinical trials in lung cancer (Mackillop *et al.*, 1986) and has revealed a widely variable acceptance rate of 11–65 per cent by physician surrogates. This result implies that many patients are asked to take part in clinical trials which a high proportion of physicians (when acting as patient surrogates) consider to be unacceptable. It would be of considerable interest to apply this same method to evaluate treatment options and current trials of bladder cancer. The differences in physician choices regarding treatment options could also be used as a basis to determine relevant goals of future clinical trials.

Explanatory and pragmatic trials

A clinical trial may be assigned to one of two distinct categories, which have been referred to as explanatory or pragmatic (Schwartz and Lellouch, 1967).

An explanatory trial would be one which seeks to investigate whether an experimental protocol has activity in bladder cancer. An example would be a phase-II trial of a new anticancer drug: such a trial is designed to determine if the drug has measurable activity and does not attempt to evaluate patient benefit which may result from general use of the drug. Conversely, a pragmatic trial is concerned with assessment of patient benefit from use of an experimental protocol. Most published trials in bladder cancer are pragmatic in intent whether they test surgery, local radiotherapy or chemotherapy. Not only are large, randomized, phase-III trials of chemotherapy pragmatic; but so also are single-arm studies which seek to assess patient benefit from use of available drugs.

The above distinction is important because the goals of each type of trial are quite different: these goals should be reflected not only in the design of clinical trials, but also in their analysis and the reporting of outcome.

An explanatory trial seeking evidence for activity of a treatment regimen may be performed with a small number of patients, and it may be appropriate to report only those patients who were treated according to protocol. For example, in testing for activity of a new drug, it may be legitimate to exclude patients from analysis if they have not received a certain minimum amount of treatment. This practice lessens the chance of rejecting an active agent prematurely but does not give information about overall patient benefit: this must be evaluated subsequently in a pragmatic trial.

The ideal design of a pragmatic trial should allow determination of the overall benefit of an experimental protocol to all eligible patients. The end-points of pragmatic trials should therefore include measures of both quality and quantity of survival. In this setting the reporting of only tumour shrinkage or disease-free interval is valid only if it is known to correlate with length of survival and/or reflects improved quality of life. The result of a pragmatic trial should apply to any group of similar patients. Thus it is important to report the outcome for all patients entered into the trial regardless of the quantity of treatment they receive, and to define carefully the criteria used to select patients for the trial in order to allow comparison of its results with other studies.

One example of a pragmatic trial might be the evaluation of cystectomy for medically fit patients in whom radiographic investigations do not reveal extracystic disease. All patients satisfying entry criteria should be evaluated and reported, including those in whom the surgery reveals unsuspected nodal disease and patients whose planned operation cannot be completed. Exclusion of such patients from analysis would bias the results and overestimate the true benefit of cystectomy to any similar group of clinically and radiologically staged patients.

Many trials of chemotherapy are undertaken with the implicit goal of providing patient benefit and are pragmatic in intent, although their results are often analysed by methods more suited to explanatory trials. Thus one finds inappropriate exclusion of patients, and end-point evaluation limited to tumour shrinkage with little information concerning quality and quantity of survival. The tacit assumption that measures of tumour shrinkage correlate with more global measures of patient benefit is not always justified, especially when the treatment is associated with morbidity.

Factors which influence the outcome of clinical trials

The factors which may have an effect on the outcome parameters of a clinical trial can be divided broadly into those which influence the true benefit of treatment (Table 11.2) and those that merely reflect poor design

Table 11.2 Parameters which influence the true benefit to patients of a particular regimen of treatment

Selection of patients
Referral pattern; single versus multi-institutional
Eligibility criteria for study
Selection of eligible patients

Characteristics of patients
Age and sex
Performance status; other medical problems
Prior treatment
Pathological type and grade of tumour
Sites of disease
Stage of disease; bulk of disease within stage

Quality of treatment
Adherence to protocol
Quality of supportive care
Expertise of attending physician(s)

of a trial or inappropriate analysis and reporting of data (Table 11.3). If these factors are reviewed with care the results of an individual trial can be placed in perspective and the true effect of a treatment can be evaluated, even when a variety of trials seem superficially to report widely different results. A recent summary of methodological guidelines for reports of clinical trials (Simon and Wittes, 1985) outlined the necessary parameters to make a complete evaluation and suggested that such guidelines could become requirements for publication. We review below the important factors that influence the outcome of clinical trials, as well as potential sources of error which may confuse their results.

Table 11.3 Sources of error in assessing the outcome of clinical trials

Inadequate number of patients
Exclusion of patients from analysis
Variable criteria of tumour response
Errors of measurement
Lack of peer review
Inappropriate controls (e.g. historical, other institutions)
Inadequate pretreatment assessment to define eligibility
Conclusions regarding efficacy of treatment based on comparison of
    responders versus non-responders

Selection of patients

The design of any clinical trial requires selection criteria to define appropriate patients for treatment. These criteria should allow readers to determine which of their own patients would be eligible for treatment. However, several factors influence the characteristics of patients who are treated in a clinical trial, so that they may not be representative of all patients who fit the entry criteria. These factors include the pattern of referral to the investigators and their institutions, and any bias which might influence an investigator in approaching patients for entry into a trial. The results of a trial are more likely to be reproducible if a high proportion of eligible patients is entered. Although the proportion of eligible patients entered and the reasons for non-entry are important, they are rarely included in reports of clinical trials.

It is often observed that studies performed in a single institution report superior results to multi-institution trials (Davis *et al.*, 1980). This is illustrated in Table 11.4, which lists response rates reported for treatment of advanced bladder cancer with cisplatin. Percentage response rates from single institutions (mean 40; range 33–47) were higher than from cooperative groups (mean 18; range 16–20). Selection of patients is probably an important component of this difference. A single institution is limited by its pattern of referral; multiple institution trials may have access to a broader cross-section of patients, although the preference of individual investigators within them may lead to accrual of a low proportion of eligible patients (Taylor *et al.*, 1984).

Characteristics of patients

Characteristics of patients which may influence the outcome of treatment are listed in Table 11.2. These include factors related to the extent of disease and to the individual patient (e.g. age and performance status). Many trials using chemotherapy have documented a dominant role for performance status in determining outcome: for example, in trials of non-small-cell lung cancer this was a more important factor than response to treatment in determining survival (Aisner and Hansen, 1981). Although less well

Table 11.4 Single-institution and cooperative-group results for treatment of patients with transitional cell carcinoma using cisplatin alone

Reference	Number of patients	Complete response (%)	Partial response (%)	Total (%)
Single institutions				
Merrin (1978)	19	5	42	47
Herr (1980)	21	14	29	43
Yagoda (1979)	28	0	36	36
Soloway *et al.* (1981)	27	0	33	33
Cooperative groups				
NBCCGA (Soloway *et al.*, 1983)	50	10	10	20
ECOG (Khandeker *et al.*, 1985)	48	2	15	17
SECSG (Troner, 1985)	43	0	16	16

documented for bladder cancer, performance status is certain to have a major role in treatment in all stages of the disease.

Several scales have been used to assess performance status: these include the 10-point Karnofsky scale, and the simpler 5-point ECOG scale (i.e. 0=normal, 1=some disability, 2=up more than 50 per cent of time, 3=in bed more than 50 per cent of time, and 4=moribund). Information concerning performance status of subjects in a clinical trial is crucial for its evaluation. To obtain objective and reliable information, medical personnel should be trained to record performance status (Coscarelli-Schag *et al.*, 1984).

The age of patients appears to have minimal influence on outcome of treatment provided that performance status is taken into account (Begg and Carbone, 1983). Age will, however, have a greater effect when using long-term survival as an end-point of primary treatment, and it may then be appropriate to use 'cause-specific' rather than crude or actuarial survival (see also Chapter 9).

Although stage of disease is a well-established prognostic factor, the influence of bulk of disease within a given stage has rarely been evaluated for patients with solid tumours; however, it may have considerable potential to influence the outcome of both local and systemic treatment. Unfortunately assessment of both stage and bulk may depend critically on the extent of the diagnostic evaluation, and errors of assignment (i.e. to different stages) may contribute to variability in results of clinical trials. Results of chemotherapy may also be influenced both by prior treatment and sites of metastases. Cross-resistance between drugs leads routinely to a lower chance of response in patients who have received previous chemotherapy, while radiation or surgery may damage vascular access to residual disease in the pelvis, or in other ways have an effect on subsequent response to chemotherapy (Yagoda, 1977).

Quality of treatment

A factor that is usually impossible to quantify in a clinical trial is the quality of care, although it may have a profound influence on outcome. Quality of care includes not only adherence to protocol and good supportive care, but also the judgement and technical skill of the physician or surgeon. This factor may be particularly important when attempting to generalize the results of a study which involves major surgery or aggressive chemotherapy: results obtained in institutions with considerable experience and a large support staff may not then be relevant to the setting of a community hospital.

Sources of error in assessing the outcome of clinical trials

There are many sources of error which can limit the validity and reproducibility of reported outcome in a clinical trial, and some of these are listed in Table 11.3. Small numbers of patients lead to wide confidence limits about the value of any outcome parameter and are likely to be associated with a large beta (type-II) error (Freiman *et al.*, 1978). This means that trials may fail to detect quite large differences in outcome of two treatments, and their results are often wrongly interpreted to suggest that the treatments have been shown to be equivalent.

Errors increase the uncertainty about a result, whereas bias may cause systematic departures from the true state. Exclusion of patients from analysis may introduce bias. Another often unrecognized source of bias may occur if data are reported in more than one publication: if subsequent reviews assume that the data are independent this leads to recycling of data, which can overestimate the success of therapy (Hillcoat, 1984). There are many other well-known causes of bias which have been reviewed elsewhere (Sackett, 1979).

Criteria of tumour response

In trials of chemotherapy it is often stated that 'standard' criteria of response have been used. However, in a recent survey of published clinical trials (Tonkin *et al.*, 1985) we documented that 'standard' criteria of response simply do not exist.

The extent to which criteria of tumour response are defined in publications reporting trials using cisplatin-based chemotherapy for bladder cancer, and in a larger series of trials for other types of tumour, is shown in Table 11.5. Most investigators stated a requirement for 'partial response' as 50 per cent shrinkage in cross-section of a measurable lesion, but many criteria that are required for full evaluation were stated infrequently; these include criteria for non-measurable disease, definition of start and end of response, frequency of assessment, and number of assessments used to define a response. There were no major differences in the information supplied in reports from cooperative groups or single institutions.

Although not usually included as an objective criterion of tumour

Table 11.5 Criteria of tumour response defined or referenced in publications reporting cisplatin-based trials of Ca bladder or in trials of chemotherapy for other solid tumours (includes data from Tonkin *et al.*, 1985)

Criterion of response	Number defined in original article (%)	
	Bladder cancer (*N*=14)	Other solid tumours (*N*=62)
Criteria for non-measurable disease	3(21)	17(27)
Requirement for shrinkage of a single lesion for PR (or disappearance for CR)	13(93)	62(100)
Criteria for multiple lesions	10(71)	43(69)
Definition of start of response	7(50)	23(37)
Definition of end of response	5(36)	20(32)
Frequency of assessment of patients	3(21)	29(47)
Number of assessments used in definition of response	1(7)	0(0)
Number of trials including all treated patients in analysis of response	3(21)	23(35)
Number of clinical trials in which exclusion criteria are stated	11(85)	40(65)

response, many authors stated the proportion of patients which appeared to satisfy criteria for 'minimal response' and 'stable disease'. The criterion for 'minimal response' (25–50 per cent shrinkage in cross-sectional area) is subject to very large errors of measurement (Moertel and Hanley, 1976; Warr *et al.*, 1984). Any tumour with a volume-doubling time in excess of 2 months (which probably applies to most bladder tumours) will satisfy some criteria of stability (i.e. less than 25 per cent increase in area in one month or more) unless treatment accelerates the disease. These criteria cannot be used as evidence for an effect of chemotherapy and should be abandoned. Even for 'partial response', errors in measurement for different types of lesion may lead to errors in estimates of response rate of up to 30 per cent, depending on the criteria employed (Warr *et al.*, 1984).

In order to evaluate the variability of criteria used in the clinical trials, we supplemented published information by contacting authors by telephone or by mail. Analysis of their replies shows that there is considerable heterogeneity in criteria used to determine tumour response (Table 11.6). Although differences in criteria of response documented in the table may appear to be subtle, we have generated a hypothetical model which illustrates how they might lead to large variation in reported response rates for a single set of data. This hypothetical example, shown in Table 11.7, leads to a potential range in rate of response of 20–75 per cent. Although the example may overestimate the variability in response rate that is due to differences in response criteria, it illustrates how subtle variations in criteria

Table 11.6 Criteria of tumour response determined from publications and from communication with the authors in trials of chemotherapy for bladder cancer and other solid tumours (includes data from Tonkin *et al.*, 1985)

Criterion of response	Number using stated criterion (%)*	
	Bladder cancer (*N*=15)	Other solid tumours (*N*=62)
Start of response		
Time of first treatment	6(40)	27(44)
First assessment as response	9(60)	26(42)
End of response		
Last assessment as response	0(0)	1(2)
First assessment as progression	14(93)	48(77)
Minimum duration of response		
$\leqslant 4$ weeks	8(53)	42(68)
> 4 weeks	3(20)	9(15)
Frequency of assessment		
$\leqslant 4$ weeks	10(67)	42(68)
> 4 weeks	4(27)	13(21)
Minimum number of assessments		
satisfying response criteria		
1	7(47)	28(45)
2 (with interval)	5(33)	17(27)

*Percentage is expressed in relation to the total sample. The total may be less than 100 per cent since complete information was not always obtained.

Table 11.7 Results of a hypothetical clinical trial on 50 patients (from Tonkin *et al.*, 1985)

Groups of 10 patients	Size of index lesion relative to the initial measurement, at weeks			
	2	4	6	8
A	<0.5	<0.5	<0.5	<0.5
B	<0.5	<0.5	~1.0	>1.5
C	<0.5	~1.0	>1.5	>1.5
D	~1.0	>1.5	>1.5	>1.5
E	No follow-up			

All authors would record group A as responders, some would record groups A and B, and some groups A, B and C. Depending on the inclusion or exclusion of group E, the recorded response rate for this single set of data could vary from 20 per cent (i.e. A/A + B + C + D + E) to 75 per cent (i.e. A + B + C/A + B + C + D).

for response may have a profound influence on the apparent results of clinical trials.

Peer review

External peer review has become recognized as an important component of the design of clinical trials, and ensures that appropriate standards for eligibility and assessment of response are maintained. The utilization of external review may contribute to the tendency for lower rates of response to be reported in trials of chemotherapy from cooperative groups.

Appropriateness of controls

Every clinical trial has an implicit control group. The most appropriate controls are obtained in prospective randomized trials which compare experimental with standard treatment. However, the expense and organizational difficulties associated with such trials limit the ability of an investigator to use this type of trial; thus single-arm studies are more often undertaken and are compared with historical controls or with results from other institutions. These comparisons suffer from many sources of error (Sacks *et al.*, 1982). Subtle differences in characteristics of patients, criteria used to determine response to treatment, and variation in assessment of outcome, may combine to give very large differences in apparent results even when patients in different institutions receive similar treatment (see Table 11.1).

Even the comparison with historical controls within an institution is subject to error because more recently treated patients usually fare better. The apparent improvements in outcome may be due in part to the use of newer diagnostic procedures (e.g. CT scans) which allow more accurate pretreatment evaluation and more accurate assignment of stage: this may lead to exclusion of patients in surgical series that might have been included in the historical control group. A new and sensitive diagnostic tool will tend to change the distribution of patients among the various stages of a disease and to increase the proportion of patients in the more advanced stages. This effect is illustrated in Fig. 11.1. The results for treatment of each stage will appear to be better than for historical controls in the same stage, but the overall results may be unchanged (Batley 1955; Bush, 1979): one has simply increased the proportion of patients in the more advanced stages.

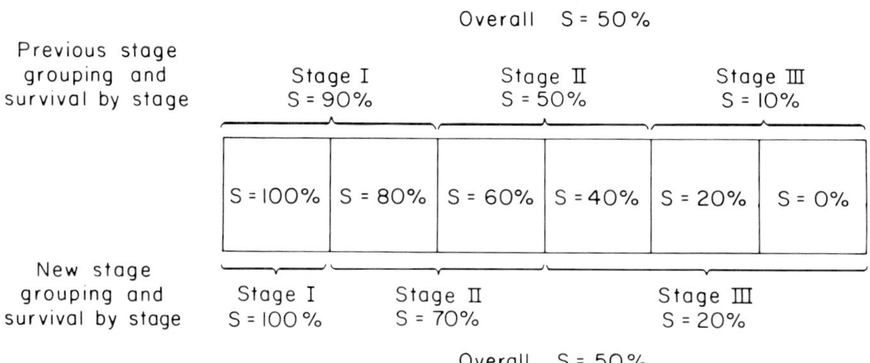

Fig. 11.1 Illustration of the paradox that a change in staging investigations may lead to the apparent improvement of results within each stage, without changing the overall results. In the example, patients may be divided into six equal groups, each with the indicated survival. Introduction of more stringent staging investigations moves patients into higher-stage groups as shown, but the overall survival of 50 per cent is unchanged. Adapted from Bush (1979)

Survival by response

In the published results of trials of cancer chemotherapy a statement is often included that the survival of responders is significantly longer than that for non-responders. This observation is frequently used as evidence for benefit from treatment. Unfortunately it is a circular argument since patients must survive for a certain minimum period before thay can be recorded as responders, and this bias may alone produce such an effect (Anderson *et al.*, 1983). This artefact may not be important in diseases where a significant proportion of durable complete remissions have been achieved, but this has not been the case in most trials for bladder cancer. Demonstration of the benefit of chemotherapy requires comparison between the entire group of treated patients and a concurrent group of untreated controls.

Some guidelines for clinical trials

The factors discussed in the preceding sections may be used to establish some guidelines for the design, analysis and reporting of clinical trials in bladder cancer. These guidelines should ensure that questions addressed by clinical trials are appropriate, that the results are meaningful and could be expected to apply to other patients, and that readers can discern from the publication exactly what was done. These guidelines would incorporate those recommended by others (Dersimonian *et al.*, 1982; Simon and Wittes, 1985) for the reporting of clinical trials. We suggest the following.

1. The parameters which we have defined in Table 11.2 are likely to

influence the true benefit to patients of a particular regimen of treatment and should be defined as carefully as possible. Thus, not only should criteria be reported for selection and exclusion of patients, but the proportion of eligible patients seen by the investigator and their institution should be stated. Reasons for non-inclusion should be given. Patient characteristics should be defined carefully, as well as the investigations that were used to define sites, stage and bulk of disease. Quality of treatment is not easily described, but should be mirrored by the quality of reporting.

2. Attempts should be made to minimize all sources of error that we have listed in Table 11.3. With the exception of pilot studies or investigations of the activity of a new drug (i.e. explanatory trials), studies with small numbers of patients place too large a confidence limit on outcome and are generally of no value. Exclusion of patients from analysis following entry into trials introduces bias and should be avoided. Peer review of all data should be incorporated into the design of clinical studies. Randomized trials are not always feasible; thus comparison with other types of controls will occur but must be undertaken with caution.

3. The criteria used to determine outcome, including both tumour response and morbidity, should be stated clearly in publications. For trials of chemotherapy criteria of tumour response should define each of the parameters listed in Table 11.5. Statements referring to standard criteria of response are inappropriate since we have shown that standard criteria do not exist.

4. Cooperative groups and editors of journals should take a leading role in developing uniform and reproducible criteria for tumour response and morbidity in clinical trials. Groups such as ECOG (Oken *et al.*, 1982) and the National Bladder Cancer Collaborative Group A (Soloway *et al.*, 1983) have established criteria with requirements for quality control. However, there are differences in their criteria for tumour response, and our group's previous study of measurement error (Warr *et al.*, 1984) suggests that some of the criteria will have poor reproducibility between observers. At a recent meeting of North American, European and Japanese physicians, consensus was achieved about the need for stringent criteria for tumour response that would be appropriate for pragmatic trials of cancer chemotherapy which seek to assess patient benefit. These criteria are summarized in Table 11.8: they include firm guidelines for the types of lesion that may be assessed for response and a requirement for at least two measurements with a 3-week interval to satisfy response criteria. These criteria are not a unique solution to irreproducibility, but should allow comparison between different clinical trials. They will require evaluation in a clinical setting to determine whether they correlate with more global measures of patient benefit.

Towards global measures of patient benefit

The goal of any treatment strategy for a patient with cancer should be to improve not only survival but also the quality of that survival. Most clinical trials include survival as an end-point, and describe the incidence of expected toxicity from treatment; but few have attempted to document the overall effect of treatment on quality of life. Clinical trials for locally invasive bladder cancer have indicated slightly better survival for patients receiving

Table 11.8 Proposed criteria for tumour response*

1.	Response should be based on bidimensionally measurable lesions. Lymph nodes and hepatic lesions defined by CT scan should have a minimum diameter of 2.5 cm before they are considered to be assessable for response.
2.	Duration of response should be measured from the time of first treatment.
3.	'Partial response' requires 50 per cent shrinkage in the sum of products of measurable lesions with no progression in any lesion. This criterion must be observed on at least two occasions at least 3 weeks apart, thus setting a minimum duration for response at 6 weeks.
4.	Where multiple lesions are present, four indicator lesions should be selected.
5.	End of response is defined by the last occasion that assessment of disease satisfied the above criteria.
6.	To avoid bias, observers should be unaware of their previous measurements when assessing a patient for response.
7.	'Complete response' (CR) requires complete clinical and radiological disappearance of disease on two occasions at least 3 weeks apart.
8.	Surgical restaging of complete responders is encouraged. Patients without pathological evidence of disease are denoted pCR.

*As proposed at the Second International Consensus Development Conference on Guidelines for Clinical Research in Bladder Cancer, Hakone, Japan, September, 1987.

both radiation and cystectomy than for those having radiation alone (Miller and Johnson, 1972; Mohiuddin and Kramer, 1981); however, the issue of patient preference between these procedures has not been evaluated.

The majority of clinical trials using chemotherapy for bladder cancer report tumour shrinkage and duration of response. These end-points do not necessarily correlate with improved quality of life as chemotherapy may palliate symptoms but may also cause significant toxicity.

The routine use of measures of quality of life as end-points for clinical trials is long overdue. Since most physicians have an inherent belief that their treatment leads to benefit, it would seem imperative that quality of life be assessed by an independent observer.

The most widely used parameters that have attempted to document quality of life are the Karnofsky and ECOG performance scales. Although observers can be trained to use these indices reproducibly (Cosgarelli-Schag *et al.*, 1984), such unidimensional scales are very limited in their ability to document the multiple factors (physical, mental, social, etc.) which contribute to patient wellbeing. More global measures of benefit have been introduced and tested in a limited number of clinical trials. Two important approaches are the use of simulated scenarios to weigh the benefit of alternative treatments, and the use of patient-directed questionnaires which evaluate multiple factors important for quality of survival.

Assessment of patient preference using simulated scenarios has been used in situations where there is a tradeoff between duration of survival and morbidity of treatment. This approach might be appropriate for trials comparing cystectomy with initial radiation therapy for locally invasive bladder cancer. In an analogous situation, McNeil *et al.* (1981) recorded that 20 per cent of a group of volunteers would opt for radiation treatment of laryngeal cancer (thus preserving speech), as compared to laryngectomy, even if surgery were to offer a 20–30 per cent higher survival. This method could be applied directly to patients with bladder cancer where acceptable options of treatment exist; however, it is limited by the ability to assign accurate probabilities for outcome parameters and morbidity.

The quality of life of patients with cancer has been assessed using either a questionnaire (e.g. Schipper *et al.*, 1984) or Linear Analogue Self-Assessment scale (LASA; e.g. Priestman and Baum 1976; Coates *et al.*, 1983; Selby *et al.*, 1984). The essential components involve questions or scales relating not only to physical but also to social and psychological aspects of quality of life. Fig. 11.2 illustrates LASA scales for three important attributes; patients are asked to mark their status on a 10 cm line joining the worst and best states with respect to each attribute. The distance of the mark from the end of the line then allows quantitation of the patient's wellbeing with respect to this attribute (see also Chapter 9).

The parameters to assess quality of life must be evaluated prior to their widespread general use. Important aspects of the validation of the above

Please score how <u>you feel</u> each of these aspects of your life was

affected by the <u>state of your health</u> during <u>today</u> (24 hrs)

   2.   Nausea

extremely severe   __________________________________ no nausea
   nausea

   13.   Physical Activity

completely unable __________________________________ normal physical
   to move my body   activity for me

   20.   Depression

   extremely   __________________________________ not depressed
   depressed   at all

Fig. 11.2 Examples of Linear Analogue Self-Assessment (LASA) scales. The patient is asked to place a vertical mark on each line to represent his or her status during a defined period of time. From Selby *et al.* (1984)

methods include determination that (1) the attributes and scales used reflect the essential components of quality of life (i.e. content and validity); (2) the assay is feasible in clinical situations; and (3) the assay is reproducible. Selby *et al.* (1984) have carefully documented each of these aspects using a 31-element LASA scale which relates to general health, frequent symptoms of disease, and morbidity of treatment in patients with breast cancer. This method is now in use in our institution as part of the end-point evaluation in trials for metastatic breast cancer.

The development and validation of patient-orientated questionnaires or the use of LASA scales to document and quantify the quality of life of patients should be given a high priority in future clinical research in patients with bladder cancer. The LASA scales developed by Selby *et al.* (1984) for breast cancer might be adapted by removing some attributes that relate specifically to carcinoma of the breast, and adding others that relate specifically to bladder cancer. A feasible list of parameters is shown in Table 11.9. If the LASA scales relating to these items were found to satisfy criteria relating to content, feasibility, reproducibility and validity, they might then become part of the outcome criteria in trials of bladder cancer. Improvement in one or more attributes, as measured by change in the distance of the patient's mark on the LASA scale from its left-hand end (Fig. 11.2), could then be used to quantitate change in these aspects of wellbeing. Such end-points might give objective weight to clinical impressions, and allow a correlation between quality-of-life measures and better-established end-point evaluation such as tumour shrinkage and length of survival.

Table 11.9 Attributes which might be appropriate for the assessment of quality of life for patients with bladder cancer

General-health-related dimensions	Dimensions related to the disease and its treatment
Mobility around home, town or country	Frequency of urination
Regular out-of-home employment	Dysuria
Self-care	Sexual relationships
Physical activity	Appearance of body
Recreation, pastimes or hobbies	Pain
Housework	Fatigue
Social life, meeting and dealing with people outside the family	Breathing
Family relationships and marriage	Nausea
Speech	Vomiting
Writing	Alopecia
Appetite (reduced or increased)	Stomatitis
Sleep (reduced or increased)	Diarrhoea
Alertness and mental function	Constipation
Anxiety	
Depression	
Anger	

Conclusions

In this chapter we have sought to evaluate critically not only factors which can influence the response and morbidity resulting from the treatment of bladder cancer, but also factors which may influence interpretation of the results of clinical trials.

Ethical issues in the design of clinical trials have been reviewed briefly, and it has been suggested that appropriate goals for future trials in bladder cancer might be defined through the use of physician surrogates.

Clinical trials can be divided into two main groups depending on whether their major goal is benefit to patients (pragmatic trials) or assessment of the activity of a new treatment (explanatory trials). These trials are different in both design and intent, and it has been emphasized that evidence for activity of a treatment does not necessarily imply benefit to patients.

Factors which influence the outcome of clinical trials include the selection of characteristics of patients and the quality of their care. Multiple factors can also introduce error and bias into the results of such trials, including small numbers of patients, inappropriate criteria for assessment of outcome, poor quality control, and inappropriate controls. The combination of these effects can lead to a large disparity in results when similar treatments are tested in different institutions. We have suggested guidelines for the design, analysis and reporting of the results of clinical trials in bladder cancer which would facilitate comparison of their results.

A major requirement in future clinical trials is the assessment of quality of life of patients who receive different treatments. We have described some global measures of patient benefit which have been evaluated in other types of cancer, which might be adapted for use in patients with bladder cancer.

References

Aisner, J. and Hansen, H. (1981). Commentary: current status of chemotherapy for non-small cell lung cancer. *Cancer Treatment Reports* **65**: 979–86.

Al-Sarraf, M., Frank, J., Smith, J.A. *et al.* (1985). Phase II trial of cyclophosphamide, doxorubicin, and Cisplatin (CAP) versus amsacrine in patients with transitional cell carcinoma of the urinary bladder: a Southwest Oncology Group study. *Cancer Treatment Reports* **69**: 189–94.

Anderson, J.R., Cain, K.C. and Gelber, R.D. (1983). Analysis of survival by tumour response. *Journal of Clinical Oncology* **1**: 710–19.

Batley, F. (1955). The problem of evaluation of cancer therapy. *Journal of the Canadian Association of Radiology* **6**: 25–8.

Begg, C.B. and Carbone, P.P. (1983). Clinical trials and drug toxicity in the elderly: the experience of the Eastern Cooperative Oncology Group. *Cancer* **52**: 1986–92.

Bush, R.S. (1979). *Malignancies of the Ovary, Uterus and Cervix*, p. 34. Edward Arnold, London.

Campbell, M., Baker, L.H., Opipari, M. and Al-Sarraf, M. (1981). Phase II trials with cisplatin, doxorubicin, and cyclophosphamide (CAP) in the treatment of urothelial transitional cell carcinoma. *Cancer Treatment Reports* **65**: 897–9.

Cassileth, B.R., Supkis, R.V., Sutton-Smith, K. and March, V. (1980). Informed consent: why are its goals imperfectly realized? *New England Journal of Medicine* **302**: 896–900.

Coates, A., Dillenbeck, F., McNeil, D.R. and Kaye, S.B. (1983). On the receiving end. II: LASA in evaluation of aspects of the quality of life of cancer patients receiving therapy. *European Journal of Cancer and Clinical Oncology* **19**: 1633–7.

Coscarelli-Schag, C., Heinrich, R.L. and Ganz, P.A. (1984). Karnofsky performance status: reliability, validity and guidelines. *Journal of Clinical Oncology* **2**: 187–93.

Davis, H.L., Multhauf, P. and Klotz, J. (1980). Comparisons of cooperative group evaluation criteria for multiple drug therapy for breast cancer. *Cancer Treatment Reports* **64**: 507–17.

Dersimonian, R., Charette, L.J., McPeek, B. and Mosteller, F. (1982). Reporting on methods in clinical trials. *New England Journal of Medicine* **306**: 1332–7.

Freiman, J.A., Chalmers, T.C. and Smith, H. (1978). The importance of beta type II error and sample size in the design and interpretation of the randomized control trial: survey of 71 'negative' results. *New England Journal of Medicine* **299**: 690–4.

Herr, H.W. (1980). Cis-diamminedichloride platinum II in the treatment of advanced bladder cancer. *Journal of Urology* **123**: 853–5.

Hillcoat, B. (1984). Data recycling and misreading: two potential errors in pooled data from small studies. *Journal of Clinical Oncology* **2**: 1047–9.

Kedia, K.R., Gibbons, C. and Persky, L. (1981). The management of advanced bladder carcinoma. *Journal of Urology* **125**: 655–8.

Khandekar, J.D., Elson, P.J., De Wys, W.D. *et al.* (1985). Comparative activity and toxicity of cis-diamminedichloroplatinum (DDP) and a combination of doxorubicin, cyclophosphamide and DDP in disseminated transitional cell carcinomas of the urinary tract. *Journal of Clinical Oncology* **3**: 539–45.

Mackillop, W.J., Ward, G.K. and O'Sullivan, B. (1986). The use of expert surrogates to evaluate clinical trials in non-small cell lung cancer. *British Journal of Cancer* **54**: 661–7.

McNeill, B.J., Weichselbaum, R. and Parker, S.G. (1981). Speech and survival: tradeoffs between quality and quantity of life in laryngeal cancer. *New England Journal of Medicine* **305**: 982–7.

Merrin, C. (1978). Treatment of advanced bladder cancer with cis-diamminedichloroplatinum (II NSC 119875): a pilot study. *Journal of Urology* **119**: 493–5.

Moertel, C.G. and Hanley, J.A. (1976). The effect of measuring error on the results of therapeutic trials in advanced cancer. *Cancer* **52**: 388–94.

Mohiudden, M. and Kramer, S. (1981). Pre-operative radiotherapy for bladder cancer: a perspective. *Urology* **17**: 515–20.

Oken, M.M., Creech, R.H., Tomey, D.C. and Morton, J. (1982). Toxicity and response criteria of the Eastern Cooperative Oncology Group. *American Journal of Clinical Oncology* **5**: 649–55.

Priestman, T.J. and Baum, M. (1976). Evaluation of quality of life in patients receiving treatment for advanced breast cancer. *Lancet* **i**: 899–901.

Sackett, D.L. (1979). Bias in analytic research. *Journal of Chronic Diseases* **32**: 51–63.

Sacks, H., Chalmers, T.C. and Smith, H. (1982). Randomized versus historical controls for clinical trials. *American Journal of Medicine* **72**: 233–40.

Samuels, M.L., Logothetis, C., Trindade, A. and Johnson, D.E. (1980). Cytoxan, Adriamycin and cis-platinum (CISCA) in metastatic bladder cancer. *Proceedings of the American Association for Cancer Research* **21**: 137.

Schipper, H., Clinch, J., McMurray, A. and Levitt, M. (1984). Measuring the quality of life in cancer patients: the Functional Living Index for cancer: development and validation. *Journal of Clinical Oncology* **2**: 472–83.

Schwartz, D. and Lellouch, J. (1967). Explanatory and pragmatic attitudes in therapeutic trials. *Journal of Chronic Diseases* **20**: 637–48.
Schwartz, S., Yagoda, A., Natale, R.B. *et al.* (1983). Phase II trial of sequentially administered cisplatin, cyclophosphamide and doxorubicin for urothelial tract tumors. *Journal of Urology* **130**: 681–4.
Selby, P.J., Chapman, J.A.W., Etazadi-Amoli, J. and Dalley, D. (1984). The development of a method for assessing the quality of life of cancer patients. *British Journal of Cancer* **50**: 13–22.
Simon, R. and Wittes, R.E. (1985). Methodologic guidelines for reports of clinical trials. *Cancer Treatment Reports* **69**: 1–3.
Smith, P.H., Child, J.A., Mulder, J.H. *et al.* (1983). Cooperative studies of systemic chemotherapy: a review of the work of the EORTC Urological Group and of the Yorkshire Urological Cancer Research Group (YUCRG). *Cancer Chemotherapy and Pharmacology* II (Suppl.): 525–31.
Soloway, M.S., Einstein, A., Corder, M.P. and Bonney, W. (1983). A comparison of cisplatin and the combination of cisplatin and cyclophosphamide in advanced urothelial cancer: a National Bladder Cancer Collaborative Group A study. *Cancer* **52**: 767–72.
Soloway, M.S., Ikard, M. and Ford, K. (1981). Cis-diamminedichloroplatinum (II) in locally advanced and metastatic urothelial cancer. *Cancer* **47**: 476–80.
Taylor, K.M., Margolese, R.G. and Soskolne, C.L. (1984). Physicians' reasons for not entering eligible patients in a randomized clinical trial of surgery for breast cancer. *New England Journal of Medicine* **310**: 1363–7.
Tonkin, K., Tritchler, D. and Tannock, I.F. (1985). Criteria of tumor response used in clinical trials of chemotherapy. *Journal of Clinical Oncology* **3**: 870–7.
Troner, M.B. (1985). Cyclophosphamide, Adriamycin and Platinol in the treatment of urothelial malignancy. *Proceedings of the American Society for Clinical Oncology* **4**: 106.
Troner, M.B. and Hemstreet, G.P. (1981). Cyclophosphamide, doxorubicin and cisplatin (CAP) in the treatment of urothelial malignancy: a pilot study of the Southeastern Cancer Study Group. *Cancer Treatment Reports* **65**: 29–32.
Warr, D., Kinney, S. and Tannock, I.F. (1984). Influence of measurement error on assessment of response to anticancer chemotherapy: proposal for new criteria of tumor response. *Journal of Clinical Oncology* **2**: 1040–6.
Yagoda, A. (1977). Future implications of phase II chemotherapy trials in ninety-five patients with measurable advanced bladder cancer. *Cancer Research* **37**: 2775–80.
Yagoda, A. (1979). Phase II trials with cis-dichlorodiammine platinum (II) in the treatment of urothelial cancer. *Cancer Treatment Reports* **63**: 1565–72.

12

Chemotherapy in bladder cancer: the North American experience

Diane C. Young and Marc Garnick

Introduction

Despite the development of radical radiotherapy and surgical approaches to the treatment of invasive bladder cancer, the prognosis of this disease remains dismal, with a 5-year survival rate of 20–50 per cent (Harker and Torti, 1983). Though these modalities have reduced local recurrence rates, the majority of patients still die of metastatic disease (Whitmore *et al.*, 1982). Patients who present with nodal involvement or distant metastases (until the reporting of some recent studies) usually survive less than one year. Systemic chemotherapy, either as primary therapy in patients with resectable or metastatic disease or in an adjuvant setting, seems to offer the best chance of improving these statistics. However, although bladder cancer is a chemotherapy-responsive tumour, optimal regimens have yet to be established.

The interpretation of the results of clinical trials in the treatment of bladder cancer has been difficult owing to a number of methodological problems (see Chapter 11). Prior to the mid-1970s most studies were drug-oriented trials involving small numbers of patients with bladder cancer. Possible prognostic factors such as stage and previous therapy were not always recorded. In addition, the accurate staging of bladder cancer and the assessment of response were more difficult before the CT scan became available (see Chapter 5). Pelvic masses, especially after surgery and radiation, can be difficult to measure by physical examination, but were often the only parameter that could be followed. Early studies also lacked standard criteria for response. Often subjective improvement or changes that would now be considered minor or mixed responses were scored as positive responses.

More recently, emphasis has been placed on using strict definitions for response. In many trials patients must have had bidimensionally measurable lesions by physical examination or radiological tests to be eligible. 'Complete response' is defined as disappearance of all evidence of disease and 'partial response' as a greater than 50 per cent reduction of the sum of the products of the perpendicular diameters of measurable lesions, without evidence of progression of disease elsewhere. An overall response rate including all complete and partial responses is generally determined. Mixed responses or 'stabilization of disease' are not considered as positive responses.

While these modifications have resulted in a more accurate and standardized reporting of results, it is important to note that the criteria for response are still changing. It has become clear that a clinically complete remission, even with the best diagnostic tests, may not be pathologically confirmed when surgical re-exploration is undertaken (Yagoda, 1983; Sternberg *et al.*, 1985). Pathologically complete remission may become the new standard for clinical trials (Yagoda, 1985). Another question is whether the category of 'partial response' should be included in the overall response (see also Chapter 11).

A final problem in interpreting bladder cancer trials is that there have been few randomized controlled studies to evaluate the advantages of chemotherapy versus non-treatment, or to compare different regimens. Thus, the relative benefits for various agents in terms of response and survival have not been established (see Chapter 17).

Single-agent trials

Despite the methodological problems, a number of drugs have been shown to be active in bladder cancer. The most effective agents are cisplatin, methotrexate, Adriamycin, cyclophosphamide, 5-fluorouracil and vinblastine (see Table 12.1).

Table 12.1 Responses to single agents in bladder cancer

Agent	Number of patients	Average CR+PR (%)
Amsacrine	59	10
Cisplatin	320	30
Cyclophosphamide	98	31
Doxorubicin	235	23
5-fluorouracil	75	35
Methotrexate	236	29
Mitomycin C	48	21
PALA	12	0
Vinblastine	38	16

Cisplatin

This is the most active single agent against bladder cancer at the present time. More than 300 patients have been treated with an average response rate (CR+PR) of 30 per cent (Yagoda, 1983). A series of 24 patients at the Memorial Sloan Kettering Cancer Center were treated with 1.25 mg/kg or 1.6 mg/kg of cisplatin every 21 days. Thirty-five per cent of patients had partial responses, lasting 5 months. In patients who had not received previous chemotherapy the partial response rate was 57 per cent (Yagoda, 1979). In trials using the same doses, similar response rates were reported by Soloway *et al.* (1981) (33 per cent) and Peters and O'Neill (1980) (50 per cent). The responses were all partial responses and generally lasted 6–8 months. Patients at Roswell Park were treated with a different schedule:

cisplatin 1 mg/kg weekly for 6 weeks, then every 3 weeks. One complete response and 8 partial responses were reported out of 19 evaluable patients (total response rate, 47 per cent). The patient with the complete response died at 6 months of a myocardial infarction, but autopsy findings were not reported (Merrin, 1978).

In two randomized trials, the response rate to cisplatin was somewhat lower. The National Bladder Collaborative Group A compared cisplatin to cisplatin plus cytoxan and found a 24 per cent response rate for the single agent and 13 per cent for the combination (Soloway *et al.*, 1983). In an Eastern Cooperative Oncology Group (ECOG) study comparing cisplatin with cisplatin, doxorubicin plus cyclophosphamide, the overall response rate to cisplatin alone was 26 per cent. Higher response rates were noted in patients with higher performance status and in those who had not had previous radiation therapy (Khandekar *et al.*, 1981). Previous chemotherapy has been associated with lower response rates in other studies (Yagoda *et al.*, 1976). Tannock *et al.* (1983) found no response to cisplatin in a group of patients who had been previously treated with methotrexate, Adriamycin and cyclophosphamide. In most of the studies, the response to cisplatin was usually seen within 2–4 weeks. Bony metastases and locoregional disease were not felt to respond as well as other sites by some investigators (Yagoda *et al.*, 1976; Soloway *et al.*, 1981). The toxicity of single-agent cisplatinum was moderate, with universal nausea and vomiting, occasional myelosuppression (especially in previously irradiated patients), and elevations of BUN and creatinine seen in one-third of patients. Obstructive uropathy was a risk factor for an elevated creatinine during therapy (Soloway, 1981). Patients required vigorous hydration and were generally given mannitol to counteract the nephrotoxic effects of cisplatin.

Methotrexate

This also appears to be an effective single agent in bladder cancer. Of 236 cases from the literature treated with a variety of doses and schedules, there was a 29 per cent response rate (Yagoda, 1983). Most of the early trials were done in Europe (Burfield, 1972; Pavone-Macaluso, 1972). A 56 per cent response rate was reported from the Royal Marsden Hospital in 61 patients treated with either methotrexate 50 mg every 2 weeks, 100 mg every 2 weeks or 200 mg with leucovorin rescue every 2 weeks. A dose–response relationship was suggested in that the response rates for the three schedules were 13 per cent, 54 per cent and 50 per cent, respectively. There were four complete responses lasting a median of 6 months. The patients in this study had advanced local disease which was not easily measurable. It was not mentioned whether previous chemotherapy had been given to these patients (Turner *et al.*, 1983). A more recent trial using 100 mg/m^2 of methotrexate plus leucovorin rescue every 2 weeks showed a 43 per cent response rate in 21 patients with measurable metastatic disease, and 28 per cent response rate in 32 patients with recurrent locoregional disease (Oliver *et al.*, 1984).

Natale *et al.* (1981) studied 49 patients with bidimensionally measurable lesions treated either with 0.5–1.0 mg/kg methotrexate weekly (40 patients) or 250 mg/m^2 methotrexate with leucovorin rescue (9 patients): 26 per cent achieved a partial remission lasting 6 months. Responses were seen in 10/33 patients receiving lower doses and only 1/9 receiving the higher dose. A 38 per cent response rate was found in a group of 16 patients without prior chemotherapy and with 90–100 per cent performance status. Response to methotrexate was usually seen within 2–3 weeks.

The principal toxicities of single-agent methotrexate are mucositis and myelosuppression, with less frequent complications including hepatotoxicity, dermatitis, pulmonary infiltrates and renal failure. Because the drug is renally excreted, careful attention needs to be paid to renal function in this patient population, especially when higher doses are given (see also Chapter 10).

Methotrexate thus appears to be an active agent in bladder cancer. It is the only single agent with significant numbers of clinical complete responses, and may be especially useful for management of locoregional disease. It is not clear whether there is any added value to higher doses with leucovorin rescue, and this may be addressed in a randomized trial.

Adriamycin

Adriamycin (doxorubicin) is also active against bladder cancer. While a review of cases prior to 1975 described a 35 per cent response rate, Yagoda (1983), using strict criteria for response, re-evaluated 223 cases and determined the response rate to be 18 per cent. Forty-two patients at Memorial Sloan Kettering Cancer Center were treated with five different schedules of Adriamycin with a 14 per cent response rate overall. A higher response rate (including some complete responses) was seen in patients treated with the schedules involving single doses given every 3 weeks versus those given 'loading doses' (frequent small doses over 10 days). Also of interest was one patient who progressed after 2 doses of $45\,mg/m^2$ every 3 weeks, then responded to $75\,mg/m^2$. Severe toxicity—especially nausea, vomiting and myelosuppression—was noted in patients receiving higher doses. It should be noted that patients in this study were heavily pretreated (50 per cent had prior chemotherapy) and had an average Karnofsky performance status of 55 per cent (Yagoda *et al.*, 1977). Gagliano *et al.* (1980, 1983) reported a 20 per cent partial remission rate in 40 patients without prior chemotherapy, treated with Adriamycin $50\,mg/m^2$ every 3 weeks; however, the duration of remission was only 14 weeks.

In a randomized study of 5-fluorouracil versus Adriamycin by the Eastern Cooperative Oncology Group, the response rate to Adriamycin $60\,mg/m^2$ every 3 weeks was only 9 per cent. These patients had not received prior chemotherapy (Knight *et al.*, 1983).

The toxicity of Adriamycin includes myelosuppression, nausea, vomiting, alopecia, and skin necrosis in the event of drug extravasation. Cardiomyopathy occurs with increasing frequency above a cumulative dose of $550\,mg/m^2$, but arrhythmias and congestive heart failure can occur at lower doses. The administration of Adriamycin in lower doses on a weekly basis may result in less cardiac toxicity than the conventional 3-week schedule (Torti *et al.*, 1983), and may allow higher cumulative doses to be given. Given the possible dose–response relationship suggested in Yagoda's study, a trial of this schedule might be worth while.

Cyclophosphamide

Insufficient data are available to determine the true effectiveness of cyclophosphamide against bladder cancer. A review of cases in the literature (Yagoda, 1980) showed a 31 per cent response rate in 98 patients treated, but this included many older trials with variable criteria for response. Critical re-evaluation in 1983 suggested that only 26 of these cases were objectively evaluable and that the response rate was only 7 per cent in these patients. There have been reports of small series in which patients treated with $1-1.2\,\text{gm/m}^2$ every 3 weeks had response rates of 40–50 per cent (Dekernion, 1977; Merrin *et al.*, 1975), but further studies are needed to confirm this.

Vinca alkaloids

Vinblastine sulphate appears to be a promising single agent for the treatment of bladder cancer. Twenty-eight extensively pretreated patients at Memorial Sloan Kettering Cancer Center were given vinblastine 0.1–0.15 mg/kg i.v. weekly; 18 per cent achieved partial responses which persisted for 2 months. Response was seen within 3–4 weeks. Patients who had not received previous chemotherapy had a better response rate than those who had (22 per cent versus 17 per cent), but the numbers in each group were small. Pulmonary and nodal metastases appeared to respond better than intra-abdominal sites. The toxicity included leucopenia in 71 per cent of courses with two episodes of nadir sepsis as well as constipation and paresthesiae (Blumenreich *et al.*, 1982).

Until recently, the activity of vincristine was unknown. A 30 per cent response rate was reported in one small series of patients treated with 25–75 mcg/kg every week (Holland *et al.*, 1972). However, the EORTC Genito-Urinary Group have completed a negative phase-II study of vincristine (see Chapter 14).

5-fluorouracil

5-fluorouracil (5-FU) is another agent whose activity is unknown despite long experience. While reviews of the literature suggest response rates as high as 35 per cent (Yagoda, 1983), more recent series are less favourable. In an Eastern Cooperative Oncology Group study which randomized patients to receive either Adriamycin or 5-fluorouracil, there were 2 complete responses and 5 partial responses among 46 patients, yielding a response rate of 15 per cent. When patients who were crossed over to 5-FU after failing Adriamycin were included, the overall response rate was 14 per cent. The dose of 5-fluorouracil in this study was $600\,\text{mg/m}^2$ i.v. weekly (Knight *et al.*, 1983). The Southeastern Cancer Study Group randomized patients to receive 5-FU or combination chemotherapy with cyclophosphamide, Adriamycin and cisplatin. They found a 26 per cent response rate to 5-FU, with remission duration greater than 3 months (Smalley *et al.*, 1981). Data were not presented in either of these studies to document whether differences in patient selection could have accounted for this disparity.

Other agents

A number of other drugs have been tested in patients with bladder cancer, but none has shown as much promise as the agents discussed above. Many of the trials have used patients who had received previous courses of chemotherapy, which may lower the response rate.

Hexamethymelamine, an agent which seems to be effective against bilharzial bladder cancer (Gad-el-Mawla *et al.*, 1978), does not appear to add much to the management of patients with transitional cell carcinoma. In a study by the Southwest Oncology Group, 29 patients who had not previously had chemotherapy were randomized to receive hexamethymelamine or the combination of 5-fluorouracil, doxorubicin and cyclophosphamide (Gagliano *et al.*, 1984). There were no responses seen to hexamethymelamine, either in the initially treated or crossover groups. Ninety per cent of the patients in this study were reportedly in a 'poor risk' category, which was defined as age over 65 or previous XRT (but these factors have not clearly been associated with poor response to chemotherapy).

Amsacrine (AMSA) has been studied in several trials. In a phase-II study by the National Bladder Cancer Collaborative Group A, involving 15 patients who had all failed previous chemotherapy regimens, there were no responses seen after two or more cycles of AMSA 90 mg/m^2 given every 3 weeks (Trump *et al.*, 1983). Natale *et al.* (1983) reported a 9.5 per cent partial response rate in 22 patients, most of whom had had chemotherapy before. The responses lasted 2–3.5 months. In a recent SWOG study which randomized patients to receive AMSA (120 mg/m^2 every 3 weeks) or cyclophosphamide and cisplatin, there was one complete and 3 partial responses in 22 patients for a response rate of 19 per cent. Responses had an average duration of 21 weeks. The side effects were tolerable, with anaemia and leucopenia being the main problems. These patients had not received prior chemotherapy (Al-Sarraf *et al.*, 1985). Thus, in the previously untreated population, AMSA may be an effective agent.

Mitomycin C has been useful in the treatment of superficial bladder tumours (see Chapter 6), but its role in systemic therapy is not clear (see Chapter 17). Early *et al.* (1973) reported a 21 per cent response rate in 19 patients given 0.25–0.5 mg/m^2 i.v. every 2 weeks. Delayed myelosuppression is the most troublesome toxicity of this drug.

Agents which have been studied in phase-II trials and are thought not to be effective include VM-26 (Qazi *et al.*, 1982), PALA (Natale *et al.*, 1982) and neocarzinostatin (Natale *et al.*, 1980). All of these series involved patients who had failed previous chemotherapy, and studies with untreated patients have not been done (see also Chapter 10).

Combination regimens

Efforts to improve the response rate in single-agent trials have led to a variety of combination regimens. Ideally, the agents involved should be non-cross-resistant and have different toxicities. Since few randomized studies have been performed, it has been difficult to demonstrate any benefit over single-agent therapy.

Cisplatin-containing regimens

The combination of cisplatin and cyclophosphamide does not appear to offer any advantage over cisplatin alone. Yagoda *et al.* (1978) treated 36 patients with advanced measurable disease with cisplatin 1.6 mg/kg and cyclophosphamide 250–1000 mg/m^2 every 3 weeks: 47 per cent of evaluable patients had partial responses lasting a median of 7 months. This was not statistically different from the response rate in their trials with cisplatin alone. In addition, they noted that many patients delayed or refused treatment because of nausea and vomiting.

A prospective multi-institutional trial done by the National Bladder Cancer Collaborative Group A (Soloway *et al.*, 1983) compared patients treated with cisplatin alone to cisplatin plus cyclophosphamide. The doses in this study were cisplatin 70 mg/m^2 and cyclophosphamide 750 mg/m^2, both given every 3 weeks. A relatively low response rate (20 per cent) was reported for cisplatin alone, and the combination had a response rate of only 11 per cent. Duration of response was similar in the two groups. Over 50 per cent of patients in this study had performance status of 2 or 3, and this may have accounted in part for the poor overall response rate in this study.

Adding Adriamycin to cisplatin may have some benefit. In the Memorial Sloan Kettering experience, there was a 54 per cent response rate of more than 3 months duration, including two complete responses in 26 evaluable patients treated with cisplatin and Adriamycin. Patients given chemotherapy previously appeared to respond as well as untreated patients to this regimen, but the numbers of patients were small in each group (Yagoda, 1979). The Southwest Oncology Group, in a prospective randomized trial comparing Adriamycin versus Adriamycin plus cisplatin showed a greater response rate for the combination (43 per cent versus 19 per cent). The combination had greater haematological and gastrointestinal toxicity than Adriamycin alone (Gagliano *et al.*, 1983). It is not clear whether the addition of 5-FU to cisplatin and Adriamycin is beneficial. One report from Indiana University showed a 58 per cent partial response rate using these three drugs, but only 17 patients were treated (Williams *et al.*, 1978).

The combination of cisplatin plus methotrexate has only been recently studied, mostly because of fears of enhanced nephrotoxicity. Trials using this combination were demonstrated to have acceptable toxicity in patients with squamous cell carcinoma of the head and neck (Jacobs *et al.*, 1983), and now there are several ongoing studies in bladder cancer patients (see Chapter 17). Data are only preliminary, but suggest a complete response rate of 20–30 per cent and an overall response rate of 40–60 per cent (Stoter *et al.*, 1985; Carmichael *et al.*, 1985; Hillcoat and Raghavan, 1986).

One interesting trial involved the combination of cisplatin (70–100 mg/m^2) and dichloromethotrexate, a halogenated analogue of methotrexate that is excreted via the hepatobiliary route, given in escalated doses. It was hoped that the possible nephrotoxicity associated with the combination of cisplatin and methotrexate could be avoided. Of 13 patients with bladder cancer there were 2 CR and 6 PR (62 per cent), although duration of response was not stated. Toxicity included myelosuppression in 40 per cent, mucositis in 30 per cent, and nephrotoxicity in 4 per cent (Natale *et al.*, 1983).

Combinations involving cisplatin, Adriamycin and cyclophosphamide (CAP or CISCA) have been studied in many centres (see Table 12.2). The initial response rates reported from M.D. Anderson Hospital were 80–90 per cent (Sternberg, 1977), but in a later series of 50 patients this was decreased to 52 per cent. Nine complete responses occurred in this group and the survival difference was significant between responders and non-responders (Samuels, 1980). It should be noted that 'survival advantage' in non-randomized studies may reflect patient characteristics rather than effects of treatment. Thirty-two patients at Memorial Sloan Kettering Cancer Center were given cisplatin 70 mg/m^2, cyclophosphamide 250 mg/m^2 and Adriamycin 45 mg/m^2 sequentially (days 1–3). Forty-six per cent of evaluable patients had responses lasting a median of 8 months. Tumour regression occurred 1–3 weeks after the first dose. The median duration of survival was 91 weeks for responders and 38 weeks for non-responders (Schwartz *et al.*, 1983).

Other smaller non-randomized trials have reported variable response rates to this regimen. Only one randomized study has been reported comparing cisplatin alone versus cisplatin, Adriamycin and cyclophosphamide. In this study by the Eastern Cooperative Oncology Group, the response rates were 24 per cent for the single agent and 37 per cent for the combination (Khandekar *et al.*, 1981).

At the University of Texas, investigators have recently reported the result of the combined intra-arterial and intravenous administration of these agents. In their experience intra-arterial chemotherapy is more effective against local disease. They studied 28 selected patients with advanced disease with or without nodal metastases, but without visceral metastases. Two different schedules of sequential intra-arterial and intravenous administration of 'CISCA' were given. Thirty-nine per cent complete responses, including one that was pathologically documented, were reported, with a median duration of 49 weeks. Further randomized studies would be necessary to establish whether this specialized technique is more effective than intravenous therapy alone.

Thus the combination of cyclophosphamide, Adriamycin and cisplatin appears to result in remissions in 40–50 per cent of carefully selected patients. 'Survival advantage' in responding patients has been implied in several studies, with responders living more than a year, and non-responders surviving only 5–20 weeks. All sites of disease respond (Schwartz *et al.*, 1983). Significant toxicity has been reported: nausea, vomiting and alopecia are universal; myelosuppression is common, but rarely fatal; and elevations of creatinine (usually reversible) occur in one-third of patients.

Methotrexate combinations

Until recently, there have been few studies of combinations of methotrexate and other drugs (see Table 12.3). Tannock *et al.* (1983) studied the combination of methotrexate, Adriamycin and cyclophosphamide with cisplatin given to patients who progressed on this regimen. Fifteen of 38 patients with bidimensionally measurable disease had responses, with a median response duration of 6 months. All sites of metastatic disease responded, and survival of responders was significantly better than of non-responders. The doses of chemotherapeutic agents were relatively low in this study: methotrexate 30 mg/m^2 on days 1–8, Adriamycin 30 mg/m^2 on day 1, and cyclophosphamide 300 mg/m^2 i.v. on day 1 with cycles given every 21 days. A trial was also undertaken of methotrexate with mitomycin C (Tannock, 1983). There were 5 partial responses in 16 patients, but only one remission lasted longer than 3 months. In addition, 6 patients had severe toxicity, including a TTP syndrome related to mitomycin C. It was concluded that this regimen would not be useful.

The combination of methotrexate and vinblastine has been reported (Needles *et al.*, 1982; Ahmed *et al.*, 1985). A 44 per cent response rate was described in 27 evaluable cases. Interestingly, 2 patients who had failed to respond to therapy with methotrexate and vinblastine as single agents responded to the combination. Toxicity included myelosuppression, mucositis, neuropathy and abnormal liver function tests. Because there have been no randomized trials comparing this or the other combinations to methotrexate alone, it is not clear whether additional drugs are conferring additional benefit.

Other combinations

Based on the synergy between Adriamycin and cyclophosphamide seen in a mouse bladder cancer model, phase-II trials of this combination were undertaken. Yagoda treated 17 patients with Adriamycin 45–60 mg/^{2} and cyclophosphamide 450–600 mg/m^2 and found only 3 partial responses (17 per cent) lasting 4–5 months. Forty-four per cent of the patients in this trial had life-threatening toxicity (Yagoda *et al.*, 1977). A 35 per cent response rate was reported among 23 patients treated with cyclophosphamide, Adriamycin and bleomycin. These were only partial responses, and there was severe skin and mucosal toxicity in 8 patients, 4 severe infections and 2 treatment-related deaths (Levi *et al.*, 1980).

The Southeastern Cancer Study Group performed a prospective randomized trial of 5-fluorouracil versus cyclophosphamide, Adriamycin and 5-fluorouracil (FAC): the response rates were 26 per cent for the single agent and 18 per cent for the combination (Smalley *et al.*, 1981). The Southwest Oncology Group found only one partial response in 15 patients treated with 'FAC', and also concluded that it was not effective therapy (Gagliano *et al.*, 1984).

New regimens

The greatest interest in the treatment of bladder cancer with chemotherapy at the present time involves the recently published results of three and four drug regimens using cisplatin, methotrexate and vinblastine with and without Adriamycin (see Table 12.4). The Northern California Oncology Group studied CMV (cisplatin 100 mg/m^2 on day 2, methotrexate 30–40 mg/m^2 on days 1 and 8, and vinblastine 4–5 mg/m^2 on days 1 and 8). Of 50 evaluable patients, 14 (28 per cent) achieved complete remissions and 14 others achieved partial remissions for an overall response rate of 56 per cent. All metastatic sites, including bone and liver, showed responses. The median duration of remission was 9 months. Three patients had complete

Table 12.2 Cisplatin, Adriamycin and Cytoxan

Institution	Drugs	Number of patients evaluable	CR	PR	CR+PR (%)	Duration	Survival advantage?
M.D. Anderson (Samuels *et al.*, 1980)	Ctx 650 mg/m^{2}d1 q 21 d ADR 50 mg/m^{2}d1 CDDP 100 mg/m^{2}d2	50	9	17	52	Not stated	Yes
SECSG (Troner and Hamsteet, 1981)	CTX 400–500 mg/m^2 q 21 d ADR 40–50 mg/m^2 CDDP 40 mg/m^2	34	3	10	38	6 months	Yes
Wayne State (Campbell *et al.*, 1981)	Ctx 600 mg/m^2 q 3–4 weeks ADR 50 mg/m^2 CDDP 75 mg/m^2	15	0	2	13	Not stated	No
Wisconsin (Citrin *et al.*, 1983)	Ctx 500 mg/m^2 d1 q 21 d ADR 40 mg/m^2 d1 CDDP 40 mg/m^2 d2 +methotrexate 40 mg/m^2 q weeks × 6 weeks	13	2	3	38	CR—13 months PR—6 months	Yes
MSKCC (Schwartz *et al.*, 1983)	CDDP 70 mg/m^2 d1 q 21 d Ctx 250 mg/m^2 d2 ADR 45 mg/m^2 d3	28	2	11	46	8 months	Yes
SWOG (Al-Sarraf *et al.*, 1985)	Ctx 600 mg/m^2 d1 q 3–4 weeks ADR 40–50 mg/m^2 d1 CDDP 75 mg/m^2 d2	36	5	10	42	7 months	Not stated

Table 12.3 Other combinations

Regimen	Drugs	Number of patients evaluable	CR	PR	Response (%)	Duration	Survival advantage?
MAC (Tannock *et al.*, 1983)	Mtx 30–40 mg/m^2 d1,8 q 21 d ADR 30 mg/m^2 d1 Ctx 300–400 mg/m^2 d1	38	2	13	38	6 months	Yes
Mtx/V1b (Needles *et al.*, 1982)	Mtx 30–40 mg/m^2 d1 q 21 d V1b 3–4 mg/m^2 q week	27	0	12	44	5 months	Not stated
Cytoxan/ADR (Yagoda *et al.*, 1977)	ADR 45–60 mg/m^2 q 21 d Ctx 450–600 mg/m^2	17	0	3	17	4–5 months	No
Cytoxan/ADR/ bleomycin (Levi *et al.*, 1980)	Ctx 500 mg/m^2 d1 q 21 d Dox. 50 mg/m^2 d1 Bleo. 30 mg/m^2 weekly	23	0	8	35	Not stated	Yes
FAC (Smalley *et al.*, 1981)	5FU 500 mg/m^2 d1, q 21 d Ctx 500 mg/m^2 d1 ADR 50 mg/m^2 d1	21	0	3	18	>3 months	No
FAC (Gagliano *et al.*, 1980)	5FU 500 mg/m^2 d1 q 21 d Ctx 500 mg/m^2 d1 ADR 50 mg/m^2 d1	15	0	1	6	7 months	No

Table 12.4 New chemotherapy programmes for patients with advanced bladder cancer

Institution	Drugs	Number of patients	CR	PR	Response (%)	Duration
NCOG	Methotrexate 30–40 mg/m^2 d1,8 q 21d					
(CMV)	Vinblastine 4–5 mg/m^2 d1,8 CDDP 100 mg^2 d2	50	14	14	56	8 months
MSKCC (MVAC)	Mtx 30 mg/m^2 d1,15,22 q 28 d VLB 3 mg/m^2 d2,15,22 CDDP 70 mg/m^2 d2 Adria. 15–30 mg/m^2 d2	45	18	12	67	>12 months

remissions confirmed surgically. In general, patients who obtained complete remissions had regression of disease by the fourth cycle of therapy and received a median of six cycles. Two patients had unmaintained remissions of 18+ and 35+ months. Toxicity was quite substantial, with significant myelosuppression, two treatment-related deaths due to sepsis and frequent renal toxicity (Harker *et al.*, 1985). Dose reductions were made in methotrexate and vinblastine, with less toxicity as a result.

Memorial Sloan Kettering Cancer Center has recently reported the results of MVAC (methotrexate 30 mg/m^2 on days 1, 15, 22, vinblastine 3 mg/m^2 on days 2, 15, 22, Adriamycin 30 mg/m^2 on day 2, and cisplatin 70 mg/m^2 on day 2 the cycle being reapeated every 28 days). Eighteen of 45 evaluable patients (40 per cent) achieved complete remissions, and 12 others had partial remissions. All sites of disease responded. Twelve of the 18 clinical complete responders were surgically explored and 4 were found to have foci of residual disease which were resected. The median duration of remission for complete responders was more than one year. As with CMV, there was significant toxicity, with 8 episodes of nadir sepsis and 3 drug-related deaths. Anorexia, nausea, vomiting, alopecia, mucositis and renal dysfunction were also common (Sternberg *et al.*, 1985). Interestingly, in this group and in the CMV-treated group, complete responders were reported who relapsed in the CNS only.

Further prospective randomized trials are needed to assess these combinations, but the high complete-response rates with these regimens are encouraging. Whether a higher complete-response rate equals improved survival is not yet known.

Chemotherapy and other modalities

The data presented indicate that metastatic bladder cancer is responsive to chemotherapeutic regimens, and that effective palliation is possible. The optimal dose and schedule have not been established, but some combinations currently being investigated seem to produce improved complete-response rates and longer remissions. It will be important to determine whether the integration of chemotherapy with surgery and radiation can increase the disease-free survival by improving local control and preventing the development of distant metastases. In the study reported by Harker *et al.* (1985) there were several cases presented in which prolonged CR status was obtained following a combined-modality approach. In 3 cases, prior treatment with CMV reduced pelvic masses or metastatic disease so that surgical resection was possible.

Most trials of combined-modality therapy have been small or non-randomized, not allowing for definite conclusions (Edlund *et al.*, 1970; Glashan *et al.*, 1977; Lundbeck and Christoferson, 1979).

The National Bladder Cancer Collaborative Group A investigated the efficacy of transurethral resection, cisplatin and radiation therapy in 27 patients with stage T2–T4 bladder cancer who were not cystectomy candidates. This study excluded patients with positive lymph nodes above the bifurcation of the common iliac arteries. They were treated with cisplatin 70 mg/m^2 every 3 weeks for 8 courses and 4500 cGy of pelvic XRT with 6480 cGy total to the tumour. Eight courses of cisplatin were planned, but less than one-third of the patients completed them owing to intolerable side effects. Evaluation was by cytoscopy. Seventy-six per cent of the patients achieved a complete response, but follow-up was insufficient to determine the long-term impact on survival. Toxicity included one episode each of renal failure, sepsis and transient small-bowel obstruction (Shipley *et al.*, 1984).

An extension of this idea is the use of chemotherapy prior to cystectomy for patients with invasive bladder cancer. The goal of these programmes is to increase survival by treating microscopic foci of metastatic disease as well as shrinking the primary lesion. Preliminary results of an Australian programme using 2 cycles of cisplatin 100 mg/m^2 followed by surgery and/or radiation therapy show a 70 per cent response rate in the primary lesion prior to surgery, and an 82 per cent complete remission rate after radiation therapy or surgery. The actuarial survival at 24 months was 82 per cent (Raghavan *et al.*, 1985). A randomized trial of 'up-front' chemotherapy plus cystectomy versus cystectomy alone is being conducted at the Dana Farber Cancer Center, and a similar study comparing chemotherapy plus radiotherapy versus radiotherapy alone is in progress in Australia (see Chapter 17).

The use of adjuvant therapy after surgery is also being explored. A series of 15 patients with stage D1 and D2 bladder cancer at Northwestern University were treated with Adriamycin and radiation therapy following surgery. With a mean follow-up period of 27 months, the survival was reported to be 68 per cent at 1 year (53 per cent free of recurrence) and 44 per cent at 2 years (41 per cent free of recurrence). When compared with historical control groups, survival appeared to be improved. Definite conclusions are difficult to draw because of small numbers patients and the variety of surgical procedures performed prior to chemoradiotherapy (Schaeffer *et al.*, 1984). Other adjuvant trials are in progress at the present time. It will be interesting to evaluate the effectiveness of combinations such as CMV and MVAC in an adjuvant setting.

Conclusions

In the past decade there have been numerous studies of chemotherapy for bladder cancer. At the present time response rates of 30–50 per cent can be expected with a variety of single agents and combinations. Combinations involving cisplatin, methotrexate and vinblastine with or without Adriamycin appear promising, although randomized prospective trials are needed to establish the true efficacy and survival benefit of these regimens.

References

Al-Sarraf, A.M., Frank, J., Smith, J.A., O'Bryan, R.M., Costanzi, J.J., Stephens, R.L., Caraveo, J. and Crawford, E.D. (1985). Phase II trial of cyclophosphamide, doxorubicin and cisplatin versus amsacrine in patients with transitional cell carcinoma of the bladder. *Cancer Treatment Reports* **69**: 189–94.

Ahmed, T., Yagoda, A., Needles, B., Scher, H.I., Watson, R.C. and Geller, N. (1985). Vinblastine and methotrexate for advanced bladder cancer. *Journal of Urology* **133**: 602–4.

Blumenreich, M.S., Yagoda, A., Natale, R.B. and Watson, R.C. (1982). Phase II trial of vinblastine sulfate for metastatic urothelial tract tumors. *Cancer* **50**: 435–8.

Burfield, G.D. (1972). Intravenous methotrexate in the treatment of advanced bladder cancer. *British Journal of Urology* **44**: 121–4.

Campbell, M., Baker, L.H., Opipan, M. and Al-Sarraf, M. (1981). Phase II trial with cisplatin, doxorubicin and cyclophosphamide in the treatment of urothelial transitional cell carcinoma. *Cancer Treatment Reports* **65**: 897–9.

Carmichael, J., Cornbleet, M., McDougall, S. *et al.* (1985). Combination cisplatin and methotrexate in the treatment of transitional cell carcinoma of the urinary tract. *British Journal of Urology* **57**: 299–303.

Carter, S.U. and Wasserman, T.M. (1975). The chemotherapy of urologic cancer. *Cancer* **36**: 729–47.

Chabner, B.A. and Myers, C.E. (1985). Clinical pharmacology of cancer chemotherapy. In *Cancer: Principles and Practice of Oncology*, pp. 287–328. Edited by DeVita, V.E., Hellman, S. and Rosenberg, S.A. Lippincott, Philadelphia.

Citrin, D.L., Hogan, T.F. and Davis, T.E. (1983). A study of cyclophosphamide, Adriamycin, cisplatinum and methotrexate in advanced transitional cell carcinoma of the urinary tract. *Cancer* **51**: 1–4.

Dekernion, J.B. (1977). The chemotherapy of advanced bladder cancer. *Cancer Research* **37**: 2771–4.

Early, K., Elias, E.G., Mittelson, A., Albert, D. and Murphy, G.P. (1973). Mitomycin C in the treatment of metastatic transitional cell carcinoma of the bladder. *Cancer* **31**: 1150–3.

Edland, R.W., Weber, J.B. and Ansfield, F.J. (1970). Advanced cancer of the urinary bladder: an analysis of the results of radiotherapy alone vs. radiotherapy and concomitant 5-fluorouracil: a perspective randomized study of 36 cases. *American Journal Roentgen* **108**: 124.

Gad-el-Mawla, N.M., Muggia, F.M., Hanza, M.R. *et al.* (1978). Chemotherapeutic management of carcinoma of the bilharzial bladder: a phase II trial with hezamethymelamine and VM-26. *Cancer Treatment Reports* **62**: 993–6.

Gagliano, R. *et al.* (1980). Randomized trial of Adriamycin vs. Adriamycin+CDDP. *Proceedings of the American Society of Clinical Oncology* **C110**: 347.

Gagliano, R.G., Levin, M., El-Bolkainy, M.N. *et al.* (1983). Adriamycin vs. Adriamycin plus CDDP in advanced transitional bladder cancer: a Southwest Oncology Group study. *American Journal of Clinical Oncology* **6**: 215–18.

Gagliano, R.G., Stephens, R.L., Costanzi, J.J., Oishi, N., Stuckey, W.J., Grozea, P.N., Frank, J. and Crawford, E.D. (1984). Randomized trial of hexamethamelamine vs. 5FU, doxorubicin and cyclophosphamide in advanced transitional cell carcinoma of the bladder: a SWOG study. *Cancer Treatment Reports* **68**: 1025–6.

Glashan, R.W. (1977). A toxicity study in the treatment of T3 bladder tumors with a combination of radiotherapy and chemotherapy. *British Journal of Urology* **49**: 669.

Harker, W.G., Meyers, F.J., Freiha, F.S., Palmer, J.M., Shortliffe, L.D., Hannigan, J.F., McWherter, K.M. and Torti, F.M. (1985). Cisplatin, methotrexate and vinblastine (CMV): an effective chemotherapy regimen on metastatic transitional cell carcinoma of the urinary tract: a Northern California Oncology Group study. *Journal of Clinical Oncology* **3**: 1463–70.

Harker, W.G. and Torti, F.M. (1983). The chemotherapy of bladder cancer: systemic therapy. *Recent Results in Cancer Research* **85**: 37–49.

Harker, W.G., Freiha, F.S., Shortliffe, L.D., Meyers, F.J., Hannigan, J.F., Flam, M.S. and Torti, F.M. (1984). Cisplatin, methotrexate and vinblastine (CMV) chemotherapy for metastatic transitional cell carcinoma of the urinary tract: evaluation of complete remissions by site. *Proceedings of the American Society of Clinical Oncology* 3: 160.

Hillcoat, B.L. and Raghavan, D. (1986). A randomized comparison of cisplatinum (C) versus cisplatinum and methotrexate (C+M) in advanced bladder cancer. *Proceedings of the American Society of Clinical Oncology* 5: 110.

Holland, J.F., Scharlan, C., Gailani, S. *et al.* (1972). Vincristine treatment of advanced cancer: a cooperative study of 392 cases. *Cancer Research* 33: 1258–64.

Khandehar, J.D., Elson, P.J., Dearp, W.D. and Slayton, R. (1981). Comparative activity and toxicity of cis-diammine dichloroplatinum (DDP) vs. cyclophosphamide (CTX), Adriamycin (ADR) and DDP (CAP) in disseminated transitional cell carcinomas of the urinary tract. *Proceedings of the American Society of Clinical Oncology* 22: 461.

Jacobs, C., Meyeers, F., Hendrickson, C. *et al.* (1983). A randomized phase III study of cisplatin with or without methotrexate for recurrent squamous cell carcinoma of the head and neck: a Northern California Oncology Group study. *Cancer* 52: 1563–9.

Knight, E.W., Pagano, A.M., Hahn, R.G. and Horan, J. (1983). Comparison of 5-fluorouracil and doxorubicin in the treatment of selected patients with invasive urothetheliol tumors. *Cancer Treatment Reports* 67: 514–15.

Levi, J.A., Aroney, R.S. and Dalley, D.N. (1980). Combination chemotherapy with cyclophosphamide, doxorubicin and bleomycin for metastatic transitional cell carcinoma of urinary tract. *Cancer Treatment Reports* 64: 1011–13.

Logothetis, C.T., Samuels, M.L., Selig, D.E., Wallace, S. and Johnson, D.E. (1985). Combined intravenous and intra-arterial cyclophosphamide, doxorubicin and cisplatin (CISCA) in the management of selected patients with invasive urothelial tumors. *Cancer Treatment Reports* 69: 33–8.

Lundbeck, F. and Christopherson, I.S. (1979). Phase II study of Adriamycin, 5FU, levamisole and irradiation in carcinoma of the bladder. *Cancer Treatment Reports* 63: 183.

Merrin, C. (1978). Treatment of advanced bladder cancer with cis-diaminodichloroplatinum (II) (NSC 119875): a pilot study. *Journal of Urology* 119: 493–5.

Merrin, C., Carbogena, R., Waxman, S., Baumgardner, C. and Murphy, G.P. (1975). Chemotherapy of bladder cancer with Cytoxan and Adriamycin. *Journal of Urology* 114: 884–7.

Natale, R.B., Wheeler, R.M., Ensminger, W. and Miller, D. (1983a). Cisplatin and dichloromethotrexate: a pharmacologically rational combination with high activity. *Proceedings of the American Association for Cancer Research* 24: 166.

Natale, R.B., Yagoda, A., Blumenreich, M.S. and Watson, R.C. (1983b). Phase II trial of amsacrine (AMSA) in urinary bladder cancer. *Cancer Treatment Reports* 67: 391–2.

Natale, R.B., Yagoda, A., Kelsen, D.P., Gralla, P.J. and Watson, R.C. (1982). Phase II trial of PALA in hypernephroma and urinary bladder cancer. *Cancer Treatment Reports* 66: 2091–2.

Natale, R.B., Yagoda, A., Watson, R.C. and Stover, P.E. (1980). Phase II trial of neocarzinostatin in patients with bladder and prostatic cancer. *Cancer* 45: 1879–88.

Natale, R.B., Yagoda, A., Watson, R.C., Whitmore, W.F., Blumenreich, M. and

Braun, G.W. (1981). Methotrexate: an active drug in bladder cancer. *Cancer* **47**: 1246–50.

Needles, B., Ahmed, T., Blumenreich, M., Yagoda, A. and Watson, R.C. (1982). Phase II trial of vinblastine (VIB) and methotrexate (MTX) in urothelial tract tumors. *Proceedings of the American Society of Clinical Oncology* **1**: 113.

Oliver, R.T.D., England, M.R., Risden, R.A. and Blandy, J.P. (1984). Methotrexate in the treatment of metastatic and recurrent primary transitional cell carcinoma. *Journal of Urology* **131**: 483–5.

Pavone-Macaluso, M. (1972). Chemotherapy of vesical and prostatic tumors. *British Journal of Urology* **43**: 701–8.

Peters, P.C. and O'Neill, M.R. (1980). Cis-diaminodichloroplatinum as a therapeutic agent in metastatic transitional cell carcinoma. *Journal of Urology* **123**: 375–7.

Qazi, R., Elson, P. and Khandehar, J.D. (1982). Phase II evaluation of VM-26 in patients with metastatic transitional cell carcinoma of the urinary tract: an ECOG study. *Cancer Treatment Reports* **66**: 405–6.

Raghavan, D., Pearson, B., Duval, P. *et al.* (1985). Initial intravenous cis-platinum therapy: improved management for invasive high-risk bladder cancer? *Journal of Urology* **133**: 399–402.

Samuels, M.L., Logothetis, C., Trindade, A. and Johnson, D.E. (1980). Cyclophosphamide, Adriamycin, and cisplatin (CISCA) in metastatic bladder cancer. *Proceedings of the American Association for Cancer Research* **21**: 137.

Schaeffer, A.J., Grayhack, J.T., Merrill, J.M., Bulkley, G.J. and Shethy, R.M. (1982). Treatment of stage D bladder cancer with adjuvant doxorubicin hydrochloride and radiation. *Urology* **20**: 393–400.

Schaeffer, A.J., Grayhack, J.T., Merrill, J.A.M., Kies, M.S., Bulkley, G.J., Shethy, R.M. and Clonick, T.S. (1984). Adjuvant doxorubicin hydrochloride and radiation in stage D bladder cancer: a preliminary report. *Journal of Urology* **132**: 1073–6.

Schwartz, S., Yagoda, A., Natale, R.B., Watson, R.C., Whitmore, W.F. and Lesser, M. (1983). Phase II trials of sequentially administered cisplatinum, cyclophosphamide and doxorubicin for urothelial tract tumors. *Journal of Urology* **130**: 681–4.

Shipley, W.U., Coombs, L.J., Einstein, A.B., Soloway, M.S., Waxman, A., Prout, G.R. and NBCCGA (1984). Cisplatin and full dose irradiation for patients with invasive bladder carcinoma: a preliminary report of tolerance and local response. *Journal of Urology* **132**: 899–908.

Smalley, R.V., Bartolucci, A.A., Hernstreet, G. and Hester, M. (1981). A phase II evaluation of a 3-drug combination of cyclophosphamide, doxorubicin and 5-fluorouracil and of 5-fluorouracil in patients with advanced bladder carcinoma or stage D prostatic carcinoma. *Journal of Urology* **125**: 191–5.

Soloway, M.S. (1978). Cis-diaminodichloroplatinum II in advanced urothelial cancer. *Journal of Urology* **120**: 716–19.

Soloway, M.S., Einstein, A., Corder, M.P., Bonney, W., Prout, G.R. and Coombs, J. (1983). A comparison of cisplatin and the combination of cisplatin and cyclophosphamide in advanced urothelial cancer. *Cancer* **52**: 767–72.

Soloway, M.S., Ikard, M. and Ford, K. (1981). Cis-diaminodichloroplatinum in locally advanced and metastatic urothelial cancer. *Cancer* **47**: 476–480.

Sternberg, C.N., Yagoda, A., Scher, H.I., Watson, R.C., Ahmed, T., Weiselberg, L.R., Geller, N., Hollander, P.S., Herr, H.W., Sogaru, P.C., Morse, M.J.

and Whitmore, W.F. (1985). Preliminary results of M-VAC (methotrexate, vinblastine, doxorubicin and cisplatin) for transitional cell carcinoma of the urothelium. *Journal of Urology* **133**: 403–7.

Sternberg, J.J., Bracken, R.B., Handel, P.B. and Johnson, D.E. (1977). Combination chemotherapy (CISCA) for advanced urinary tract carcinoma: a preliminary report. *JAMA* **238**: 2282–7.

Sternberg, C.N., Yagoda, A., Scher, H.I., Watson, R.C., Hollander, P.S., Herr, H.W., Sogani, P.C., Morse, M.J., Fair, W.R. and Whitmore, W.F. (1985). M-VAC: update of methotrexate, vinblastine, Adriamycin and cisplatin for urothelial tract cancer. *ASCO Abstracts* #C-409, p. 105.

Stoter, G., Fossa, S.D., Kline, J.G.M. *et al.* (1985). Combination chemotherapy with cisplatin (DDP) and methotrexate (Mtx) in advanced bladder cancer: an EORTC phase II study. *Proceedings of the American Society of Clinical Oncology* **4**: 106.

Tannock, I.F. (1983). Methotrexate and mitomycin for patients with metastic transitional cell cancer of the urinary tract. *Cancer Treatment Reports* **67**: 503–4.

Tannock, I.F., Gospodarowicz, M. and Evans, W.K. (1983). Chemotherapy for metastatic transitional cell cancer of urinary tract. *Cancer* **51**: 216–219.

Torti, F.M., Bristow, M.R., Howes, A.E. *et al.* (1983). Reduced cardiotoxicity of doxorubicin delivered on a weekly schedule. *Annals of International Medicine* **99**: 745–9.

Trump, D.L., Loening, S., Ahmed, S.W. and Waxman, A. (1983). Phase II study of amsacrine in previously treated patients with advanced TC cancer of urothelium: a NBC collaborative group A study. *Cancer Treatment Reports* **67**: 845–6.

Turner, A.G., Hendry, W.F., Williams, G.B. and Bloom, H.J.G. (1977). The treatment of advanced bladder cancer with methotrexate. *British Journal of Urology* **49**: 673–8.

Wallace, S., Chuang, V.P., Samuels, M. and Johnson, D. (1982). Transcatheter intra-arterial infusion of chemotherapy in advanced bladder cancer. *Cancer* **49**: 640–5.

Weisenthal, L.M., Lalude, A.O. and Miller, J.B. (1983). *In vitro* chemosensitivity of human bladder cancer. *Cancer* **51**: 1490–6.

Whitmore, W.F., Batata, M.A., Ghoneim, M.A. and Gradstald, H. (1977). Radical cystectomy with or without prior irradiation in the treatment of bladder cancer. *Journal of Urology* **120**: 716–19.

Williams, S.D., Rohn, R.J., Donohue, J.P. *et al.* (1978). Chemotherapy of bladder cancer with cis-diamminodichloroplatinum, Adriamycin and 5-fluorouracil. *Proceedings of the American Society of Clinical Oncology* **19**: 316.

Yagoda, A. (1979). Phase II trials with cis-dichlorodiammeplatinum (II) in the treatment of urothelial cancer. *Cancer Treatment Reports* **63**: 1565–1572.

Yagoda, A. (1980). Chemotherapy of metastatic bladder cancer. *Cancer* **45**: 1879–88.

Yagoda, A. (1983). Chemotherapy for advanced urothelial cancer. *Seminars in Urology* **1**: 60–74.

Yagoda, A. (1985). Progress in the treatment of advanced urothelial tract tumors. *Journal of Clinical Oncology* **3**: 1448.

Yagoda, A., Watson, R.C., Gonzalez-Vitale, J.C., Grabstald, H. and Whitmore, W.F. (1976). Cis-dichlorodiamminoplatinum (II) in advanced bladder cancer. *Cancer Treatment Reports* **60**: 917–23.

Yagoda, A., Watson, R.C., Grabstald, H., Barzell, W.E. and Whitmore, W.F.

(1977). Adriamycin and cyclophosphamide in advanced bladder cancer. *Cancer Treatment Reports* **61**: 97–9.
Yagoda, A., Watson, R.C., Whitmore, W.F., Grabstald, H., Middleman, M.P. and Krakoff, I.H. (1977). Adriamycin in advanced urinary tract cancer. *Cancer* **39**: 279–85.

13

The management of bladder cancer in Scotland

S.B. Kaye, R.H. MacDougall, R.P. Symonds and D.A. Tolley

Introduction

Bladder cancer is a common problem in Scotland, affecting one in six thousand adults each year. The majority of patients are treated in the two largest referral centres, at Glasgow and Edinburgh, and in this chapter management policies over the past decade are reviewed. The data indicate that for both superficial and invasive disease, a more selective approach to treatment may lead to optimal results. However, these results remain far from satisfactory in certain subgroups, and the use of chemotherapy holds some promise for further improvements.

In order to assist in the development of new treatment strategies in this and other urological cancers, a Scottish Urological Oncology Group was formed in 1983, representing urologists and oncologists in most parts of the country.

Patient assessment

The assessment and management of patients with bladder cancer requires a multidisciplinary approach, and this is facilitated in Edinburgh by means of a combined weekly cystoscopy clinic, first set up by Duncan, Selby-Tulloch and Newsam, and now routinely attended by urologists and radiation oncologists. This system has led to improvements in accurate staging and assessment of the disease (Hindmarsh *et al.*, 1983). Cystourethroscopy with resection of the exophytic part of the tumour and deep biopsies of the base in invasive cases is performed routinely, and pre- and post-resection bimanual examinations under the same general anaesthetic are carried out by both urologist and radiation oncologist. An essential aspect of this examination is that patients are fully relaxed, allowing the insertion of 2 fingers into the rectum for proper disease evaluation. Weekly clinicopathological meetings which have included histopathologists have been an important means for ensuring uniform baseline assessment, and in this way, management has been determined. Increased collaboration between units, by means of computerized records, may lead to a better understanding of the natural history of the disease.

The Edinburgh group has also established that bone scintigraphy is not indicated as a routine investigation in patients with bladder cancer without symptoms of metastases (Davey *et al.*, 1985), while lymphography does predict prognosis but at present has no therapeutic implications (Rodger *et al.*, 1980).

Superficial tumours

The majority of patients with bladder cancer have superficial tumours, and while many of these are easy to treat by endoscopic resection, tumour recurrence occurs after complete resection in about 70 per cent of patients (Green *et al.*, 1973; England *et al.*, 1982). Many tumours recur with a higher degree of malignancy than the primary tumour (Green *et al.*, 1973). The 5-year survival rate following endoscopic management only is about 72 per cent (Williams *et al.*, 1977) and in 10 per cent of patients the tumour will progress to invasive carcinoma (Green *et al.*, 1973). The reason for this high recurrence rate is unknown but may be due to implantation of tumour cells during primary endoscopic management; recurrent tumours might develop as new primary tumours in an already unstable urothelium.

Superficial bladder cancer therefore carries a significant risk to the patient and repeated follow-up cystoscopies are required. In an elderly population, this in itself can cause significant morbidity and check cytoscopies for bladder cancer form a large part of the workload of a department of urology.

Superficial bladder tumours are readily accessible to the direct action of anticancer drugs instilled via a urethral catheter, and, in an attempt to reduce recurrence rate, intravesical chemotherapy was first used in 1961 (Jones and Swinney, 1961). Easy accessibility permits a high concentration of chemotherapeutic agents with minimal local systemic toxicity. There is now clear evidence that intravesical chemotherapy reduces the recurrence rate after primary transurethral resection (Jacobi, 1982; Schulman, 1982). It may also delay the development of invasive bladder cancer (Kurth *et al.*, 1983; Green *et al.*, 1983).

Many urologists in Scotland, and indeed throughout the United Kingdom, use transurethral resection and repeated cytoscopies to control most superficial bladder tumours, but the formation of the Scottish Urological Group in 1983 has provided an opportunity for collaborative studies to assess the role of intravesical chemotherapy in the management of superficial bladder cancer. Three units also collaborate with the Medical Research Council, which undertakes collaborative studies within the United Kingdom.

This section reports our experience with these trials and gives a schema for the management of patients with superficial bladder cancer in the Department of Urology, Edinburgh Royal Infirmary.

MRC studies

The Medical Research Council's working party on bladder cancer activated a protocol for the study of thiotepa in superficial bladder cancer in October 1981, and the results of study were published (MRC Working Party, 1985). All patients with previously untreated superficial (Ta or T1) transitional cell carcinomas of the bladder were treated by routine transurethral resection. The patients were then randomized to receive either no thiotepa or a single dose of thiotepa (30 mg) immediately after resection, while a third group received a further instillation of thiotepa at each 3-monthly check cystoscopy for one year. Four hundred and seventeen patients with newly diagnosed superficial tumours were entered from 15 centres throughout the UK, and regular check cystoscopies revealed no significant difference in the rate at which tumours recurred in the three groups ($p=0.4$, $p=0.7$ for control versus thiotepa given once and 5 times respectively).

It was concluded that neither thiotepa regimen produces sufficient improvement to justify its use in this group of patients, and a further MRC study was started in March 1984 in which mitomycin C was substituted for thiotepa. This study has recruited over 250 patients from many participating centres and there are now three participating units in Scotland.

The Scottish Urological Oncology Group recently completed a phase-II study to judge the efficacy of mitomycin C when used for primary therapy in patients with superficial bladder cancer (McFarlane *et al.*, 1985). There were four collaborating centres.

Twenty-five patients with primary or recurrent multifocal transitional cell carcinoma of the bladder (TIS, Ta or T1) which could no longer be controlled endoscopically were entered into the study. Patients received 7 weekly instillations of 40 mg mitomycin C in 40 ml sterile water via a urethral catheter. The solution was retained in the bladder for 2 hours. Cytoscopic assessment was carried out at 4, 8 and 12 weeks after the initial treatment and biopsy of any remaining tumours together with endoscopic destruction was carried out at the 12-week cystoscopy.

The overall response rate was 70 per cent (complete response 43 per cent, partial response 27 per cent), which was rather lower than that reported in previous studies using a more intensive (thrice-weekly) schedule (Harrison *et al.*, 1983).

Two other important observations were noted. First, there was a higher response rate in patients with Ta tumours than in those with T1 tumours for whom more intensive treatment may be more appropriate. Second, in those patients who responded to treatment, the response was evident at 8 weeks and there seems to be little point in continuing with therapy after this time if no response is seen.

Although intravesical chemotherapy is undoubtedly an effective treatment modality for patients with superficial tumours, our knowledge of the optimum dose and timing of administration and identification of the most suitable patients is as yet limited. To this end there is collaboration between urologists in Scotland and the EORTC, whose studies are described in further detail in Chapter 14.

If progress is to be made in the treatment of this condition, there is need for continuing collaboration on both a national and international scale. The management plan indicated in Fig. 13.1 which we have adopted provides us with the greatest opportunity for collaboration.

An alternative approach to the management of certain groups of patients with superficial bladder cancer is the use of radiotherapy. External-beam irradiation has been used for patients with multiple, well-differentiated T1 tumours, but in the experience of the Edinburgh group (Quilty and Duncan, 1986) it is doubtful whether radiotherapy makes any significant contribution, since local control at 5 years is only 16 per cent.

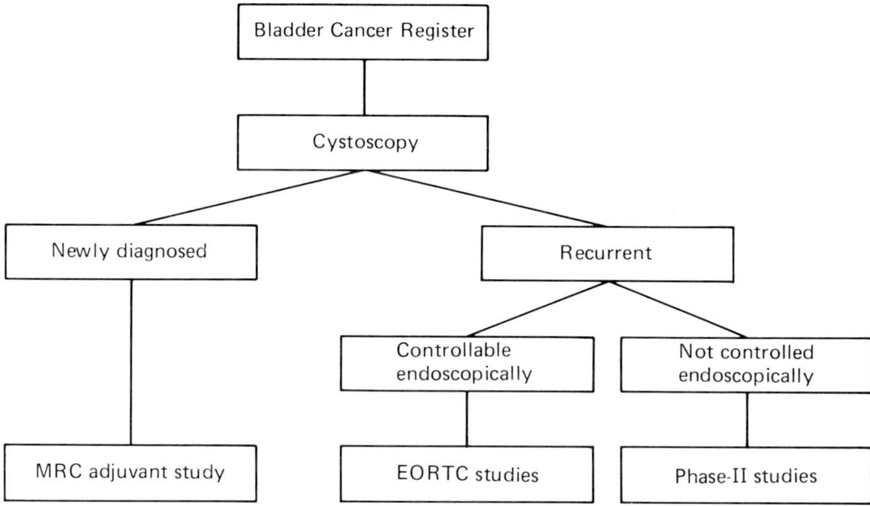

Fig. 13.1 Schema for the management of superficial bladder cancer in the Royal Infirmary, Edinburgh

In contrast, patients with poorly differentiated (grade III) T1 or pT2 tumours are prone to recur after endoscopic resection, and radiotherapy has a major place in their management. Quilty and Duncan (1985) indicated a 5-year local control rate of 55.6 per cent in such patients. No patients with grade-III T1 cancer had either local recurrence or distant metastases between 5 and 10 years after treatment, suggesting long-term cure. They concluded that although radical radiotherapy offered little probability of control of T1 tumours of grades I and II, it was clearly useful for grade-III superficial transitional cell carcinoma. As well as offering a high degree of local control, it appears to reduce the risk of subsequent metastases, and is recommended as the treatment of choice in that group.

In Glasgow, solitary tumours of this poorly differentiated type under 4 cm in diameter were in the past treated with a permanent radioactive implant using radioactive gold (Au^{198}) seeds. The 5-year survival for patients treated this way between 1969 and 1974 was 68 per cent. However, this technique is no longer used, chiefly because of improved endoscopic techniques and the greater availability of megavoltage irradiation. Because patients with these tumours have an unstable urothelium, the whole bladder is treated with a margin of normal tissue around the tumour, using external irradiation as in Edinburgh.

Radiotherapy for invasive tumours

For practical purposes, T2 and T3 tumours are often grouped together, since it is difficult to distinguish them clinically (Chisholm *et al.*, 1980), and since in some (but not all) studies the prognosis for grade-III T2 and T3 tumours treated by radiotherapy is very similar (Blandy *et al.*, 1980).

In Scotland the standard treatment for invasive bladder cancer remains radical primary radiotherapy with retrieval surgery. However, the technique differs in the two referral centres.

In Glasgow the view has been taken that pelvic lymph nodes should be included within the irradiated volume. This approach, however, is not shared by some other centres, including Edinburgh (see below) and Manchester, England (Pointon, 1985), which advocate treatment of the bladder alone. It is perhaps noteworthy that no randomized trial in T3 bladder cancer comparing treatment volumes has yet been performed, and comparison of different series can clearly be misleading.

The basis for the Glasgow technique is the observation by Bloom (1980) that 40–50 per cent of surgically treated T3 cases have pelvic lymph node metastases. Furthermore, analysis of the Institute of Urology trial (Bloom *et al.*, 1982) indicated that the most favourable results were obtained in those patients receiving preoperative irradiation in whom sterilization of pelvic lymph nodes was demonstrated surgically, in association with pathological downstaging of primary tumour.

The radiation field encompasses lymph nodes below the iliac bifurcation, since involvement of lymph nodes above this point is associated with more distant spread and complications are more likely when a larger volume is treated. The tolerance of surrounding normal tissue limits the radiation dose which can be given to any tumour. The tolerance of small bowel limits the dose which can be given to the true pelvis, but the dose of 40–50 Gy in 4–5 weeks is sufficient to control small lymph node metastases. However, it is insufficient to eliminate bulky bladder tumours and a higher dose must be given as a boost to the bladder.

A trial of radiotherapy in hyperbaric oxygen conducted in Glasgow provided considerable insight into the radiation tolerance of the bladder (Kirk *et al.*, 1976). Twenty-seven patients were randomly allocated to receive radiotherapy (60 Gy in 24 fractions over 5 weeks), in either air or hyperbaric oxygen. Treatment was given by an anterior and two anterior oblique fields, but only two fields were treated each day. No differences in toxicity or tumour control were noted in the two arms, but a total of 9 patients developed severe high-dose effects requiring surgery (8 required cystectomy and one required transplantation of the ureters). No tumour could be found in the excised specimens.

Although all patients received the same modal dose, analysis using the 'cumulative radiation effect' (CRE) formula revealed unsuspected high-dose areas in the bladder, and a close correlation between the development of high-dose effects and the maximum CRE value was found. The CRE is an isoeffect formula developed in Glasgow which attempts to estimate the biological effect on normal connective tissue of differing radiation schedules (Kirk *et al.*, 1971). High-dose effects were not seen below a maximum value of 1910 radiation equivalent units (reu), which seems to be the tolerance value for the whole bladder.

A clear relationship between tumour control and radiation dose was elegantly demonstrated by Morrison (1975). He treated patients with bladder cancer at doses of 42.5 to 62.5 Gy over 4 weeks (CRE values of 1435–2110 reu). Tumour control rose from 37 to 80 per cent with increasing dose, but at the highest level of local control a 37 per cent serious-complication rate was noted. Detailed analysis using the CRE formula has shown that the complication rate rose sharply when a CRE value of 1910 reu was exceeded.

This CRE analysis has been the basis of the radiation schedule used in Glasgow since 1982 for patients with T3 bladder cancer. A total dose of 42.5 Gy is given in 20 fractions over 4 weeks to the true pelvis followed by a boost to the bladder of 21.5 Gy in 10 fractions. The total modal dose is 64 Gy in 6 weeks (1900 reu). To date complications have been negligible, and 43 out of 46 evaluable patients (93 per cent) have shown no evidence of tumour when cystoscoped 3 months after radiotherapy. Subsequently 7 (15 per cent) have developed a local recurrence and 7 (15 per cent) distant metastases with no local recurrence. Eight patients are dead from tumour and 2 have died from ischaemic heart disease whilst in remission. Currently 27 patients (59 per cent) are tumour-free with a mean follow-up time of 17 months. These results are superior to those achieved during 1980–82. During this period 60 Gy was given in 6 weeks (1766 reu). Using that technique 41 out of 61 (67 per cent) achieved complete tumour control and 36 per cent are currently tumour-free with a mean follow-up time of 42 months.

Between 1969 and 1974 the overall 5-year survival of all cases of transitional cell carcinoma treated in the Western Infirmary, Glasgow, by radiotherapy was 32 per cent. Preliminary data suggest that an increase in dose to 64 Gy may lead to an increased survival rate, but these results are probably the best that can be obtained using conventional fractionated megavoltage radiotherapy. Additional methods, including the use of the radiosensitizer misonidazole or hyperbaric oxygen, have not led to increased survival. It is possible that the use of chemotherapy together with radiother-apy may improve local control and ultimately survival (see below). In addition, radiation treatment of large fields might not be necessary if effective chemotherapy were available to eradicate disease in involved regional lymph nodes.

In contrast to the Glasgow approach, the radiotherapy technique used in Edinburgh is a 3-field beam-directed technique in which the whole bladder is irradiated within the pelvis to a modal target dose of 55 Gy delivered in 20 fractions over 4 weeks. Field size is normally 10×10 cm. Duncan and Quilty (1986) have reviewed the experience of treating 963 patients in this way over a 10-year period, and this allowed a retrospective stratification into various subgroups. These included T stage, and analysis showed that the 5-year survival rates were: 61 per cent for T1 (190 patients); 40 per cent for T2 (284 patients); 26 per cent for T3 (333 patients); and 12 per cent for T4 (82 patients). Subsequently, a detailed multivariate analysis (Quilty *et al.*, 1986) has identified prognostic variables which can be used to identify the patients most likely to respond well to radiotherapy. Age, T stage, tumour size and haemoglobin level at diagnosis were found to be independent covariates and combined to give a prognostic index. The 'good prognosis' group comprised 26 per cent of patients. By selecting for treatment patients with T1 and T2 tumours who are under 75 years of age, have a tumour size of less than 5 cm and a normal haemoglobin level, impressive 5-year survival rates of 70 per cent can be achieved by the routine radiotherapy technique described above. Using the above prognostic index, a 'moderate prognosis' group (compris-ing 32 per cent of the total) had a 5-year survival of 47 per cent; a 'fair prognosis' group (32 per cent of the total) had a 5-year survival of 31 per cent; while a 'poor prognosis' group (10 per cent of the total) had a 5-year survival of only 6 per cent. Previous trials and comparisons between other treatment modalities in bladder cancer have not taken these factors into account and misleading impressions have been obtained.

Local control was also analysed in the same way. T stage, grade, haemoglobin and urea level at diagnosis were found to be significant covariates and combined to derive a tumour control index. This type of analysis is important because when results of radiotherapy are reported in terms of survival alone a misleading impression may be given of its success in disease control.

Quilty *et al.* (1986) suggested that both the prognostic index and the local tumour control index should be used in decision making about optimum management. They are based on simple data which should normally be available soon after the initial assessment at cystoscopy, biopsy and bimanual examination under general anaesthesia. This points the way to a selective approach to treatment and subsequent benefits to the individual patient. In summary, the results of treatment in Glasgow and Edinburgh are broadly similar, but remain less than satisfactory.

Neutron therapy of bladder cancer

In 1976, a cyclotron was provided by the Medical Research Council for evaluation by the Department of Radiation Oncology in Edinburgh. Invasive transitional cell carcinoma of the bladder was one of the areas examined in a randomized controlled trial to study the effects of neutron therapy compared with megavoltage x-ray therapy. One hundred and thirteen patients were recruited to this trial. The overall tumour control rate was 43 per cent in both treatment groups and was related to T stage. There was no statistically significant difference in the control rates between the two treatment groups by T stage.

The actuarial 5-year survival rate, however, was 12 per cent for the neutron group and 45 per cent for the photon (megavoltage) group. This difference is highly significant and is principally due to the high late radiation morbidity affecting bowel and bladder seen in the neutron group and subsequent high late radiation mortality in this group. It is concluded that there is no therapeutic advantage in neutron therapy for bladder cancer (Duncan *et al.*, 1985). Of interest is the observation that the survival rates for the control (photon-treated) group in this randomized study are superior to those in the earlier retrospective series. The supportive care of the patients in this study (prompt treatment of urinary infection, regular blood transfusions, etc.) was intensive, and this could partly explain the difference, which might also be partly due to differences in staging.

Chemotherapy

As described elsewhere in this volume, activity has been demonstrated for a range of cytotoxic drugs in advanced bladder cancer. However, as single agents, response rates have been relatively low and response duration modest. Combinations of drugs have sometimes yielded higher response rates, but results have been variable, and there are no randomized studies clearly indicating superiority over single agents. Moreover, in advanced disease the toxicity of treatment may outweigh the benefits in terms of palliation, although it is clearly important to identify active combinations for use at an earlier stage (see below).

Against this background, some of the recent reports of combinations which include cisplatinum have been particularly encouraging. The combination of cisplatinum with vinblastine, Adriamycin and methotrexate, used at the Memorial Sloan Kettering Cancer Center, is reported to yield an overall response rate of 76 per cent (including 36 per cent complete responses) among 69 evaluable patients with advanced disease (Sternberg *et al.*, 1985). Moreover, the responses seemed durable, with a median response duration of over a year for complete responders. However, the four-drug combination certainly leads to substantial toxicity, probably to a greater extent than the two-drug combination of methotrexate and cisplatinum which has been assessed in several studies (see Chapters 14, 15 and 17).

In Scotland the combination of methotrexate and cisplatinum has received attention both in Glasgow and Edinburgh. Because of the possibility of enhanced drug toxicity using this combination of nephrotoxic drugs together, a pharmacokinetic study was carried out in Glasgow to exclude the possibility that cisplatinum-induced renal damage might enhance methotrexate toxicity (Kaye *et al.*, 1984). Five patients with advanced bladder cancer received treatment with methotrexate ($50 \, mg/m^2$) every two weeks, and with every alternate course cisplatinum ($50 \, mg/m^2$) was given simultaneously with appropriate hydration diuresis. Methotrexate clearance was measured in a total of 12 courses, by means of serial plasma measurements using the EMIT assay.

The results indicated that the use of simultaneously administered cisplatinum did not affect methotrexate clearance in 4 patients with normal renal function, while in one patient in whom the clearance of methotrexate was delayed when given alone, there was actually an improvement when methotrexate was given with cisplatinum (together with hydration). There was no evidence of enhanced methotrexate toxicity (e.g. mucositis or myelosuppression) in any patient in the study. Thus it appears that when using methotrexate and cisplatinum together in patients with bladder cancer simultaneous administration is a safe method of treatment.

Meanwhile in Edinburgh, the combination of methotrexate and cisplatinum was given to 19 patients with recurrent or metastatic bladder cancer, albeit using a slightly different schedule: methotrexate $200 \, mg/m^2$ as a 24-hour infusion with cisplatin $100 \, mg/m^2$ given 3-weekly (Carmichael *et al.*, 1985). An objective response rate of 68 per cent was obtained, including 21 per cent complete responders. The median duration of response was 21 weeks, median survival 54 weeks and the most responsive disease sites were lung (73 per cent objective response) and lymph nodes (100 per cent).

Cisplatinum, although clearly active in bladder cancer (Yagoda, 1979), possesses significant toxicity, particularly gastrointestinal, and it has therefore been appropriate to attempt to replace it with a less toxic but equally effective analogue. Carboplatin (JM8) has been identified as one of the current cisplatinum analogues with a more favourable toxicity profile (Calvert *et al.*, 1982) (see Chapter 10). As the first of a series of studies the Chemotherapy Sub-Committee of the MRC Bladder Cancer Group have therefore performed a phase-II study of carboplatin in 48 patients with measurable metastatic bladder cancer, with the support of members of the Scottish Urological Oncology Group (MRC Working Party, 1987). Of the 48 patients (mean age 62 years) treated with carboplatin, 30 had received no prior chemotherapy. For patients with normal renal function, a dose of 400 mg/m^2 as a 1-hour infusion was given, although this was reduced to 300 mg/m^2 for patients aged over 65 years and also reduced to 100–200 mg/m^2 in the presence of significantly impaired renal function (present in 14 of the 48 patients). Carboplatin was repeated at 4-weekly intervals for 3 cycles before reassessment took place.

Treatment was reasonably well tolerated, the only significant side effects being minor myelosuppression, nausea and vomiting. With respect to myelosuppression, a WBC of less than 2.0×10^9/l was recorded on a total of only four occasions, and a platelet count of less than 50×10^9/l on only nine occasions, including all 3 cycles in all 48 patients. Vomiting was described as severe in only 8 of the 48 patients, and 2 of these withdrew from treatment, which was generally better tolerated than cisplatinum.

Unfortunately the response rate was significantly lower than had previously been reported for single-agent cisplatinum. No complete responses were seen, and only three partial responses (6 per cent) were confirmed out of a total of 48 patients. Further studies with carboplatin are in progress elsewhere, and although it remains possible that a higher response rate will be achieved using higher doses of carboplatin (associated with more severe myelosuppression), for the present cisplatinum remains a major component of current protocols.

The MRC Bladder Cancer Group Sub-Committee has now turned its attention to new cytotoxic agents of different classes, and is currently performing a phase-II study of mitozolomide, a new nitrosourea developed at Aston University in Birmingham, which is well absorbed orally and has demonstrated high levels of preclinical activity in tumour xenografts (Hickman *et al.*, 1985).

Combined modalities

The survival data cited in this chapter for patients receiving radical radiotherapy for invasive bladder cancer confirm that the overall outlook for patients with T3 and T4 disease remains poor. At least in part this reflects the inability of this treatment to prevent the emergence of metastatic disease, despite adequate local control. Thus increasing attention has turned towards combined modality approaches. In view of the responses seen in patients with metastatic disease for several cytotoxic agents, earlier studies examined the role of these drugs given as part of primary therapy for invasive bladder cancer. The aim was to attempt therapy for micrometastatic disease at an early stage and also to induce shrinkage in the local tumour prior to local irradiation. This approach was first used in Glasgow in 1979, when a pilot study in 17 patients with T3 bladder cancer was initiated (Kaye *et al.*, 1985). The study was designed to assess the feasibility and impact on survival of a course of chemotherapy (4 cycles of cyclophosphamide, methotrexate and 5-fluorouracil) prior to radical radiotherapy (60 Gy in 6 weeks). In addition it was hoped that data on the effect of chemotherapy on the primary tumour (as opposed to the previously published data on the effect on metastatic disease) would become available. This three-drug combination (CMF) was chosen because each agent had previously been reported to be active in bladder cancer (Turner *et al.*, 1977; de Kernion, 1977), although the reported response rates would probably not be reproduced using modern criteria.

A total of 17 patients entered this initial study, which closed for trial entry in 1981. Follow-up data are now available for a minimum of 3 years after entry. It was possible to conclude that, although the use of chemotherapy as primary therapy was feasible and did not lead to increased toxicity, there was no survival advantage in comparison with earlier series of patients treated with radiotherapy alone for invasive bladder cancer; 13 of the 17 patients have died and the median survival for patients in the study was 27 months, with a 3-year survival rate of 26 per cent. Disease recurrence occurred both locally and in metastatic sites. Four patients remain alive and disease-free, at 44, 68, 69 and 71 months.

The study served to emphasize that assessment of response to chemotherapy as initial treatment for the primary bladder tumour was very difficult, partly because of the variable extent of the initial diagnostic biopsy. Assessment was attempted using bimanual examination, cystoscopy and ultrasound examination, and in no case was a clear response in a measurable primary tumour documented prior to radiotherapy.

The conclusion of the study was that if chemotherapy is used as part of initial treatment other drug combinations would be necessary, probably incorporating cisplatinum. In addition, careful assessment of tumour response is required, including ultrasound or CT scans of the pelvis after the initial biopsy, but prior to the start of chemotherapy.

Combined modality programmes involving cisplatinum-containing chemotherapy regimens together with radiotherapy are discussed elsewhere in the volume (see Chapter 15). In some studies cisplatinum has been given simultaneously with radiotherapy, in order to capitalize on its experimental properties as a radiosensitizer (Soloway *et al.*, 1979). Although response rates using this approach have been reported to be high, the possibility of enhanced normal tissue damage is a major consideration. Experience in Glasgow of one patient treated with cisplatinum (30 mg/m^2) during a course of radical radiotherapy for T3 bladder cancer was noteworthy, in that major post-treatment problems of early radiation damage led to the patient's death. On the other hand, experience in other diseases with the use of cisplatinum prior to radiotherapy has been much more favourable. In a pilot study in stage III and stage IV cervical cancer, 22 patients received 2 courses of vincristine, bleomycin and cisplatinum prior to active radiotherapy to the pelvis (Symonds *et al.*, 1985). Local control rates have been very high, and at this stage there are no signs of enhanced radiation toxicity. With this background a study is now underway under the auspices of the M.R.C. in patients with previously untreated invasive bladder cancer whereby initial treatment comprises 2 courses of methotrexate, vinblastine and cisplatinum, which is one of the most effective combinations in metastatic bladder cancer (Harker *et al.*, 1985). Adriamycin is omitted because of potential interaction with subsequent radiotherapy. Disease will be reassessed by means of cystoscopy, repeat ultrasound and CT scans and repeat examination under anaesthetic. Responding patients will receive 2 further courses of chemotherapy prior to radical radiotherapy. The aim of the study is to assess the feasibility of such a combined modality approach, and if early results are encouraging a randomised M.R.C. study in invasive bladder cancer would be appropriate, whereby patients would receive radiotherapy with or without initial chemotherapy comprising methotrexate, vinblastine and cisplatinum.

References

Bloom, H.J.G. (1980). Pre-operative intermediate dose radiotherapy and cystectomy for deeply invasive carcinoma of the bladder: rationale and results. In *Bladder Cancer: Principles of Combination Therapy*, p. 151. Edited by Oliver, R.T.D., Hendry, W.F. and Bloom, H.J.G. Butterworth, London.

Bloom, H.J.G., Hendry, W.F., Wallace, D.M. and Skeet, R.G. (1982). Treatment of T3 bladder cancer: controlled trial of pre-operative radiotherapy and radical cystectomy versus radical radiotherapy. *British Journal of Urology* **54**: 136–51.

Carmichael, J., Cornbleet, M.A., MacDougall, R.H., Allan, S.G., Duncan, W., Chisholm, G.D. and Smyth, J.F. (1985). Cis-platin and methotrexate in the treatment of transitional cell carcinoma of the urinary tract. *British Journal of Urology* **57**: 299–302.

Calvert, A.H., Harland, S.J., Newell, D.R., Siddik, Z.H., Jones, A.C., McElwain, T.J., Raju, S., Wiltshaw, E., Smith, I.E., Baker, J.M., Peckham, M.J. and Harrap, K.R. (1982). Early clinical trials with cis-diamine-1,1-cyclobutane dicarboxylate platinum II. *Cancer Chemotherapy and Pharmacology* **9**: 140–47.

de Kernion, J.B. (1977). The chemotherapy of advanced bladder cancer. *Cancer Research* **37**: 2771–4.

Davey, P., Merrick, M.V., Duncan, W. and Redpath, A.T. (1985). Bladder cancer: the value of routine bone scintigraphy. *Clinical Radiology* **36**: 77–9.

Duncan, W., Arnott, F.J., Jack, W.J.L., MacDougall, R.H., Quilty, P.M., Rodger, A., Kerr, G.R. and Williams, J.R. (1985). A report of a randomised trial of d(15)+Be neutrons compared with megavoltage x-ray therapy of bladder cancer. *International Journal of Radiation Oncology, Biology and Biophysics* **11**: 2043–9.

Duncan, W. and Quilty, P.M. (1986). The results of a series of 963 patients with invasive transitional cell carcinoma of the urinary bladder primarily treated by radical megavoltage x-ray therapy. *Radiotherapy and Oncology* **7**: 299–310.

England, H.R., Blandy, J.P. and Harris, A.M.I. (1982). The treatment of single and multiple papillary tumours of the bladder. In *Bladder Tumours and Other Topics in Urological Oncology*, pp. 343–5. Edited by Pavone-Macaluso, Smith and Edsmyre. Plenum Press, New York.

Green, L.F., Hanash, K.A. and Farrow, G.M. (1973). Benign papilloma of papillary carcinoma of the bladder. *Journal of Urology* **110**: 205–7.

Green, D.F., Smith, P.H., Melvyn, R.G., Glashan, R., Newling, D. and Dalesio, O. (1983). Does intravesical chemotherapy prevent invasive bladder cancer? *AUA Las Vegas*, abstract 315.

Harker, W.G., Meyers, F.J., Freiha, F.S., Palmer, J.M., Shortliffe, L.D., Hannigan, J.F., McWhirter, K.M. and Torti, F.M. (1985). Cisplatin, methotrexate and vinblastine: an effective chemotherapy regimen for metastatic transitional cell carcinoma of the urinary tract. *Journal of Clinical Oncology* **3**: 1463–70.

Harrison, G.S., Green, D.F., Newling, D.W., Richards, B., Robinson, M.R. and Smith, P.H. (1983). Phase II study of intravesical mitomycin C in the treatment of superficial bladder cancer. *British Journal of Urology* **55**: 676–8.

Hickman, J.A., Stevens, M.F., Gibson, N.W., Langdon, S.P., Fizames, C., Lavelle, F., Atassi, G., Lunt, E. and Tilson, R.M. (1985). Experimental antitumour activity against murine tumour model systems of 8-carbamoyl-3-imidazo-tetrazin-4-one (mitozolomide), a novel broad-spectrum agent. *Cancer Research* **45**: 3008–13.

Hindmarsh, J.R., Theodourou, C., Hargreave, T.B., Webb, J., Busuttil, A., Newsam, J.E. and Chisholm, G.D. (1983). Diagnosis, management and treatment of superficial bladder cancer. *British Journal of Urology* **55**: 676–8.
follow-up of patients with bladder cancer. *Journal of the Royal College of Surgeons of Edinburgh* **28** (3): 135–40.

Jacobi, G. (1982). Chemotherapy for urinary bladder cancer: developments, trends and future perspectives. In *Clinical Bladder Cancer*, pp. 93–105. Edited by Denis, L., Smith, P. and Pavone-Macaluso, M. Plenum Press, New York.

Jones, H.C. and Swinney, J. (1962). Thiotepa in the treatment of tumours of the bladder. *Lancet* **2**: 615–16.

Kaye, S.B., MacFarlane, J.R., McHattie, I. and Hart, A.J. (1985). Chemotherapy before radiotherapy for T3 bladder cancer: a pilot study. *British Journal of Urology* **57**: 434–7.

Kaye, S.B., McWhinnie, D., Hart, A., Deane, R.F., Billiaert, P., Welsh, J., Milsted, R., Stuart, J.F.B. and Calman, K.C. (1984). The treatment of advanced bladder cancer with methotrexate and cisplatinum: a pharmaco-kinetic study. *European Journal of Cancer* **20**: 249–52.

Kirk, J., Gray, W.M. and Watson, E.R. (1971). Cummulative radiation effect. I: Fractionated treatment regimes. *Clinical Radiology* **22**: 145–55.

Kirk, J., Wingate, W.H. and Watson, E.R. (1976). High dose effects in the treatment of carcinoma of the bladder under air and hyperbaric oxygen conditions. *Clinical Radiology* **27**: 137–44.

Kurth, K.H., Maksimovic, P.A., Hop, W.C.J., Schroder, F.R. and Bakker, N.J. (1983). Single-dose intravesical Epodyl after TUR of Ta transitional cell bladder carcinoma. *World Journal of Urology* **1**: 89–93.

McFarlane, J.R., Tolley, D.A., and the Scottish Urological Oncology Group (1985). Report of a multicentre phase II study. *British Journal of Urology* **57**: 37–9.

MRC Working Party on Urological Cancer (1985). The effect of intravesical thiotepa on the recurrence rate of newly diagnosed superficial bladder cancer. *British Journal of Urology* **57**: 680–85.

M.R.C. Working Party on Urological Cancer (1987). A phase II study of carboplatin in metastatic transitional cell carcinoma of the bladder. *European Journal of Cancer and Clinical Oncology* **23**: 375–7.

Morrison, R. (1975). The results of treatment of cancer of the bladder: a clinical contribution to radiology. *Clinical Radiology* **26**: 67–75.

Pointon, R.C.S. (1985). The genito-urinary tract. In *Radiotherapy of malignant disease*, pp. 316–46. Edited by Easson, E.C. and Pointen, R.C.S. Springer-Verlag, New York.

Quilty, P.M. and Duncan, W. (1986). The treatment of superficial (T1) tumours of the bladder by radical radiotherapy. *British Journal of Urology* **58**: 147–52.

Quilty, P.M., Kerr, G.R. and Duncan, W. (1986) Prognostic indices for bladder cancer: an analysis of patients with transitional cell carcinoma of the bladder primarily treated by radical megavoltage x-ray therapy. *Radiotherapy and Oncology* **7**: 311–21.
Rodger, A., Wild, S.R. and Duncan, W. (1980). Bipedal lymphography in the management of bladder cancer. *Clinical Radiology* **31**: 555–8.
Soloway, M.S., Morris, C.R. and Sudderth, B. (1979). Radiation therapy and cis-platinum in transplantable and primary murine bladder cancer. *International Journal of Radiation Oncology, Biology and Physics* **5**: 1355–61.
Sternberg, C.N., Yagoda, A., Scher, H.I., Watson, R., Hollander, P.S., Herr, H.W., Sogani, P., Morse, M., Fair, W. and Whitmore, W.F. (1985). Update of methotrexate, vinblastine, Adriamycin and cisplatin for urothelial tract cancer. *Proceedings of the American Society of Clinical Oncology* **4**: 105.
Stoter, G., Fossa, S.D., Klein, J.G., Denis, L., Splinter, T., Jones, W.G., Keizer, J. and Sylvester, R. (1985). Combination chemotherapy with cisplatin and methotrexate in advanced cancer: an EORTC phase II study. *Proceedings of the American Society of Clinical Oncology* **4**: 106.
Symonds, R.P., Habeshaw, T., Kaye, S.B. and Watson, E.R. (1985). Combination chemotherapy prior to radical radiotherapy for stage III and IV carcinoma of cervix. In *Third European Conference on Clinical Oncology*, p. 462 (abstract). Stockholm.
Turner, A.G., Hendry, W.E., Williams, G.B. and Bloom, H.J.G. (1977). The treatment of advanced bladder cancer with methotrexate. *British Journal of Urology* **49**: 673–8.
Williams, J.L., Hammonds, J.C. and Saunders, J. (1977). T1 bladder tumours. *British Journal of Urology* **49**: 663–8.
Yagoda, A. (1979). Phase II trials with cis-dichlorodiaminine platinum in the treatment of urothelial cancer. *Cancer Treatment Reports* **63**: 1565–72.

14

Current status of bladder cancer protocols in the EORTC Genito-Urinary Tract Cancer Cooperative Group

L. Denis, K.H. Kurth, C. Bouffioux, M. Robinson, F. Debruyne, G. Stoter, R. Sylvester, M. De Pauw, and members of the EORTC Genito-Urinary Group

Introduction

The EORTC Genito-Urinary Tract Cancer Cooperative Group is one of the 31 clinical groups and working parties within the EORTC (European Organization for Research on Treatment of Cancer). This group has thus far conducted 33 clinical trials on urological cancers, involving approximately 5000 patients entered by investigators from 92 institutions located in 12 different European countries. These clinical trials consist of phase-II studies in bladder, prostate and renal cancer and phase-III studies in bladder, prostate and testicular cancer. Almost 60 per cent of all patients entered in the group's studies are included in bladder trials.

Phase-II studies are conducted in patients with bidimensional *measurable* disease and their response evaluated according to the WHO criteria. Differences in clinical activity and toxicity between several competing therapies are investigated in randomized phase-III studies.

The phase-III studies in bladder cancer focus on the comparison of different intravesical treatments (Sylvester, 1985) and their schedules in superficial disease.

In this report, we summarize the current status of EORTC GU Group trials in the management of bladder cancer. Protocols are numbered as follows. The prefix 30 designates the GU group; the two following numbers indicate the year of writing of the study (e.g. 80 refers to 1980); the last two numbers refer to the number of the study for that year.

Phase-II trials

Single-agent chemotherapy studies

Protocol 30797:
Phase-II trial of vincristine in advanced bladder carcinoma
Study coordinator: B. Richards, York
Activated: March 1978

Closed to follow-up: June 1981
Number of patients entered: 43

Treatment scheme: Vincristine (VCR) 1 mg/m^2 per week intravenously for an induction course of 8 weeks and 2-weekly thereafter.

Results: Of the 23 evaluable patients with measurable metastatic disease, one patient with lung metastases showed a complete remission which lasted for 7 months. Stable disease was noted in 8 patients and progression in 14 patients. Among the 14 evaluable patients with measurable primary tumours, there were 2 partial remissions, 2 no changes and 10 progressions. Vincristine was thus rejected as an active single agent in the treatment of advanced bladder cancer.

Publication: Richards *et al.* (1983).

Protocol 30823:

Phase-II study of mitoxantrone in advanced transitional cell carcinoma
Study coordinator: A. Van Oosterom, Leiden
Activated: April 1982
Closed to follow-up: March 1984
Number of patients entered: 29

Treatment scheme: Mitoxantrone 12 mg/m^2 intravenously every 3 weeks.

Results: No responses were observed among the 28 evaluable patients.

Publication: Van Oosterom *et al.* (1985).

Combination chemotherapy studies

Protocol 30771:

Phase-II trial of cisplatin+Adriamycin+cyclophosphamide (CAP) in advanced bladder carcinoma
Study coordinator: J. Mulder, Rotterdam
Activated: March 1978
Closed to follow-up: November 1985
Number of patients entered: 52

Treatment scheme: Cisplatin (CDDP) 40 mg/m^2, Adriamycin (ADM) 40 mg/m^2 and cyclophosphamide (CTX) 400 mg/m^2, all on day 1, intravenously every 3 weeks.

Results: The 12 per cent complete remissions and the 20 per cent partial remissions observed among 42 evaluable patients with measurable disease were judged to be equivalent to the results of CDDP as a single agent.

Publication: Mulder *et al.* (1982).

Protocol 30802:

Phase-II trial of cisplatin+VM-26 in advanced urothelial cancer
Study coordinator: G. Stoter, Amsterdam
Activated: January 1981
Closed to follow-up: November 1985
Number of patients entered: 57

Treatment scheme: Cisplatin (CDDP) 70 mg/m^2 on day 1, and VM-26 100 mg/m^2 on days 1 and 2, every 3 weeks.

Results: Of the 41 evaluable patients with measurable disease, the overall response rate was 51 per cent (10 per cent complete remissions and 41 per cent partial remissions). Again, it was concluded that these results were no better than the results obtained with CDDP alone.

Publication: Stoter *et al.* (1984).

Protocol 30821:

Phase-II study of cisplatin and methotrexate in advanced transitional cell carcinoma

Study coordinators: G. Stoter, Amsterdam, J.A. Child, Leeds and B. Richards, York

Activated: June 1982

Closed to follow-up: November 1985

Number of patients entered: 53

Treatment schedule: Cisplatin (CDDP) 70 mg/m^2 on day 1, and methotrexate (MTX) 40 mg/m^2 on days 8 and 15, intravenously every 3 weeks.

Results: The overall response rate in the 43 evaluable patients was 46 per cent, including 23 per cent complete responses with a median duration of 50 weeks and 23 per cent partial responses. The reported toxicity prohibited the utilization of this scheme in an adjuvant programme and a less toxic treatment regimen was advocated (see protocol 30842).

Publication: Stoter *et al.* (1985).

Protocol 30842:

Phase-II study of a combination of cisplatin and methotrexate in patients with advanced transitional cell carcinoma of the urinary tract

Study coordinator: G. Stoter, Amsterdam

Activated: June 1984

Open to patient entry

Number of patients entered: 63

Treatment scheme: Cisplatin (CDDP) 70 mg/m^2 on day 1, and methotrexate (MTX) 40 mg/m^2 on days 1 and 15, intravenously every 3 weeks.

Remark: In this study, the dose of MTX has been changed from day 8 to day 1 in the hope of decreasing the toxicity. Since this study is ongoing, results are not available for publication.

Protocol 30851:

Phase-II study of a combination of cisplatin and methotrexate in patients with T$_{3-4}$N$_{0-x}$M$_0$ transitional cell carcinoma of the bladder

Study coordinator: T. Splinter, Rotterdam

Activated: December 1985

Open to patient entry

Treatment scheme: Cisplatin (CDDP) 70 mg/m^2 on day 1, and methotrexate (MTX) 40 mg/m^2 on days 1 and 15, intravenously every 3 weeks.

Remarks: Patients receive two cycles of chemotherapy. If they achieve partial or complete response they receive another two cycles, while if stable or progressive disease is obtained the chemotherapy is stopped. The treatment to be given after chemotherapy is optional.

Phase-III superficial, prophylactic trials

Protocol 30781:
Pyridoxine (vitamin B_6) versus placebo in the management of superficial bladder cancer
Study coordinators: M. Robinson, Castleford and D. Newling, Hull
Activated: January 1979
Closed to patient entry: November 1981
Number of patients entered: 291

Treatment scheme: One week following complete resection of all Ta and T1 tumours, patients were randomized to receive either placebo or pyridoxine tablets (20 mg a day) on a double-blind basis for a minimum of 3 years.

Obectives: The objectives of the trial were to determine the incidence of abnormal tryptophan metabolites in the urine of these patients and to assess whether pyridoxine decreases the recurrence rate for these tumours.

Results: No significant differences between the treatment arms with respect to treatment efficacy were detected. The most important prognostic factors were the type of tumour (primary or recurrent), the number of tumours present at the time of randomization, and the previous recurrence rate. The sum of the values of the tryptophan metabolites kynurenin and acetyl kynurenin before treatment was also of prognostic value.

Publication: Newling *et al.* (1984).

Protocol 30782:
Thiotepa versus Adriamycin versus cisplatin in the management of superficial bladder cancer
Activated: February 1979
Closed to patient entry: September 1983
Number of patients entered: 356
Study coordinator: L. Denis, Antwerp

Treatment scheme: This study was designed to compare the effectiveness of these three drugs in preventing recurrence, progression and death from cancer in patients with superficial bladder tumours. Only patients with recurrent Ta and T1 tumours were eligible. Randomization was carried out after TUR. The first instillation treatment had to be given within 14 days of TUR. Treatment was given every week for the first 4 weeks and then once every 4 weeks for a total duration of one year.

Objectives: To compare the three treatment groups with respect to recurrence rate, time to first recurrence, progression to a higher stage of the disease and toxicity.

Results: There was no significant difference between the three treatment groups with respect to treatment efficacy. The most important prognostic factors were the number of tumours at entry and the size of the largest tumour. The most important side effect was an anaphylactic reaction to CDDP which consisted of rash and hypotension in 7 of 67 patients. This experience and a similar report in the literature prompted us to drop the CDDP arm in this protocol.

Publication: Denis (1983).

Protocol 30790:
Adriamycin versus Epodyl versus TUR only in the management of super-
ficial bladder cancer
Study coordinator: K.H. Kurth, Rotterdam
Activated: November 1979
Closed to patient entry: September 1983
Number of patients entered: 443

Treatment scheme: This study was reserved for patients presenting with
primary and recurrent Ta/T1 tumours. The treatment regimen started
within 14 days after TUR and compared the efficacy of Adriamycin 50 mg
versus Epodyl 1.13 g versus no treatment. Drug instillations were given
every week for 4 weeks and then once every 4 weeks for 11 months.

Objectives: To compare the disease-free interval, tumour recurrence rate
and the increase in tumour stage or grade of recurrent tumours.

Results: In 1982 the control arm (TUR alone) was closed to further entry
because the tumour recurrence rate was significantly higher after TUR
alone than in the adjuvantly treated patients. Currently the recurrence rate
is significantly higher in patients treated by TUR alone as compared with
Adriamycin or Epodyl. There is no significant difference between these two
adjuvant treatments. Instillations were stopped because of excessive toxicity
in 6 patients, 3 on each treatment. Only mild systemic side effects like nausea
and diarrhoea were seen after instillation of either Adriamycin or Epodyl.
The most important prognostic factors were the number of tumours at entry
on-study, the prior recurrence rate and tumour grade.

Publication: Kurth *et al.* (1984).

Protocols 30831 and 30832:
Randomized studies to assess the prophylactic value of immediate versus
delayed administration of mitomycin C (MMC 30831) and Adriamycin
(ADM 30832), and to assess the value of maintenance versus no-
maintenance treatment in superficial TCC of bladder
Study coordinators: (30831) C. Bouffioux, Liege; (30832) K.H. Kurth,
Rotterdam
Activated: September 1983
Still open to patient entry
Number of patients required for each study: 400

Treatment scheme: The treatment regimen consists of 4 weekly instillations
of ADM 50 mg or MMC 30 mg followed by 5 monthly instillations (total 9
instillations) for a total of 6 months. A second randomization assigns the
patient to a further 6 instillations or no additional treatment.

Objectives: To determine if early administration of MMC or ADM after
TUR (within 6 hours) gives better results than delayed instillation (7–10 days
after TUR) and to determine if 6 months' treatment gives the same results as
12 months' treatment. Results will be analysed in terms of disease-free
interval, recurrence rate, increase in stage of recurrent tumour, the incidence of carcinoma-in-situ and the frequency of side effects.

Remark: Up to May 1985, 463 patients had been randomized in the MMC
study. Of the 1923 instillations with MMC there had been 3 per cent of

bacterial cystitis and 5 per cent of chemical cystitis, indicating a very good local tolerance. The occurrence of chemical cystitis was not higher in patients treated with early instillation than in patients with delayed instillation.

In the ADM study a total of 361 patients had been randomized up to May 1985. The occurrence of chemical cystitis was 2 per cent and of bacterial cystitis 6 per cent. Again the percentage of chemical cystitis was not higher in patients treated by early instillation. Results are not yet available.

Protocol 30845:
Comparative study of intravesical instillation of mitomycin C and instillation of BCG-RIV in primary and recurrent Ta–T1 papillary carcinoma and primary carcinoma-in-situ of the urinary bladder
Study coordinator: F. Debruyne, Nijmegen
Activated: January 1985
Still open to patient entry
Number of patients required for the study: 234

Treatment scheme: Seven to 15 days after TUR, patients are randomly allocated to receive intravesical BCG-RIV (once a week for 6 weeks followed by an additional 6 weeks if recurrence at 3 months) or intravesical mitomycin C (once a week for 4 weeks and then monthly for a total of 6 months).

Objectives: The treatments will be compared with respect to recurrence rate, disease-free interval, rate of progression to a higher stage of disease, and the incidence and severity of side effects.

Remarks: No results are as yet available.

Discussion

The phase-III intravesical trials outlined above have shown no difference in efficacy or side effects between thiotepa, Adriamycin and Epodyl, and these drugs are thus currently recommended as the treatments of choice. Cisplatin has proved too toxic and should not be used in intravesical treatment. Mitomycin C and BCG are both under investigation in current EORTC trials and it is still too early to judge their efficacy.

Two intravesical trials were recently initiated (30831 and 30832) to study the questions of treatment timing (immediate versus delayed instillations) and treatment duration (6 versus 12 months). The answers obtained from these trials will be of considerable importance in shaping future research.

In the various intravesical trials carried out by the EORTC, two prognostic factors have constantly revealed themselves to be of major importance: the number of tumours at entry on study and the patient's previous recurrence rate (Dalesio *et al.*, 1983). Since patients have very different prognoses based on these two factors, and can be divided into two subgroups of good and poor prognoses, future EORTC trials will study these two subgroups separately. The aggressiveness of the treatments studied will be based on the patient's prognosis.

Separate studies will also be carried out in patients with carcinoma-in-situ, starting with phase-II trials to answer basic questions relating to response rate. Similarly, phase-II intravesical, chemoresection trials will also be started in patients presenting with papillary, multifocal lesions.

In patients with locally advanced, invasive disease, a new trial has been started to study the effect of combination chemotherapy on the primary tumour. As more promising single and combination chemotherapies evolve from phase-II trials, the prospects for more new innovative trials in patients with invasive disease will present themselves and, it is to be hoped, solve the existing controversies concerning the relative value of cystectomy, radiotherapy and chemotherapy in this disease.

The search for effective, less toxic drugs at the phase-II level will continue, with the goal of providing new, effective treatment regimens which pose the least burden possible to the patient at all stages of the disease.

References

Dalesio, O., Schulman, C., Sylvester, R., De Pauw, M., Robinson, M., Denis, L., Smith, P., Viggliano, G. and members of the EORTC (1983). Prognostic factors in superficial bladder tumours: a study of the EORTC Genito-Urinary Tract Cancer Cooperative Group. *Journal of Urology* **129**: 730–33.

Denis, L. (1983). Letter to the Editor: Anaphylactic reactions to repeated intravesical instillation with cisplatin. *Lancet*, 18 June, 1378–9.

Kurth, K., Schröder, F.H., Tunn, A., Ay, R., Pavone-Macaluso, M., Debruyne, F., De Pauw, M., Dalesio, O., Ten Kate, F. and members of the EORTC (1984). Adjuvant chemotherapy of superficial transitional cell bladder carcinoma: preliminary results of an EORTC randomized trial comparing doxorubicin hydrochloride, ethoglucid and TUR alone. *Journal of Urology* **132**: 258–62.

Mulder, J.H., Fossa, S.D., De Pauw, M. and Van Oosterom, A.T. (1982). Cyclophosphamide, Adriamycin and cisplatin combination chemotherapy in advanced bladder carcinoma: an EORTC phase II study. *European Journal of Cancer and Clinical Oncology* **18**: 111–12.

Newling, D., Robinson, M.R.G., Lockwood, R., Stevens, I., Byar, D., Sylvester, R. and members of the Yorkshire Urological Cancer Research Group (1984). Tryptophan metabolites in superficial bladder cancer: the background to and preliminary report on EORTC trial 30781. In *Controlled Clinical Trials*, pp. 269–72. Edited by Denis, L., Murphy, G., Prout, G. and Schröder, F. Raven Press, New York.

Richards, B., Newling, D., Fossa, S., Bastable, J.R.G., Denis, L., Jones, W.B., DePauw, M. and members of the EORTC (1983). Vincristine in advanced bladder cancer: an EORTC phase II study. *Cancer Chemotherapy Reports* **67**: 575–7.

Stoter, G., Fossa, S.D., Klein, J.G.M., Denis, L., Splinter, T., Jones, W.G., Keizer, J. and Sylvester, R. (1985). Combination chemotherapy with cisplatin (DDP) and methotrexate (MTX) in advanced bladder cancer: an EORTC phase II study. *Proceedings of the American Society of Clinical Oncology* **4**: C413.

Stoter, G., Van Oosterom, A.T., Mulder, J.H., De Pauw, M. and Fossa, S. (1984). An EORTC phase II study of combination chemotherapy with cisplatin and VM-26 in patients with advanced transitional cell carcinoma of the bladder. *European Journal of Cancer and Clinical Oncology* **20**: 315–17.

Sylvester, R. (1985). The analysis of results in prophylactic superficial bladder cancer studies. In *Superficial Bladder Tumors*, EORTC Genito-Urinary

Group monograph 2, part B, pp. 3–11. Edited by Schröder, F.H. and Richards, B. Alan R. Liss, New York.

Van Oosterom, A.T., Fossa, S.D., Mulder, J.H., Calciati, A., De Pauw, M. and Sylvester, R. (1985). Mitoxantrone in advanced bladder carcinoma: a phase II study of the EORTC Genito-Urinary Tract Cancer Cooperative Group. *European Journal of Cancer and Clinical Oncology* **21**: 1013–14.

15

First-line intravenous chemotherapy for invasive bladder cancer

Derek Raghavan

Introduction

The cure of invasive (T2–T4) non-metastatic bladder cancer remains a major problem in management. With the exception of some of the data reported from Rotterdam (van der Werf Messing, 1979), the 5-year survival of patients treated by radiotherapy for stages T2 to T4 transitional cell carcinoma (TCC) of the bladder has usually been less than 50 per cent (see Chapter 8). Similarly the results obtained with radical cystectomy or a combination of the two modalities have been disappointing (Chapters 4 and 7).

From clinical and autopsy data, it appears that micrometastases are often present at the time of first diagnosis (Cummings *et al.*, 1979; Skinner, 1980). Recurrence or metastasis is usually documented within 12–18 months, the bladder bed and pelvis being the commonest sites of recurrence. Metastases may be detected in the para-aortic or supraclavicular nodes, in bone, liver, lung, brain, or less frequently in other sites (Cummings *et al.*, 1979; Skinner, 1980; Raghavan, 1985).

As discussed elsewhere in this volume, cytotoxic chemotherapy has been used in the management of recurrent and metastatic TCC for more than a decade, with variable success (see Chapters 10–13). Although response rates in the range of 10 to 40 per cent have been reported with the use of methotrexate, doxorubicin, cisplatin and the vinca alkaloids, long-term survival has been relatively uncommon (Yagoda, 1980).

More recently, combination cytotoxic regimens have been reported to yield response rates of 60–70 per cent, with complete remission rates of about 30 per cent, and with corresponding survival rates in excess of two years (Harker *et al.*, 1985; Sternberg *et al.*, 1985). However, the first enthusiastic report of combination chemotherapy for metastatic bladder cancer, using cisplatin, doxorubicin and cyclophosphamide, was published a decade ago (Sternberg *et al.*, 1977) and has not withstood critical random-ized evaluation (Chapter 11). It is thus not clear whether the newer combination regimens reflect a real increase in survival, or are merely a function of careful selection of patients. On balance, however, it is possible that the MVAC regimen (Sternberg *et al.*, 1985) will yield a survival benefit in view of the documented responses in bone (a distinctly uncommon phenomenon). Randomized trials are currently in progress to define the role of combination cytotoxic regimens in the treatment of metastatic and recurrent bladder cancer. Until the role of these combinations has been proved in such trials, their use earlier in management schedules will remain controversial. In our institution and in other centres, the role of single-agent intravenous cytototoxic chemotherapy has been evaluated in the management of clinically non-metastatic disease. More recently, other investigators have begun to study combination chemotherapy in this context.

First-line intravenous chemotherapy: rationale

In an attempt to improve the cure rate for invasive bladder cancer, programmes of first-line intravenous chemotherapy have been devised in which cytotoxic agents are administered as the first step in management, followed by 'definitive' treatment (radiotherapy and/or cystectomy). This approach is based on the following concepts:

1. Downstaging of a bladder cancer by radiotherapy before cystectomy appears to confer a survival benefit (Whitmore, 1980; Bloom *et al.*, 1982).
2. The optimal time to treat micrometastases is probably when their volume is minimal (Steel, 1977).
3. Cisplatin may act as a radiosensitizer when administered some hours to some days before irradiation (Luk *et al.*, 1979).
4. Tumours often contain hypoxic regions which are relatively resistant to radiotherapy and in which the cells may predominantly be in the G0 phase or only slowly progressing through the cell cycle (Kennedy *et al.*, 1980); these areas may be more sensitive to the effects of cytoxic agents than to radiotherapy.
5. The use of intravenous chemotherapy before the completion of irradiation may avoid the reduction of access to the tumour that occurs as a result of radiation-induced vascular sclerosis.

In the early attempts to apply these principles, intravenous cisplatin was used as the sole modality of first-line treatment of invasive bladder cancer. However, these studies were characterized by a high local failure rate (Soloway *et al.*, 1981). Subsequently, programmes have been developed in which initial chemotherapy has been used as an adjunct to definitive treatment, the so-called approach of 'neoadjuvant chemotherapy'.

Neoadjuvant chemotherapy of bladder cancer: experience at Royal Prince Alfred Hospital, Sydney

Patients and methods

Fifty patients with invasive, clinically non-metastatic TCC (stages $T_{2-4}N_XM_0$) were treated between August 1981 and November 1983, allowing a minimum follow-up of 3 years. An additional 20 cases were treated in the subsequent year. The characteristics of the patients and of their tumours are summarized in Table 15.1.

Each patient underwent an intensive staging programme of 'non-invasive' tests, including a detailed history and examination, cystoscopy, biopsy and examination under anaesthesia, biochemical screening, assessment of

Table 15.1 Details of patients and tumours

Characteristic	First series (N=50)*	Quality of life survey	Total series (N=70)†
Patients			
Age: Median	65	64	65
Mean ± SD	63.4 ± 8.4	64 ± 7.1	63.5 ± 8.2
Range	29–79	51–77	29–79
Sex: Male	40	25	54
Female	10	4	16
Smokers	86%	85%	85%
Analgesic abuse	25%	29%	25%
Hydroneph/renal dysfunction	50%	44%	50%
Prior radiotherapy	0	0	0
Prior i.v. chemotherapy	0	0	0
Tumours			
Stage: T2	14%	28%	29%
T3	62%	51%	50%
T4	24%	21%	21%
Grade: I	0	0	0
II	12%	7%	14%
III	88%	93%	86%
TCC	100%	100%	100%
Pure SCC	0	0	0
Pure AD CA	0	0	0

*Raghavan *et al.* (1985).
†Pearson and Raghavan (1985).

tumour markers (carcinoembryonic antigen, human chorionic gonadotrophin), CAT scan of abdomen and pelvis, and chest x-ray (Raghavan *et al.*, 1984, 1985; Pearson and Raghavan, 1985). An increased T stage was not allocated on the basis of CAT scan alone; thus the scans merely confirmed the results of clinical staging and served to demonstrate distant metastases. Enlarged pelvic nodes visualized by CAT scan did not preclude the patient from entry into the study.

The protocol of treatment has been reported in detail elsewhere (Raghavan *et al.*, 1984, 1985, 1986; Pearson and Raghavan, 1985). In brief, patients received two doses of cisplatin (100 mg/m² i.v. every 3 weeks), with appropriate reduction of dose in the presence of severe renal dysfunction. Active hydration with forced diuresis, requiring meticulous nursing and medical supervision, was used. Patients received mannitol and frusemide.

After two doses of cisplatin, patients underwent reassessment, including cystoscopy, biopsy and examination under anaesthesia. A reduction of apparent tumour mass on CAT scan alone did not constitute a 'response'. Patients subsequently received definitive treatment (radiotherapy alone in 55 cases; cystectomy±radiotherapy in 15 cases), depending on the referring clinician's preference. The end-point of this pilot study was the assessment of the safety and efficacy of first-line cisplatin, and hence no attempt was made to influence the choice of definitive treatment. The standard regimen of irradiation consisted of 45–50 Gy to the pelvis, with a boost yielding a total of 60 Gy to the bladder itself. Planning for radiotherapy was carried out with the aid of CAT scan localization. The predominance of patients who received radiotherapy alone reflects the pattern of urological practice in our referral area.

Further restaging of the tumours was carried out upon completion of the treatment programme. Although there are no perfect criteria of objective assessment of response in the bladder by non-invasive means, we attempted to assess whether tumour reduction was achieved, using previously reported criteria (Raghavan *et al.*, 1985). This approach may be associated with a substantial risk of understaging due to the false-negative error rates of CAT scan and endoscopy, compared with cystectomy.

The toxicity of the treatment regimen was assessed in several ways. To document acute side effects, patients were examined after receiving treatment and a detailed history was taken. In addition, nursing and medical records were monitored.

The assessment of delayed toxicity was made in part by the referring clinicians who were responsible for monitoring the patients' progress by physical and cystoscopic examination. In addition, long-term survivors were asked to complete a questionnaire which included multiple-choice questions and linear analogue self-assessment (LASA) scales (Grundy *et al.*, 1987). Twenty-nine of 38 patients (76 per cent) responded to the survey (male:female=25:4; mean age 64 years, range 51–77, standard deviation 7.1). The distribution of patient and tumour characteristics was similar to that of the total series of treated patients (Table 15.1).

Self-administered questionnaires were mailed to the patients with a detailed explanatory letter. The questionnaire was developed specifically for this population group, based on previously validated models (Spitzer *et al.*, 1981; Coates *et al.*, 1983; Selby *et al.*, 1984). In addition to questions relating to the general aspects of lifestyle, illness and toxicity of treatment, specific issues with regard to bladder cancer and its treatment were addressed (Grundy *et al.*, 1987). Eight major features were studied, including physical wellbeing, symptoms of the disease, side effects of treatment, functional status, social and sexual interactions, satisfaction with treatment and overall quality of life.

The results were analysed for each feature. The percentage response was calculated for each answer in the multiple-choice sections; responses on LASA scales were measured on a 10 cm scale which was divided into five equal sections; a numerical value was assigned for each response, allowing the expression of a mean value (± standard deviation).

Results

All patients were assessed for the toxicity of first-line intravenous cisplatin and of the subsequent treatment programme. 'Objective response' was assessed in 66 patients (in 4 cases, different urologists performed the pre- and post-treatment cystoscopies). Mature 3-year survival data are now available for the first 50 patients, with follow-up extending to more than 5 years in some cases.

Acute toxicity

The pattern of acute toxicity is summarized in Table 15.2. Nausea and vomiting were almost universal, although in most instances they lasted less than 2–3 days. The auditory side effects (tinnitus, high-tone hearing loss or changes on audiometry) were mild in most instances; one patient continued to be troubled by subjective high-tone hearing loss for several months. In the majority of cases, renal dysfunction consisted of an asymptomatic rise of serum creatinine to less than twice the upper limit of normal; in only one instance, the serum creatinine rose to eight times the upper limit of normal (in an asymptomatic patient) and resolved spontaneously over the succeeding three weeks. In no case was dialysis required.

Table 15.2 Toxicity of neoadjuvant cisplatin programme (objective)

Side effect	Number of patients
Nausea	65
Vomiting	60
Colitis*	10
Cystitis*	10
Auditory	8
Renal†	8
Diarrhoea‡	5
Myelosuppression	5
Infection	2
Subacute bowel obstruction	2
Haematemesis	1
Stomatitis	1
Dehydration (diabetic)	1
Inappropriate ADH production	1
Subendocardial infarction	1
Atrial fibrillation	1
Total	70

*Chronic, post-radiotherapy.
†Creatinine less than twice upper limit of normal (one patient with transient level 8 × normal).
‡Acute post-chemotherapy.

The spectrum of toxicity after radiotherapy was unremarkable and the preceding administration of cisplatin did not compromise the dosage or schedules of irradiation. In patients who underwent cystectomy, there were no unusual complications that could be related to the preceding chemotherapy, nor was the frequency of postoperative complications increased. There were no deaths related to treatment with cisplatin plus radiotherapy.

Delayed toxicity and quality of life

The long-term side effects of this regimen have been relatively mild, as assessed by the referring clinicians. The major chronic toxicities have been post-radiation colitis (15 per cent) and cystitis (15 per cent), the prevalence having increased with time over the first 2 years. However, no patients have required colostomy, and the symptoms of colitis have usually resolved quickly with prednisolone enemas, oral steroids or other conservative measures. In two cases, patients have suffered episodes of subacute bowel obstruction which have resolved with conservative treatment. Chronic clinically significant ototoxicity, neurotoxicity and renal dysfunction have not been observed.

Similar data have been obtained from the formal assessment of quality of life in long-term survivors. The results of this study are summarized in Table 15.3 and have been analysed in detail elsewhere (Grundy *et al.*, 1987).

Of particular interest, one-third of respondents suffered two or more episodes of nocturia per night and 15 per cent suffered frequent diarrhoea. One-third of patients noted a substantial decrease in sexual function after radical radiotherapy (and another third refused to answer questions on this subject). Nevertheless, the majority of patients claimed to have a satisfactory quality of life and level of activity.

Table 15.3 Quality of life in long-term survivors after neoadjuvant programme*

| | *Response* (%) | | |
Index	Yes	No	No response
Nocturia (>2/night)	35	50	15
Troubled by nocturia	9	85	6
Difficulty micturating	12	73	15†
Frequent diarrhoea	15	85	0
Troubled by diarrhoea	25	75	0
Good/normal appetite	96	0	4
Auditory problems	30	70	0
Prior auditory problems	27	73	0
Hobbies and interests maintained	84	16	0
Capable of unassisted self-care	100	0	0
Active outside home	85	15	0
Deterioration in sexual function	35	31	34
Deterioration in social interactions	4	81	15
Satisfied with results of treatment	96	0	15
Should a friend have this treatment if required for bladder cancer?	100	0	0
Normal/good quality of life	76	8	15

*Adapted from Grundy *et al.* (1987).
†Post-cystectomy.

Response

After two doses of cisplatin, 40 patients (57 per cent) showed an apparent reduction in tumour mass, notwithstanding the inaccuracies of non-invasive assessment (Raghavan *et al.*, 1985). In three patients, tumour progression occurred during the period of chemotherapy—in one case, an increase in the size of the primary tumour, and in two others, the development of distant metastases (supraclavicular node; liver). Upon completion of definitive treatment, 84 per cent of the patients had responded.

An unanticipated feature of the reponses was the speed with which the symptoms of malignant cystitis (strangury, frequency, dysuria, nocturia) resolved; more than 70 per cent of symptomatic patients reported an improvement within 3 weeks of the commencement of chemotherapy.

Survival

The 3-year survival figures for the first 50 patients (entered before December 1983) are now mature. Twenty-seven patients (54 per cent) have died of cancer or tumour-related causes, and three have died of intercurrent disease (myocardial infarctions without evidence of cancer). Thus the true 3-year survival is 40 per cent (including stages T2–T4). As can be seen in Fig. 15.1, the actuarial 5-year survival is also 40 per cent, although the true 5-year survival is likely to be less.

Patterns of relapse and its treatment

To date, 44 of the 70 patients (62 per cent) have relapsed, the commonest site being the bladder bed/pelvis (42 patients). However, in six of these cases only superficial TCC was present at the time of relapse. Other sites of relapse included bone (10 patients), distant lymph nodes (9), liver (7), vagina (4), brain (2), lung (2), abdomen (2) and skin (1).

Ten patients have undergone salvage cystectomy, 12 have been treated with radiotherapy and 18 have received salvage chemotherapy. In 11 instances, no active treatment was administered for relapse. Details of salvage chemotherapy are summarized in Table 15.4.

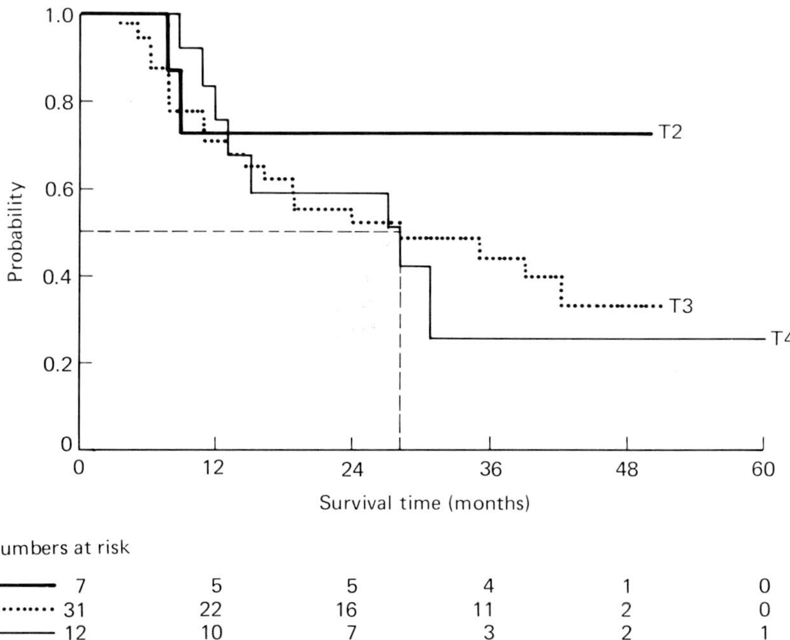

Fig. 15.1 Graphical portrayal of survival results at the Royal Prince Alfred Hospital

Table 15.4 Salvage chemotherapy after failure of RPAH neoadjuvant programme

Regimen	Complete remission	Partial remission	Total
A–M	1	3	7
MTX	0	2	9
CDDP	0	1	3
MVAC	0	1	1
DMDR	0	0	1

A–M:	Adriamycin 40–50 mg/m^2 q 3 weekly Mitomycin C 10–15 mg/m^2 q 6 weekly
MTX:	Methotrexate 100–200 mg/m^2 q 2–3 weekly
CDDP:	Cisplatin 100 mg/m^2 q 3 weekly
MVAC:	See text
DMDR:	Demethoxydaunorubicin phase-II study.

Neoadjuvant chemotherapy of bladder cancer: results from other institutions

The utility of first-line intravenous chemotherapy for the management of invasive bladder cancer has been assessed in several single-arm clinical trials. In the majority of these studies, cisplatin has been combined as a single agent (70–100 mg/m^2 i.v.) with radiotherapy or cystectomy (see Table 15.5). Where radiotherapy has been the definitive treatment, cisplatin has been administered beforehand (Fagg *et al.*, 1984) or concurrently (Shipley *et al.*, 1984; Jakse *et al.*, 1985). In a preliminary study, Oliver (1981) demonstrated that first-line intravenous methotrexate is a safe and potentially useful adjuvant before radiotherapy. In all of these studies, the acute toxicity has been relatively minor and high response rates (50–80 per cent) have been demonstrated. However, long-term survival data have not been published.

More recently, the use of combination cytotoxic regimens has been evaluated in the context of neoadjuvant chemotherapy (see Table 15.6). Kaye *et al.* (1985) (see also Chapter 13) reported an unsuccessful attempt to increase long-term survival with a first-line regimen of cyclophosphamide, methotrexate and 5-fluorouracil. Although the side effects were relatively mild, only 4 of 17 patients with T3 tumours survived longer than 30 months. However, in this study, the lack of efficacy may have been due to an inactive cytotoxic regimen (rather than failure of neoadjuvant treatment *per se*) as no objective responses were seen.

By contrast, high objective response rates have been reported with the use of methotrexate–cisplatin (Calais da Silva and Denis, 1987), the MVAC regimen (Sternberg *et al.*, 1987; Simon and Srouji, 1986 and the combination of cisplatin, doxorubicin, VM-26 and 5-fluorouracil (Francini *et al.*, 1987). Not surprisingly, the toxicity of the combination regimens has been greater than that reported for single agents, although a randomized trial in this context has not been reported. Whether these regimens will ultimately yield a survival benefit is not clear at present.

Table 15.5 Neoadjuvant chemotherapy for invasive non-metastatic bladder cancer: single agents

Number treated	Number assessed	M:F ratio	Age Median	Mean	Range	Stage	Response rate (%)	Toxicity	Median survival (months)	Other treat-ment	Series
Cisplatin, 70 mg/m²											
13	13	?	?	?	?	Invasive	30	?	15	0	Soloway *et al.* (1981)
27	17	21:6	69	?	46–87	T2–T4	76*	N,V,D,C, R,SBO,In.	>24	RT	Shipley *et al.* (1984)
24	24	?	?	?	?	T3–T4	38†	'0'	>24	RT+S	Herr (1985)
30	30	24:6	?	67	45–85	T3–T4	77‡	N,V,R,D,C	>23 (mean)	RT	Jakse *et al.* (1985)
Cisplatin, 100 mg/m²											
17	17	16:1	?	63.8	58–73	T2–T4	65	N,V,D,R, Ot,M,Ne	>12	RT	Fagg *et al.* (1984)
70	70	54:16	65	63.5	29–79	T2–T4	60	Table 15.2	28§	RT(±S)	Raghavan *et al.* (1986)
Methotrexate, 100 mg/m²+leucovorin											
19	19	?	?	?	?	T2–T4	50?	St	>12	RT	Oliver (1981)

* Note response not defined in 10/27 cases; † tumour downstaging at cystectomy; ‡ after chemotherapy and radiotherapy; § first 50 patients (treated before December 1983).
RT—radiotherapy; S—surgery; N—nausea; V—vomiting; D—diarrhoea; R—renal; C—cystitis; St—stomatitis; Ot—ototoxicity; M—myelosuppression; Ne—neurotoxicity; In—infection; SBO—small bowel obstruction.

Table 15.6 Neoadjuvant chemotherapy for invasive non-metastatic bladder cancer: combination regimens

Regimen	Assessed/ treated ratio	M:F ratio	Age			Stage	Response rate (%)	Toxicity	Median survival (months)	Other treat- ment	Series
			Median	Mean	Range						
M–C	19/42	36:6	?	64	50–80	T2–T4	64	N,V,R, St,M,In.	>17	S	Calais da Silva and Denis (1987)
CyMF	12/17	12:5	?	63.8	44–79	T3	0	N,C,D.	27	RT	Kaye *et al.* (1985)
CAFT	13/13	12:1	56	?	42–65	T3–T4	71	N,V,R,M.	?	S	Francini *et al.* (1987)
MVAC	31/?	25:6	63	?	35–74	T3–T4	42	?	>6	S	Sternberg *et al.* (1987)

M: Methotrexate
C: Cisplatin
F: 5-fluorouracil
A: Doxorubicin (Adriamycin)
Cy: Cyclophosphamide
T: VM-26 (Teniposide).
N: nausea; V: vomiting; R: renal; St: stomatitis; M: myelosuppression; In: infection; C: cystitis; D: diarrhoea.

Discussion

At present, it is not possible to define the true role of first-line intravenous chemotherapy in the management of invasive TCC of the bladder. There appears to be a reasonable basis for the enthusiasm generated by the initial cautious reports of high response rates and actuarial 2-year survival rates of 70–80 per cent (Fagg *et al.*, 1984; Shipley *et al.*, 1984; Raghavan *et al.*, 1984, 1985). However, the decline in the survival curves seen at 4 and 5 years (Raghavan *et al.*, 1986; Fig. 15.1) mandates the completion of randomized trials. Factors such as patient selection, inadvertent overstaging, and stage-migration (in which improved staging techniques may alter the distribution of tumour stages over a period of time) may have contributed to the apparent improvement of survival of these patients compared with historical controls.

However, these randomized trials may be difficult to complete. Patient accrual may suffer from the current wave of enthusiasm in which some clinicians believe that it is unethical to withhold first-line intravenous chemotherapy because of the excellent preliminary data. Paradoxically, others who intuitively do not believe in the use of randomized trials may choose not to enter patients on the basis of the early failures in neoadjuvant programmes.

Another problem is raised by the lack of consensus with regard to the optimal definitive treatment—cystectomy versus radiotherapy versus combined-modality treatment (as discussed elsewhere in this volume). This issue is further complicated by the uncertainty regarding the most appropriate cytotoxic regimen for use in a neoadjuvant setting. As noted previously, there is considerable controversy regarding the relative merits and problems associated with the use of single agents as compared with combination cytotoxic programmes. To date, randomized trials have not demonstrated a clinically significant survival benefit from the use of combination regimens in the management of recurrent and metastatic disease (Soloway *et al.*, 1983; Hillcoat and Raghavan, 1986). Whether it is appropriate, rational or ethical to use the more toxic, yet unproven, combination regimens in the phase-II assessment of neoadjuvant chemotherapy remains to be seen. As noted before, the concerns raised by the widely varying reported response rates for the 'CAP' regimen (13–82 per cent, see Chapter 11) can also be translated to the use of such regimens as MVAC, CMV and others. By contrast, however, the question also remains as to whether a negative neoadjuvant study using cisplatin as a single agent can imply that a combination neoadjuvant programme will also fail: clearly the answer is 'no'.

Conclusions

The following points can be concluded from the available information.

1. The use of cisplatin or methotrexate as single agents for neoadjuvant chemotherapy of invasive TCC is safe and reasonably well tolerated by patients. The use of combination cytoxic regimens in this setting is associated with greater toxicity and *possibly* a higher initial response rate.

2. Rapid improvement in the symptoms of malignant cystitis can be achieved by the use of cisplatin in this fashion, although it is not clear

whether this is solely due to the activity of the drug or is a function (at least in part) of the high intravenous fluid load with resulting 'flushing' of the bladder.

3. Long-term survival of patients with T3–4 bladder cancer can be achieved in 45–50 per cent of cases treated with neoadjuvant cisplatin plus radiotherapy. However, the majority of long-term survival figures for radiotherapy alone antedate the routine use of CAT scanning, and hence a direct comparison of the results of neoadjuvant programmes with historical series is not valid (Raghavan, 1988).

4. It is unlikely that the randomized trials that are currently in progress will define the optimal management of invasive bladder cancer. Some of these studies are examining specific combined modality regimens in a single-arm, non-randomized fashion and will not be comparable to the published historical data. Others will yield relatively limited information: for example, the parallel studies in the United Kingdom and Australia which compare radiotherapy alone versus the combination of first-line cisplatin plus radiotherapy, and which will not yield information regarding the role of combination cytotoxic regimens nor of radical cystectomy.

I believe that a format will be required in which direct comparisons can be made between single and combination cytotoxic regimens in a neoadjuvant context, and between radiotherapy, cystectomy and combinations of these as definitive treatment. This will only be achieved in a stepwise fashion, and this will require first the completion of those randomized trials currently in progress that ask simple questions. In view of the practical difficulty of randomizing patients to receive radiotherapy or cystectomy (with substantial differences in the pattern of side effects), it may be necessary to evolve an innovative format of clinical trial in which patients are treated according to standard institutional policies (with documentation of all patients treated as well as those that are excluded) after common staging protocols, with a direct comparison of the end results. Although a flawed design, this approach may yield the most accurate answer to the question regarding the optimal definitive treatment of invasive bladder cancer.

To abandon the logical and systematic approach inherent in two-armed randomized trials in favour of a series of phase-II, multi-drug, combined modality programmes is not likely to resolve the therapeutic problem posed by the fact that half of the patients with deeply invasive bladder cancer still die within 5 years of presentation.

References

Bloom, H.J.G., Hendry, W.F., Wallace, D.M. and Skeet, R.G. (1982). Treatment of T3 bladder cancer: controlled trial of pre-operative radiotherapy and radical cystectomy versus radical radiotherapy (second report and review). *British Journal of Urology* **54**: 136–51.

Calais da Silva, F. and Denis, L. (1987). Preoperative chemotherapy and cystectomy in invasive bladder cancer. In *Treatment of Advanced Bladder Cancer: EORTC Monograph 5*. Edited by Smith, P.H. and Pavone-Macaluso, M. Alan. R. Liss, New York.

Coates, A.S., Fischer, Dillenbeck, C., McNeill, D.R. *et al.* (1983). On the receiving end. II: Linear analogue self-assessment (LASA) in evaluation of aspects of the quality of life of cancer patients receiving therapy. *European Journal of Cancer and Clinical Oncology* **19**: 1633–7.

Cummings, K.B., Shipley, W.U., Einstein, A.B. and Cutler, S.J. (1979). Current concepts in the management of patients with deeply invasive bladder carcinoma. *Seminars in Oncology* **6**: 220–8.

Fagg, S.L., Dawson-Edwards, P., Hughes, M.A., Latief, T.N., Rolfe, E.B. and Fielding, J.W. (1984). Cis-diammine dichloroplatinum (DDP) as initial treatment of invasive bladder cancer. *British Journal of Urology* **56**: 296–300.

Francini, M., Veronesi, A., Dal Bo, V., Carbone, A. and Monfardini, S. (in press). Neo-adjuvant chemotherapy in locally advanced bladder carcinoma. In *Treatment of Advanced Bladder Cancer: EORTC Monograph 5*. Edited by Smith, P.H. and Pavone-Macaluso, M. Alan R. Liss, New York.

Grundy, R., Raghavan, D., Lancaster, L., Duval, P. and Pearson, B. (submitted for publication). Assessment of quality of life in long-term survivors after neoadjuvant chemotherapy for invasive bladder cancer.

Harker, W.G., Meyers, F.J., Freiha, F.S. *et al.* (1985). Cisplatin, methotrexate, and vinblastine (CMV): an effective chemotherapy regimen for metastatic transitional cell carcinoma of the urinary tract: a Northern California Oncology Group study. *Journal of Clinical Oncology* **3**: 1463–70.

Herr, H.W. (1985). Preoperative irradiation with and without chemotherapy as adjunct to radical cystectomy. *Urology* **25**: 127–34.

Hillcoat, B.L. and Raghavan, D. (1986). A randomised comparison of cisplatinum (C) versus cisplatinum and methotrexate (C+M) in advanced bladder cancer. *Proceedings of the American Society of Clinical Oncology* **5**: 110 (abstract).

Jakse, G., Fritsch, E. and Frommhold, H. (1985). Combination of chemotherapy and irradiation for non-resectable bladder carcinoma. *World Journal of Urology* **3**: 121–5.

Kaye, S.B., MacFarlane, J.R., McHattie, I. and Hart, A.J.L. (1985). Chemotherapy before radiotherapy for T3 bladder cancer: a pilot study. *British Journal of Urology* **57**: 434–7.

Kennedy, A.K., Feicher, B.A., Rockwell, S. and Sartorelli, A.C. (1980). The hypoxic tumor cell: a target for selective cancer chemotherapy. *Biochemical Pharmacology* **29**: 1–8.

Luk, K.H., Ross, G.Y., Phillips, T.L. and Goldstein, L.S. (1979). The interaction of radiation and cis-diamminedichloroplatinum (II) in intestinal crypt cells. *International Journal of Radiation Oncology, Biology and Biophysics* **5**: 1417–20.

Oliver, R.T.D. (1981). Methotrexate as salvage or adjunctive therapy for primary invasive carcinoma of the bladder. *Cancer Treatment Reports* **65** (Suppl. 1): 179–81.

Pearson, B.S. and Raghavan, D. (1985). First-line intravenous cisplatin for deeply invasive bladder cancer: update on 70 cases. *British Journal of Urology* **57**: 690–3.

Raghavan, D. (1985). First-line intravenous cis-platinum for invasive clinically non-metastatic bladder cancer. In *Genitourinary Cancer*, pp. 193–207. Edited by Garnick, M.B. Churchill Livingstone, Edinburgh.

Raghavan, D. (1988). First-line (neoadjuvant) intravenous chemotherapy for invasive bladder cancer: *British Journal of Urology* **61**: in press.

Raghavan, D., Pearson, B., Coorey, G. *et al.* (1984). Intravenous cis-platinum for invasive clinically non-metastatic bladder cancer: safety and feasibility of a new approach. *Medical Journal of Australia* **140**: 276–278.

Raghavan, D., Pearson, B., Duval, P. *et al.* (1985). Initial intravenous cisplatinum therapy: improved management for invasive high risk bladder cancer? *Journal of Urology* **133**: 399–402.

Raghavan, D., Pearson, B. and Duval, P. (1986). First line intravenous cisplatin in the treatment of invasive, non-metastatic bladder cancer. In *Neo-Adjuvant Chemotherapy*, pp. 693–700. Edited by Jacquillat, C., Weil, M. and Khayat, D. INSERM/John Libbey Eurotext, London.

Selby, P.J., Chapman, J.A.W., Etazadi-Amoli, J., Dalley, D. and Boyd, N.F. (1984). The development of a method for assessing the quality of life of cancer patients. *British Journal of Cancer* **50**: 13–22.

Shipley, W.U., Coombs, L.J., Einstein, A.B., Soloway, M.S., Wajsman, Z., Prout, G.R. and National Collaborative Bladder Cancer Group A (1984). *Journal of Urology* **132**: 899–903.

Simon, S.D. and Srougi, M. (1986). Neo-adjuvant M-VAC chemotherapy in invasive transitional cell carcinoma of the bladder: a pilot study. In *Neo-Adjuvant Chemotherapy*, pp. 701–4. Edited by Jacquillat, C., Weil, M. and Khayat, D. INSERM/John Libbey Eurotext, London.

Skinner, D.G. (1980). Current perspectives in the management of high grade invasive bladder cancer. *Cancer* **45**: 1866–74.

Soloway, M.S., Einstein, A., Corder, M.P., Bonney, W., Prout, G.R. and Coombs, J. (1983). A comparison of cisplatin and the combination of cisplatin and cyclophosphamide in advanced urothelial cancer. *Cancer* **52**: 767–72.

Soloway, M.S., Ikard, M. and Ford, K. (1981). Cis-diamminedichloro-platinum (II) in locally advanced and metastatic urothelial cancer. *Cancer* **47**: 476–80.

Spitzer, W.O., Dobson, A.J., Hall, J. *et al.* (1981). Measuring the quality of life of cancer patients: a concise QL-index for use by physicians. *Journal of Chronic Diseases* **34**: 585–97.

Steel, G.G. (1977). *Growth Kinetics of Tumours*, pp. 5–55 and 217–307. Oxford University Press, Oxford.

Sternberg, C.N., Yagoda, A., Scher, H.I. *et al.* (1985). Preliminary results of M-VAC (methotrexate, vinblastine, doxorubicin and cisplatin) for transitional cell carcinoma of the urothelium. *Journal of Urology* **133**: 403–7.

Sternberg, C.N., Yagoda, A., Scher, H.I. *et al.* (1987). Neo-adjuvant M-VAC chemotherapy trials in transitional cell carcinoma: perspectives for first line chemotherapy. In *Treatment of Advanced Bladder Cancer: EORTC Monograph 5*. Edited by Smith, P.H. and Pavone-Macaluso, M. Alan R. Liss, New York.

Sternberg, J.J., Bracken, R.B., Handel, P.B. and Johnson, D.E. (1977). Combination chemotherapy (CISCA) for advanced urinary tract carcinoma: a preliminary report. *Journal of the American Medical Association* **238**: 2282–7.

Van der Werf Messing, B. (1979). Preoperative irradiation followed by cystectomy to treat carcinoma of the urinary bladder category $T_3N_{x,0-4}M_0$. *International Journal of Radiation Oncology, Biology and Physics* **5**: 394–401.

Whitmore, W.F. (1980). Integrated irradiation and cystectomy for bladder cancer. *British Journal of Urology* **52**: 1–12.

Yagoda, A. (1980). Chemotherapy of metastatic bladder cancer. *Cancer* **45**: 1879–88.

16

Cancer of the upper urothelial tract

L.T. Malden, D. Raghavan, D. Eisinger and B.S. Pearson

Introduction

Carcinoma of the bladder cannot be considered in isolation. Urothelium lines the entire urinary tract, and tumours may occur synchronously or metachronously in multifocal sites, as illustrated by our experience at Royal Prince Alfred Hospital (see Table 16.1). Nevertheless, tumours of the renal pelvis and ureter are relatively uncommon, accounting for less than 10 per cent of urinary tract malignancy (Bloom *et al.*, 1970; Williams and Mitchell, 1973a,b; Johansson *et al.*, 1974). These tumours occur in a ratio for renal pelvis:ureter:bladder of 1:1–3:20–60 (Williams and Mitchell, 1973a,b; Bengtsson *et al.*, 1978; Chasko *et al.*, 1981; McCredie *et al.*, 1982). In the case of ureteric tumours, the lower third is the commonest site of occurrence (Babaian and Johnson, 1980; Werth *et al.*, 1981).

Table 16.1 Royal Prince Alfred Hospital series: site and sex distribution

Site	Male	Female	Associated bladder cancer
Ureter	12	2	43%
Renal pelvis	15	25	30%
Both	9	9	44%

Pathology

Histologically most of the tumours of the upper urinary tract are identical to the transitional cell carcinomas that occur in the bladder, rather than resembling tumours of the renal parenchyma. The spectrum of malignancy, as in the bladder, ranges from benign papillomas to highly anaplastic, invasive cancers (Benington and Beckwith, 1976; Chasko *et al.*, 1981). Occasional squamous carcinomas or adenocarcinomas of the upper tracts have been reported, and rarely melanomas and sarcomas (Benington and Beckwith, 1976; Chasko *et al.*, 1981; Booth *et al.*, 1980). In our experience of 72 cases seen between 1970 and 1984, 64 consisted of pure transitional cell carcinoma (TCC), 5 squamous carcinoma (SqCC) and three patients had mixed TCC and SqCC.

The systems for classifying these tumours with respect to grade and stage are similar, in principle, to those for primary bladder cancer (see Chapters 2 and 4). However, it should be remembered that the absence of a significant surrounding layer of muscle or fat is associated with a reduced barrier to the spread of upper tract tumours (see Table 16.2). In our experience, there is a

Table 16.2 Staging of upper tract urothelial tumours (modified from Cummings, 1980)

Extent of tumour	Jewett system	TNM system
Carcinoma-in-situ	0	T0
Non-invasive		Ta
Invasion of lamina propria	A	T1
Superficial invasion of muscle layer	B1	T2
Deep invasion of muscle without extension through adventitia	B2	T3
Extension through adventitia of pelvis, ureter or kidney capsule	C,D	T4 (N$_+$M0–1)

correlation between high-grade (less differentiated) and advanced-stage tumours (Table 16.3), notwithstanding the bias from our referral pattern of patients with invasive and metastatic disease. Similarly, we have noted correlations between high-grade histological patterns and the presence of multifocal disease and prior abuse of analgesic compounds (see below) (Table 16.4). However, a similar correlation has not been demonstrated between stage at presentation and either multifocal disease or prior analgesic abuse (Table 16.5).

Table 16.3 RPAH series: stage and grade of tumours

Stage	Grade				
	1	2	3	X	Total
0	2	2	0	0	4
A	1	3	1	0	5
B	0	2	1	0	3
C	0	6	9	3	18
D	0	6	13	9	28
X	0	3	4	7	14
Totals	3	22	28	19	72

X denotes 'unknown'.

Table 16.4 RPAH series: patterns of differentiation in multifocal disease and among analgesic abusers

Characteristic	Grade			
	1	2	3	X
Multifocal disease	1	14	18	8
Analgesic abuse	2	5	14*	8
Totals	3	22	28	19

*All females.

Table 16.5 RPAH series: stage at presentation in multifocal disease and among analgesic abusers

Characteristic	Stage					
	0	A	B	C	D	X
Multifocal disease	3	3	3	8	14	10
Analgesic abuse	2	2	2	7	11	5
Total in series	4	5	3	10	28	22

Epidemiology

Upper tract urothelial cancer is a disease of older age groups, occurring most commonly in the fifth to eighth decades, with a mean age at presentation of 60–65 years (Babaian and Johnson, 1980; Booth *et al.*, 1980; Werth *et al.*, 1981; Malden *et al.*, submitted). The sex distribution varies somewhat with the population under study. However, in most series, the male to female ratio is 1–2 : 1, in contrast to the marked male predominance in primary bladder cancer. The increased representation of females is associated particularly with the excessive intake of phenacetin-containing analgesic compounds (Table 16.4).

From 1918 until the 1960s, a common practice among the lower socio-economic classes, and in particular in female factory workers, was to take excessive amounts of phenacetin-containing analgesic compounds in order to experience a transient 'high'. It appears that the practice originated at the time of an influenza epidemic in Huskvarna, Sweden. In the 1950s and 60s, extensive data were reported that linked this social habit to the development of so-called 'analgesic nephropathy', characterized by renal papillary damage and the development of chronic renal failure. In 1965, Hultengren *et al.* described epithelial renal pelvic tumours in six such patients. A series of subsequent reports from Sweden and Australia (the two countries in which the prevalence of this social phenomenon has been unusually high) has provided unequivocal evidence of a causal relationship between the excessive ingestion of these compounds and the subsequent development of TCCs, with lag periods of 4–42 years (Adam *et al.*, 1970; Bengtsson *et al.*, 1968, 1978; McCredie *et al.*, 1982). In our series of patients, half of the 55 patients for whom data regarding analgesic consumption were available had taken excessive quantities at some time (Malden *et al.*, 1987). The majority of these patients were women.

Another association has been described between Balkan endemic nephropathy and cancer of the renal pelvis (Petkovic *et al.*, 1975), although the common aetiological factor is unknown.

Other potential aetiological factors include cigarette smoking (Schmauz and Cole, 1974; Werth *et al.*, 1981; Malden *et al.*, 1987), the leather industry (Schmauz and Cole, 1974), dye working (McAlpine, 1947) and possibly coffee drinking (Armstrong *et al.*, 1976). Congenital renal tract anomalies have also been reported in patients with upper tract TCCs (Booth *et al.*, 1980).

Diagnosis

Presentation

Macroscopic haematuria is the presenting feature in about 70 per cent of cases, and was the only symptom in 75 per cent of these patients in our series (Malden *et al.*, 1987). Less common presentations include flank pain (38 per cent), abdominal pain, weight loss, urinary symptoms (frequency, dysuria, nocturia) and occasionally paraneoplastic or metabolic syndromes (Bourne *et al.*, 1964; Wagle *et al.*, 1974; Batata *et al.*, 1975; Mazeman, 1976; Murphy *et al.*, 1981; Kakizoe *et al.*, 1980). In our experience, 6 per cent of patients had the diagnosis made during a routine clinical assessment.

Investigation

Initial assessment

As outlined in Chapter 4, thorough clinical assessment, including a detailed history and physical examination, is required to reveal the possible local and systemic effects of the disease. In view of the uncertainty regarding the aetiology of the disease, features that should be documented include occupational history, social aspects (cigarette smoking, intake of analgesic compounds), ethnic origin and family history, and history of other malignancies.

The classical triad of gross haematuria, a palpable mass and impaired renal function on intravenous urogram is uncommon (Ochsner *et al.*, 1974; Fraley, 1978). Although there is no great difference in presentation between pelvic and ureteric tumours, it has been suggested that urinary tract infections are more commonly associated with tumours of the renal pelvis (Resseguie *et al.*, 1978).

The initial evaluation of such patients should include at least a baseline assessment of renal and hepatic function, measurement of serum uric acid and calcium, and a full blood count (screening for the anaemia of chronic renal failure or for acute infection). In some patients, assay of carcinoembryonic antigen or human chorionic gonadotrophin may provide a marker of subclinical disease, although rarely of clinical benefit in our experience (see also Chapters 1 and 2).

Urine samples should be sent for culture and sensitivity and for cytological assessment for malignant cells. In patients who have been treated with antibiotics for urinary tract infection, haematuria may mistakenly be ascribed to resolving infection, and a follow-up examination is mandatory. Similarly, sterile pyuria must be investigated further to exclude coincidental occult malignancy of upper and lower urinary tract.

Intravenous urography

The commonest finding in patients with tumours of the renal pelvis is a constant, irregular, radiolucent filling defect. Calcification may be present in up to 70 per cent of patients. Obstruction associated with non-function of the kidney has been reported in about 30 per cent of renal pelvic tumours and in up to 45 per cent of ureteric lesions (Williams and Mitchell, 1973a,b; Batata *et al.*, 1975; Murphy *et al.*, 1981; Malden *et al.*, 1987; Fig. 16.1).

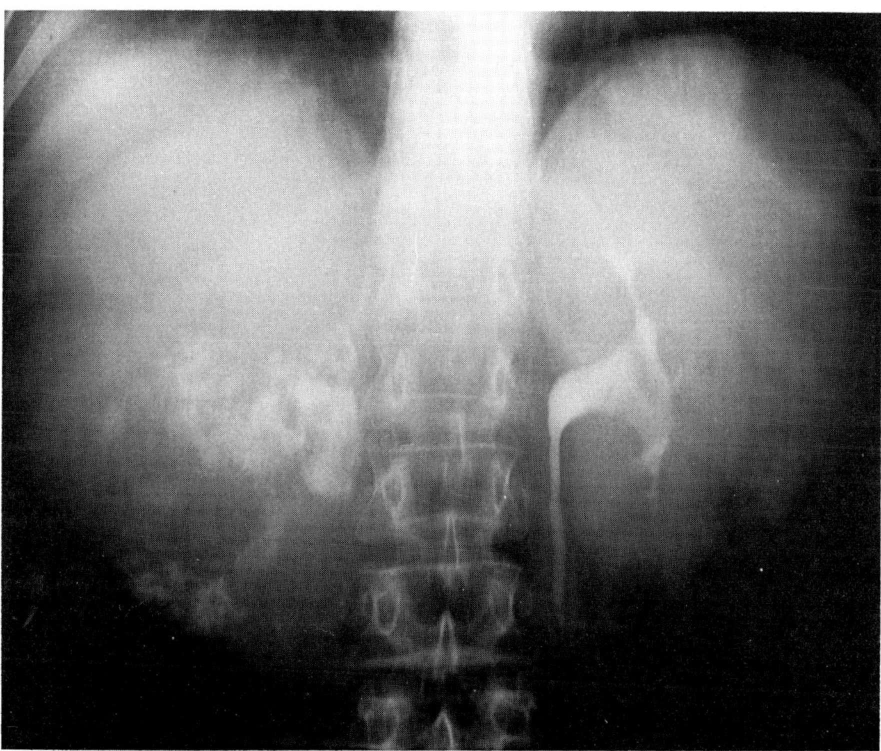

Fig. 16.1 Intravenous pyelogram showing a large right-sided tumour of the renal pelvis

Plain x-rays

Simple radiological investigations, such as plain x-rays of chest and abdomen, may be useful in staging the tumour. The loss of the psoas shadow may reveal an extensive retroperitoneal tumour extending from the renal pelvis or ureter. Aberrant patterns of calcification may be noted in a plain x-ray of the abdomen. Occasionally lytic or sclerotic metastases will be revealed in the vertebrae or pelvis. Similarly pulmonary metastases may occasionally be demonstrated in a chest x-ray, although these are uncommon as a presenting feature of upper tract tumours.

Retrograde urography

A bulb catheter or 5 French gauge catheter ureteropyelogram will reveal a filling defect in more than 80 per cent of cases (Murphy *et al.*, 1980). Typical findings are illustrated in Figs. 16.2 and 16.3. Diluted contrast, small injection volumes (1–2 ml) or double-contrast studies using contrast/air may be helpful in elucidating uncertain filling defects. Signs that suggest the presence of a tumour include coiling of the catheter beneath the tumour (Bergman's sign) or the 'goblet' produced by localized ureteric dilatation at the site of the tumour. This investigation is combined with cystoscopy (see

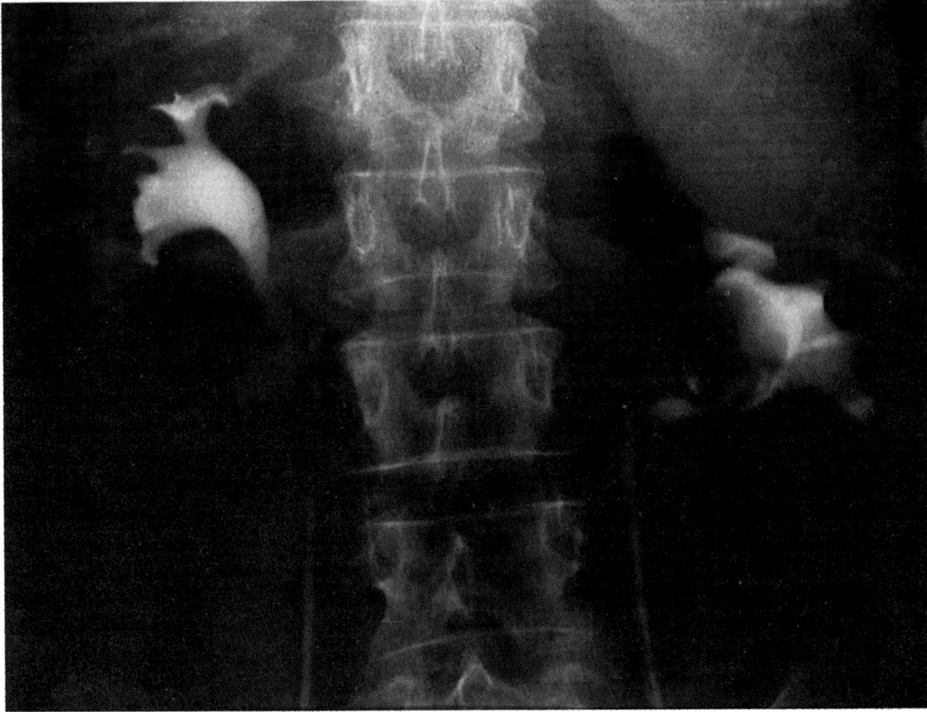

Fig. 16.2 Retrograde pyelogram showing filling defect in left renal pelvis

below) to exclude other causes of haematuria, such as coexistent lower tract tumours, which may be present in up to 45 per cent of cases (Mazeman *et al.*, 1976; Kakizoe *et al.*, 1980) (see also Table 16.1). Cytological assessment, brush or basket biopsy, or ureterorenoscopy may be performed at the same time (see below).

Computerized tomography
Computerized tomographic (CT) scanning may be used to determine the nature of a filling defect, and is particularly useful in differentiating a radiolucent stone from a tumour. In TCC, CT scanning may show intrusion into the renal pelvis, infiltration of the renal parenchyma (Figs. 16.4 and 16.5) or invasion of the perinephric space. Thickening of the ureteric wall or periureteric infiltration may also be seen. The technique is also of value in staging the tumour, with the demonstration of enlarged lymph nodes, hepatic metastases or other sites of apparent involvement (see Chapter 5).

Angiography
The overall accuracy of angiography in defining the nature of a filling defect may be as high as 60–75 per cent in expert hands (Eklund and Tothlin, 1976). However, because of the 25–40 per cent rate of error, the invasiveness of the procedure, and the ready availability of CT scanning, angiography is not routinely used in the evaluation of upper tract TCCs in our

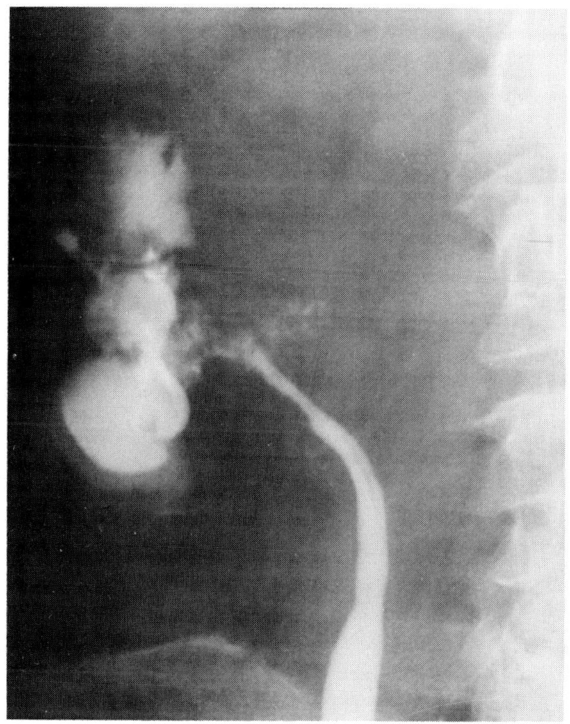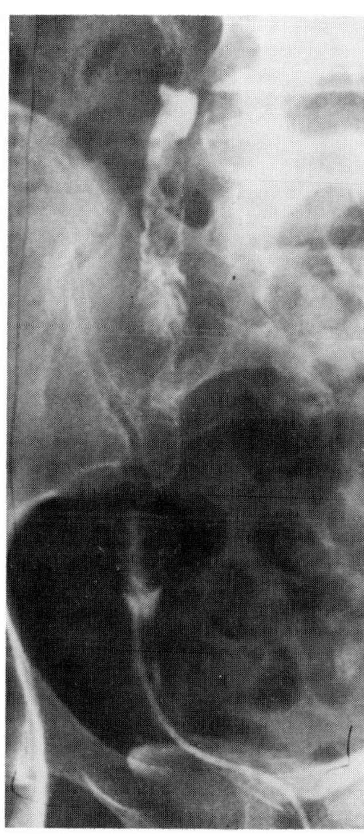

Fig. 16.3 (a) Retrograde pyelogram showing a large tumour of the right renal pelvis. (b) Retrograde pyelogram showing extensive tumour of the right ureter

institution. Small tumours often fail to have arterial abnormalities. In advanced tumours, such as those that extend beyond the renal capsule, arteriography may show the tumour circulation and the extent of the tumour (Fig. 16.6), which may help in the planning of surgery. In addition, more extensive tumours may be characterized by decreased branching of the interlobar arteries, giving the 'pruned-tree' appearance (Mitty *et al.*, 1969). Renal venography has also been reported to aid in the diagnosis and staging of these tumours (Bernath *et al.*, 1981).

Cystoscopy, ureterorenoscopy and biopsy

Earlier studies suggested that endoscopy was of only limited value in patients with upper tract TCCs (Hvidt and Feldt-Rasmussen, 1973). However, in view of the potential for field defects and multifocal sites of involvement (especially in patients who have been analgesic abusers), we believe that this procedure is integral to management. In addition to cystoscopy and bimanual examination under anaesthesia, retrograde pyelography has an important role in diagnosing and assessing the extent of tumour (see above). Similarly, retrograde brushing provides material for both cytological and histological examination (Gill *et al.*, 1979). Catheters that can be 'steered' are now available and can increase the yield from this procedure (Lieberman *et al.*, 1984), with a reported diagnostic accuracy as

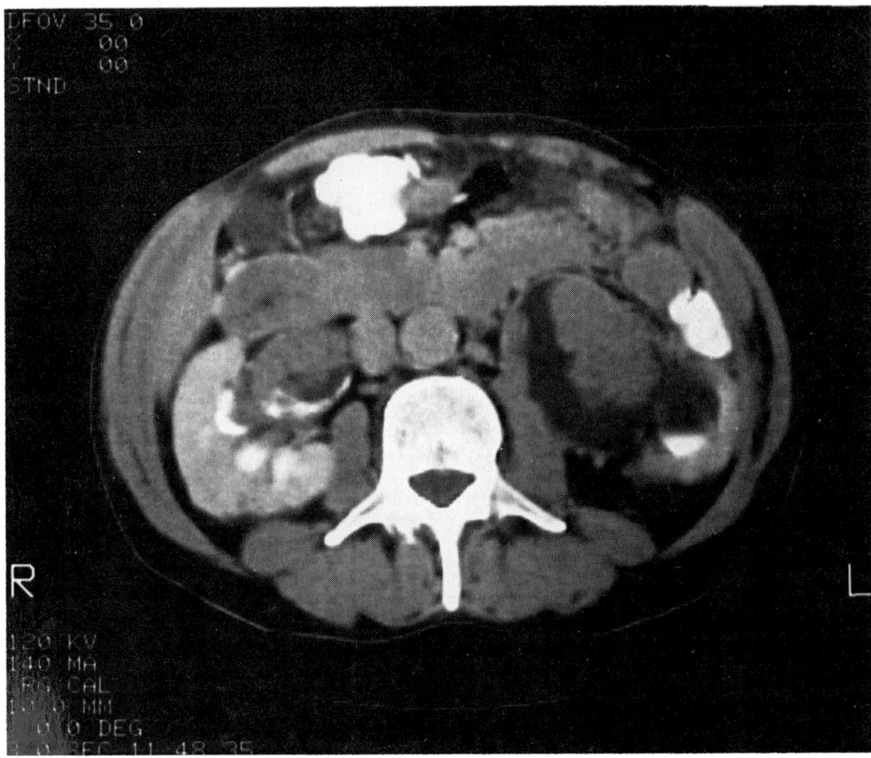

Fig. 16.4 CAT scan showing large left-sided tumour of the renal pelvis, with impaired renal function

high as 80 per cent. Tissue for diagnosis can also be obtained using a wire basket, introduced under fluoroscopic control (Kiriyama *et al.*, 1975).

More recently, the IIF rigid ureterorenoscope has been introduced into clinical practice, and enables visualization of the entire length of ureter and renal pelvis. Biopsy can be performed with forceps or a basket. However, ureterorenoscopy carries a risk of perforation and severe haemorrhage, and must be performed with caution.

In some instances, excellent cytological preparations can be obtained by ureteric catheterization without barbotage (with less disruption of the architecture of the exfoliated cells). However, barbotage is associated with the highest yields of tumour cells. The accuracy of cytological examination varies greatly with the method of specimen collection, the experience of the cytologist, and the clinical situation (grade of the tumour, prior radiotherapy or chemotherapy). The overall reported accuracy ranges from 40 to 70 per cent (Sarnacki *et al.*, 1971; Zincke *et al.*, 1976). False-negative results may be due to inadequate collection techniques, ureteric obstruction, a non-functioning kidney, or inexperience of the cytologist.

Fine-needle aspiration biopsy
A useful alternative for obtaining a tissue diagnosis has become available

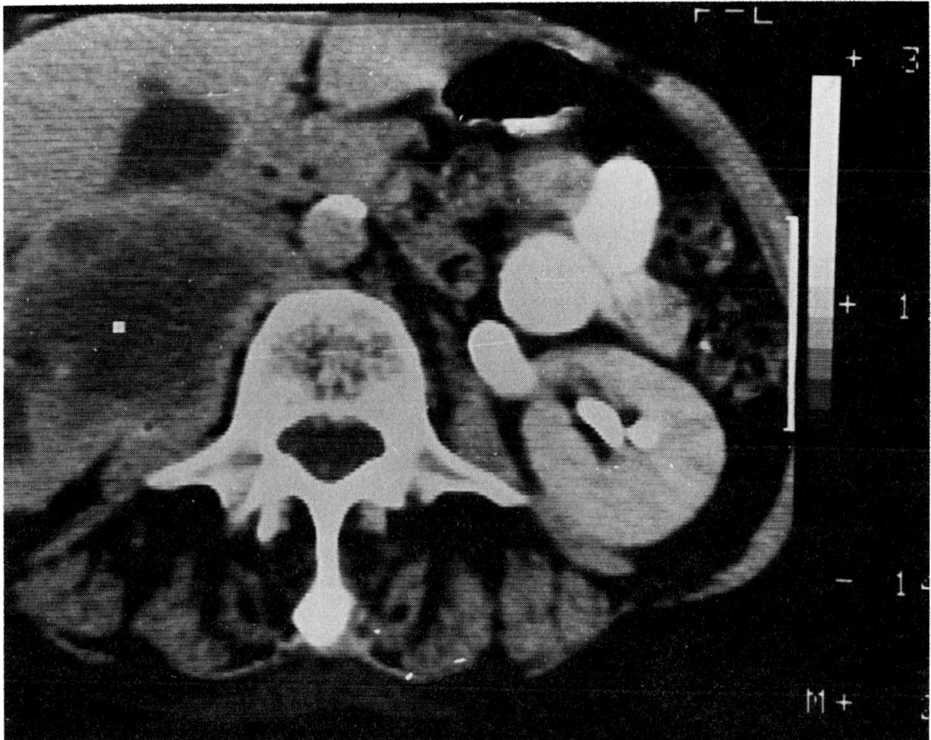

Fig. 16.5 CAT scan showing large tumour of the right renal pelvis with extension into the parenchyma

with the introduction of fine-needle aspiration biopsy into routine clinical practice. This procedure, in which a narrow-gauge biopsy needle is introduced percutaneously into the suspected tumour mass, is often performed under CT scan control. An experienced cytologist must be available to assess the specimen at the time of the procedure to ensure optimal sampling and diagnostic yield. However, there is a potential risk of tumour seeding along the needle tract (Gibbons *et al.*, 1977), and the technique should only be used by experienced personnel.

Treatment

Surgery

Nephroureterectomy is the treatment of choice for TCCs of the upper urinary tract (Williams and Mitchell, 1973a; Wagle *et al.*, 1974; Booth *et al.*, 1980; Werth *et al.*, 1981). It has been demonstrated that subsequent bladder recurrence can be reduced if a cuff of bladder is removed with the lower end of the ureter (Williams and Mitchell, 1973a; Strong and Pearse, 1976; Cummings, 1980). All such patients should be monitored regularly by cystoscopy (as if the original tumour had been in the bladder) because of the

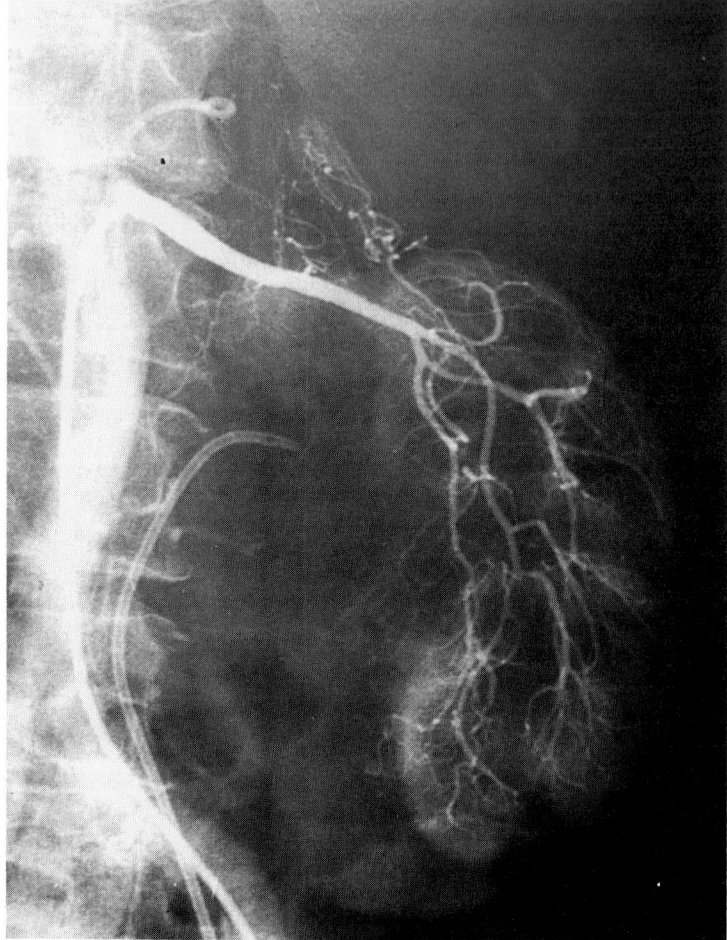

Fig. 16.6 Renal arteriogram demonstrating extrarenal extension from a large TCC of the left renal pelvis

multifocal nature of the disease. The results of treatment depend on the grade and stage of the disease. For example, in renal pelvic tumours, Williams and Mitchell (1973a) demonstrated a 5-year survival of 48 per cent in superficial disease, compared with 11 per cent for invasive tumours. Similar survival figures have been reported for ureteric tumours, depending on the extent of invasion (Bloom *et al.*, 1970; Heney *et al.*, 1981).

Conservative surgery, with local excision of superficial tumours of the renal pelvis (Vest, 1945) or ureter (Petkovic, 1972b) and conservation of the kidney, has been advocated intermittently for more than 40 years. Numerous approaches have been used, including partial ureterectomy, partial excision of the renal pelvis and partial nephrectomy, sometimes preceded or followed by radiotherapy. The indications for conservative surgery have included renal failure, solitary kidneys, poor general medical condition of the patient, or bilateral tumours (Petkovic, 1972a; Brown and Roumani, 1974; Cummings, 1980). In the case of renal pelvic tumours, it is generally recommended that conservative approaches should be reserved for small tumours with a narrow pedicle. The optimal management of tumours of the ureter is more controversial. However, criteria that have been cited as prerequisites for local resection include:

1. good potential function of the ipsilateral kidney;
2. a polypoidal filling defect in the ureter, which can be demonstrated radiologically or endoscopically to be localized;
3. at operation, the ureteric wall should not be indurated (the subject of considerable debate).

The issue of conservative versus radical surgery has not yet been resolved (Gittes, 1980; Cummings, 1980). The pendulum appears to be swinging in favour of conservatism, at least in highly selected cases, based on several arguments:

1. With the improvements in the techniques for diagnosis and staging (e.g. cytology, ureterorenoscopy, and percutaneous nephroscopy), low-stage and low-grade tumours can be identified more confidently—these are associated with a good prognosis after local excision.
2. Similar techniques can be used for monitoring after local excision to detect any recurrences early.
3. High grade, high stage tumours appear to be associated with a poor prognosis whatever surgical approach is used (Gittes, 1980).
4. Conservative surgery may be indicated in some patients with high risk or metastatic disease, in whom sacrifice of the kidney is not essential to obtain adequate clearance of tumours. These patients may then be spared dialysis for the remainder of their lives (particularly in the case of bilateral tumours or solitary kidneys), or may achieve improved renal function without dialysis in the short term, facilitating the use of cytotoxic chemotherapy to achieve tumour control.

However, the advocates of a radical approach emphasize that the good results of conservative surgery reflect careful patient selection in expert hands, the natural history of low-grade, low-stage disease, and may also be a function of a failure to report poor results (Batata and Grabstald, 1976). Patients with tumours of intermediate and high grade and stage have been reported to have a longer survival after radical surgery (Booth *et al.*, 1980; Cummings, 1980; Murphy *et al.*, 1981). However, it should be noted that these studies reflect non-randomized clinical trials, and the differences may be due, in part, to patient selection; for example, the more robust patients may undergo radical surgery, while the medically unfit patients receive conservative treatment.

An important problem in interpreting the available data in order to define an optimal policy of management is the prevalence of bias in reporting. For example, the development of contralateral tumours in 10–20 per cent of patients has been cited variously in support of conservatism (Petkovic, 1972a,b) and of radical surgery (Batata and Grabstald, 1976).

Ideally this issue is one that might be resolved by a well-designed, randomized multicentre trial. However, in view of the low incidence of upper tract tumours, such a study might not be feasible owing to problems with accrual of patients. In the absence of unequivocal data, our routine approach for intermediate and high-grade invasive tumours is to perform a nephroureterectomy with removal of a cuff of bladder. Such patients are then monitored regularly by cystoscopy with intermittent retrograde pyelography, as well as urinary cytology, depending on the preference of the individual clinician. For patients who present an unduly high operative risk because of their general physical condition, nephrectomy alone may be performed, accepting the risk of ureteric stump recurrence in order to reduce the extent of the operation. The approach to low-grade, low-stage tumours is individualized, and conservative techniques are often employed (especially in patients with chronic renal failure, analgesic nephropathy with the associated risk of metachronous contralateral tumours, or those with solitary kidneys after prior surgery for cancer or chronic infection). Opening the renal pelvis in a conservative procedure carries a risk of local tumour implantation. Although it has been suggested that appropriate packing, suction applied to the ureteric catheter and irrigation with agents such as 0.25% eusol, sterile water or nitrofurazone solution (Fraley, 1978) may reduce this risk, local recurrences still may occur (Tomera *et al.*, 1982). The selection of cases for conservative surgery is important. For example, it appears that a higher relapse rate is characteristic of tumours of the renal pelvis than in ureteric tumours (Mazeman, 1976; Zincke and Neves, 1984).

At the present time, the impact of radiotherapy, the newer cytotoxic agents and the advances in technology (such as fibreoptic endoscopes and photodynamic therapy) has not been assessed in the context of conservative management of upper tract tumours. In view of the uptake of haematoporphyrin derivatives by superficial TCC and by carcinoma-in-situ, and its fluorescence under laser beam, the combination of intraoperative or percutaneous renoscopy and the use of laser fibres may provide an effective means of obtaining local tumour control in highly selected patients. Similarly, the introduction of innovative cytotoxic regimens with higher apparent response rates (see also Chapters 10 and 12) may facilitate the use of conservative surgical techniques with adjuvant chemotherapy in an effort to improve overall survival. However, such an approach would require validation in formal clinical trials.

Another investigational approach that is being evaluated in Sweden represents an attempt to conserve the kidney without loss of surgical tumour clearance (Pettersson *et al.*, 1984). In this study, patients have undergone nephroureterectomy, followed by renal autotransplantation and pyelocystostomy. Five of seven patients have remained free of tumour for periods between 1 and 3 years, and two patients have died without evidence of local recurrence. It should be noted, however, that the majority of these cases represented low-grade low-stage tumours, and further data will be required before an accurate assessment of the validity and cost-effectiveness of this programme can be achieved.

Radiotherapy

The role of radiotherapy, either as definitive treatment or as an adjunct to surgery, has not been well defined. With regard to the use of irradiation as definitive treatment for tumours of the renal pelvis and ureter, there are the important problems owing to the limitations of non-invasive staging or tumour localization and the limited tolerance of the kidney to doses of irradiation greater than 2000 cGy.

Nevertheless, Brady *et al.* (1968) have reported the use of radiotherapy as the primary treatment in six patients with cancer of the ureter, three of whom survived more than 5 years. Two of these patients were treated for recurrent cancer and four for tumours that were unresectable at operation.

Postoperative radiotherapy has been studied to a limited extent. Holz (1962) reported a series of 20 cases of ureteric carcinoma and suggested that a prognostic benefit is derived from postoperative irradiation, a view supported in other reports (Batata *et al.*, 1975; Babaian and Johnson, 1980). By contrast, in earlier studies it has been concluded that radiotherapy should be reserved for the palliation of recurrences or metastases (Scott, 1943; Bergman *et al.*, 1961). However, it must be noted that these are dated, and were produced in an era of highly inaccurate non-invasive staging; in this context, it is not surprising that the investigators concluded that radiotherapy had only a limited role.

The role of preoperative irradiation also remains uncertain. Almgaard *et al.* (1973) initiated a study to evaluate the efficacy and toxicity of this approach. However, to our knowledge, follow-up data have not been reported.

In our own institution, preoperative irradiation is not used for the management of upper tract tumours. Occasionally, patients with involved lymph nodes demonstrated at laparotomy will undergo adjuvant radiotherapy, with a field including the para-aortic chain (after a nephroureterectomy) with shielding of the contralateral kidney.

Chemotherapy

There are extensive data regarding the efficacy of cytotoxic chemotherapy in the management of urothelial tumours in general (see Chapters 10, 11, 12, 15 and 17). However, there is scant information available with respect to response and survival of patients receiving chemotherapy for upper tract tumours *per se*. In most instances, reports of the use of chemotherapy for urothelial cancer incorporate occasional upper tract tumours amongst large numbers of bladder cancers, without dissecting out the respective response rates and survival. As a result, it has been impossible to make a definitive statement regarding the role of cytotoxic drugs in the management of upper tract urothelial tumours.

The situation has been complicated by two important factors:

1. Upper tract urothelial tumours are associated with chronic renal failure and analgesic nephropathy. Thus a population of less-fit patients with impaired metabolic function, who are less able to adhere to cytotoxic protocols, may be selected.

2. There is a reduced barrier to the spread of upper tract cancer because of the absence of thick layers of muscle and fat, accompanied by a high lymphatic and vascular investment. Hence tumours of the upper tracts are often more advanced and widespread at diagnosis, which may be associated with a worse prognosis.

Nevertheless, from the available literature, it is clear that upper tract tumours do, in fact, sometimes respond to cytotoxic chemotherapy, although it is not possible to determine the comparative sensitivities of bladder and upper tract tumours (Sternberg *et al.*, 1977; Von Eyben *et al.*, 1979; Kotake *et al.*, 1983; Sternberg *et al.*, 1985). The drugs that appear active in the management of upper tract tumours include cisplatinum, methotrexate, Adriamycin and vinblastine (see Table 16.6).

Table 16.6 Cytotoxic drugs that occasionally induce objective responses in upper tract urothelial cancer

Single agents
Vinblastine
Methotrexate
Cisplatinum
Adriamycin
CCNU?
Neocarzinostatin?

Combination regimens
Methotrexate/vinblastine/Adriamycin/Cisplatinum (MVAC)
Cyclophosphamide/Adriamycin/5-fluorouracil (CAF)
Cyclophosphamide/Adriamycin/Cisplatinum (CAP)
Vinblastine/CCNU

Note: There are insufficient data available to list response rates for upper tract tumours.

In our experience (Table 16.7), responses have been documented after treatment with cisplatinum, the combination of cisplatinum and methotrexate, Adriamycin plus mitomycin C, and after 5-fluorouracil (a heavily pretreated patient). Contrary to the experience from the Memorial Sloan Kettering Cancer Center, where a series of reports have implied common sensitivity of bladder and upper tract tumours, our only two patients with upper tract tumours who were treated with the MVAC regimen (see Chapter 12) failed to respond. In each instance the patient experienced severe toxicity.

Case 1: A 45-year-old Yugoslav underwent a nephrectomy for a poorly differentiated transitional cell and squamous cell carcinoma of the right renal pelvis. Two months later, he was referred with locoregional recurrence and metastases in lymph nodes, liver and bone. No tumour was demonstrated in the bone marrow. The patient's renal function was normal. He was treated with the MVAC regimen (Sternberg *et al.*, 1985) in standard doses, but with the addition of folinic acid rescue. He suffered grade-3 vomiting, despite antiemetics, and subsequently developed grade-4 stomatitis, grade-4 neutropenia, and mild thrombocytopenia. Despite controlling these complications, the patient gradually deteriorated, becoming hypercalcaemic, with tumour progression and the development of a subacute bowel obstruction. He died 4 weeks after the commencement of treatment.

Case 2: A 58-year-old Australian woman, with a past history of analgesic abuse, underwent a right nephroureterectomy for an infiltrating grade-III TCC of ureter. Histological examination of the kidney revealed nephrotic changes and interstitial fibrosis. She was referred 2 months later with local recurrence and lymph node metastases. Her renal function was at the upper limit of normal. Other staging tests were normal. She was treated with the MVAC regimen with folinic acid rescue (in view of her prior history). Twenty days after treatment, she developed grade-4 neutropenia and thrombocytopenia, septicaemia and grade-4 stomatitis. Her condition deteriorated, she developed a large abdominal mass and subacute bowel obstruction, and died 4 months after treatment had begun.

These cases serve merely to illustrate that the MVAC regimen does not necessarily constitute the 'state of the art' in the management of recurrent or metastatic upper tract tumours. As outlined elsewhere in this volume (Chapters 15 and 17), further randomized studies will be required to define the exact place for this regimen in routine management.

Table 16.7 RPAH series: chemotherapy of upper tract urothelial cancer

Cytotoxic drug	Number of patients	Response
Cisplatinum	6	1 PR
Cisplatinum/methotrexate	4	1 PR
Methotrexate	7	0
Adriamycin	6	1 PR*
5-fluorouracil	1	1 PR

*Response occurred in relapsed patient who previously responded to cisplatinum/methotrexate.

We share a concern expressed by others that upper tract urothelial tumours may be somewhat less sensitive than those arising in the bladder. Nevertheless, it is clear that sustained remissions can be achieved by cytotoxic chemotherapy for recurrent or metastatic upper tract tumours. Our current practice is to treat these patients according to protocols established for urothelial tumours that arise from any site. Particular attention is required for patients with a past history of analgesic abuse: documentation of renal function (including creatinine clearance), monitoring of hydration, careful choice of cytotoxic agents and doses. Specific reporting of the results of treatment of these tumours (within the larger randomized trials for bladder cancer) will be required in order to define the optimal plan of chemotherapeutic management of cancer of the upper tracts.

References

Adam, W.R., Dawborn, J.K., Price, C.G., Ridell, J. and Story, H. (1970). Anaplastic transitional cell carcinoma of the renal pelvis in association with analgesic abuse. *Medical Journal of Australia* **1**: 1108–9.

Almgaard, L.E., Freedman, D. and Ljungqvist, A. (1973). Carcinoma of the ureter. *Scandinavian Journal of Urology and Nephrology* **7**: 165–7.
Armstrong, B., Garrod, A. and Doll, R. (1976). A retrospective study of renal cancer with special reference to coffee and animal protein consumption. *British Journal of Cancer* **33**: 127–36.
Babaian, R.J. and Johnson, D.E. (1980). Primary carcinoma of the ureter. *Journal of Urology* **123**: 357–9.
Batata, M.A. and Grabstald, H. (1976). Upper urinary tract urothelial tumors. *Urologic Clinics of North America* **3**: 70–86.
Batata, M.A., Whitmore, W.F., Hilaris, B.S., Tokita, N. and Grabstald, H. (1975). Primary carcinoma of the ureter: a prognostic study. *Cancer* **35**: 1626–32.
Bengtsson, U., Angervall, L., Ekman, H. and Lehmann, L. (1968). Transitional cell tumours of the renal pelvis in analgesic abusers. *Scandinavian Journal of Urology and Nephrology* **2**: 145–50.
Bengtsson, U., Johansson, S. and Angervall, L. (1978). Malignancies of the urinary tract and their relation to analgesic abuse. *Kidney International* **13**: 107–13.
Bennington, J.L. and Beckwith, J.B. (1975). Tumors of the kidney, renal pelvis and ureter. In *Atlas of Tumor Pathology*, Armed Forces Institute of Pathology, Fascicle 12, second series, Washington, D.C.
Bergman, H., Friedenberg, R.M. and Sayegh, V. (1961). New roentgenologic signs of carcinoma of the ureter. *American Journal of Roentgenology* **86**: 707–17.
Bernath, A.S., Addonizio, J.C., Kinkhabwala, M. and Thelmo, W. (1981). Renal venography in diagnosis of infiltrating transitional cell carcinoma of renal pelvis. *Urology* **18**: 164–6.
Bloom, N.A., Vidone, R.A. and Lytton, B. (1970). Primary carcinoma of the ureter: a report of 102 new cases. *Journal of Urology* **103**: 590–98.
Booth, C.M., Cameron, K.M. and Pugh, R.C.B. (1980). Urothelial carcinoma of the kidney and ureter. *British Journal of Urology* **52**: 430–35.
Bourne, H.E., Tremblay, R.E. and Ansell, J.S. (1964). Stupor, hypercalcemia and carcinoma of the renal pelvis. *New England Journal of Medicine* **271**: 1005–6.
Brady, L.W., Gislason, G.H., Faust, D.S., Kazem, I., Antoniades, J. and Davis, J.A. (1968). Radiotherapy: a valuable adjunct in the management of carcinoma of the ureter. *Journal of the American Medical Association* **206**: 2871–4.
Brown, H.E. and Roumani, G.K. (1974). Conservative surgical management of transitional cell carcinoma of the upper urinary tract. *Journal of Urology* **112**: 184–7.
Chasko, S.B., Gray, G.F. and McCarron, J.P. (1981). Urothelial neoplasia of the upper urinary tract. *Pathology Annual* **16/2**: 127–53.
Cummings, K.B. (1980). Nephroureterectomy: rationale in the management of transitional cell carcinoma of the upper urinary tract. *Urologic Clinics of North America* **7**: 569–78.
Eklund, L. and Tothlin, J. (1976). Angiography in carcinoma of the renal pelvis and the ureter. *Acta Radiologica Diagnostica* **17**: 676–82.
Fraley, E.E. (1978). Cancer of the renal pelvis. In *Genitourinary Cancer*, pp. 134–49. Edited by Skinner, D.G. and DeKernion, J.B. W.B. Saunders, Philadelphia.
Gibbons, R.P., Bush, W.H. and Burnett, L.L. (1977). Needle tract seeding following aspiration of renal cell carcinoma. *Journal of Urology* **118**: 865–7.
Gill, W.B., Lu, C.-T. and Bibbo, M. (1979). Retrograde brush biopsy of

the ureter and renal pelvis. *Urologic Clinics of North America* **6**: 573–586.

Gittes, R.F. (1980). Management of transitional cell carcinoma of the upper tract: case for conservative local excision. *Urologic Clinics of North America* **7**: 559–68.

Heney, N.M., Nocks, B.N., Daly, J.J., Blitzer, P.H. and Parkhurst, E.C. (1981). Prognostic factors in carcinoma of the ureter. *Journal of Urology* **88**: 380–85.

Holtz, F. (1962). Papillomas and primary carcinoma of the ureter: report of 20 cases. *Journal of Urology* **88**: 380–85.

Hultengren, N., Lagergren, C. and Ljungqvist, A. (1965). Carcinoma of the renal pelvis in renal papillary necrosis. *Acta Chirurgica Scandinavica* : 314–20.

Hvidt, V. and Feldt-Rasmussen, K. (1973). Primary tumours in the renal pelvis and ureter with particular attention to the diagnostic problems. *Acta Chirurgica Scandinavica* **43** (Suppl.): 91–101.

Johansson, S., Angervall, L., Bengtsson, U. and Wahlquist, L. (1974). Uroepithelial tumours of the renal pelvis associated with abuse of phenacetin-containing analgesics. *Cancer* **33**: 743–53.

Kakizoe, T., Fujita, J., Murase, T. *et al.* (1980). Transitional cell carcinoma of the bladder in patients with renal pelvic and ureteral cancer. *Journal of Urology* **124**: 17–19.

Kiriyama, T., Hironaka, H. and Fukada, K. (1975). Six years of experience with retrograde biopsy of intraureteric carcinoma using the Dormia stone basket. *Journal of Urology* **116**: 308–10.

Kotake, T., Usami, M., Miki, T. *et al.* (1983). Combination chemotherapy including Adriamycin for advanced transitional cell carcinoma of the urinary tract. *Cancer Chemotherapy and Pharmacology* **11** (Suppl.): 38– 42.

Lieberman, R.P., Cummings, K.B. and Leslie, W.B. (1984). Sheathed catheter systems for fluoroscopically guided retrograde catheterization, and brush and forceps biopsy of the upper urinary tract. *Journal of Urology* **131**: 450–3.

Malden, L.T., Raghavan, D., Philips, J. *et al.* (1987). Urothelial cancer of the upper tracts: a report of 72 cases, including responses to chemotherapy.

Mazeman, E. (1976). Tumours of the upper urinary tract calyces, renal pelvis and ureter. *European Urology* **2**: 120–28.

McAlpine, J.B. (1947). Papilloma of the renal pelvis in dye workers: two cases, one of which shows bilateral growth. *British Journal of Surgery* **35**: 137–40.

McCredie, M., Ford, J.M., Taylor, J.S. and Stewart, J.S. (1982). Analgesics and cancer of the renal pelvis in New South Wales. *Cancer* **49**: 2617–25.

Mitty, H.A., Baron, M.G. and Feller, M. (1969). Infiltrating carcinoma of the renal pelvis. *Radiology* **92**: 994–8.

Murphy, D.M., Zincke, H. and Furlow, W.L. (1980). Primary grade-I transitional cell carcinoma of the renal pelvis and ureter. *Journal of Urology* **123**: 629–31.

Murphy, D.M., Zincke, H. and Furlow, W.L. (1981). Management of high grade transitional cell cancer of the upper urinary tract. *Journal of Urology* **125**: 25–9.

Ochsner, M.G., Brannan, W., Pond, H.S. and Collins, H.T. (1974). Transitional cell carcinoma of the renal pelvis and ureter. *Urology* **4**: 392–6.

Petkovic, S.D. (1972a). Conservation of the kidney in operations for tumours of the renal pelvis and calyces: a report of 26 cases. *British Journal of Urology* **44**: 1–8.

Petkovic, S.D. (1972b). A plea for conservative operation for ureteral tumors. *Journal of Urology* **107**: 220–23.

Petkovic, S.D. (1975). Epidemiology and treatment of renal pelvic and ureteral tumours. *Journal of Urology* **114**: 858–65.

Pettersson, S., Brynger, H., Henriksson, C., Johansson, S.L., Nilson, A.E. and Ranch, T. (1984). Treatment of urothelial tumors of the upper urinary tract by nephroureterectomy, renal autotransplantion and pyelocystostomy. *Cancer* **54**: 379–86.

Resseguie, J.L., Nobrega, G., Farrow, G.M., Timmons, J.W. and Worobec, T.G. (1978). Epidemiology of renal and ureteral cancer in Rochester, Minnesota, 1950–1974, with special reference to clinical and pathologic features. *Mayo Clinic Proceedings* **53**: 503–10.

Sarnacki, C.T., McCormack, L.J., Kiser, W.S. *et al.* (1971). Urinary cytology and the clinical diagnosis of urinary tract malignancy: a clinicopathologic study of 1400 patients. *Journal of Urology* **106**: 761–4.

Schmauz, R. and Cole, P. (1974). Epidemiology of cancer of the renal pelvis and ureter. *Journal of the National Cancer Institute* **52**: 1431–4.

Scott, W.W. (1943). Review of primary carcinoma of the ureter: presenting two cases. *Journal of Urology* **50**: 45–64.

Soloway, M.S., Ikard, M. and Ford, K. (1981). Cis-diamminedichloro-platinum (II) in locally advanced and metastatic urothelial cancer. *Cancer* **47**: 476–80.

Sternberg, C.N., Yagoda, A., Scher, H.I. *et al.* (1985). Preliminary results of M-VAC (methotrexate, vinblastine, doxorubicin and cisplatin) for transitional cell carcinoma of the urothelium. *Journal of Urology* **133**: 403–7.

Sternberg, J.J., Bracken, R.B., Handel, P.B. and Johnson, D.E. (1977). Combination chemotherapy (CISCA) for advanced urinary tract carcinoma. *Journal of the American Medical Association* **238**: 2282–7.

Strong, D.W. and Pearse, H.D. (1976). Recurrent urothelial tumours following surgery for transitional cell carcinoma of the upper urinary tract. *Cancer* **38**: 2178–83.

Tomera, K.M., Leary, F.J. and Zincke, H. (1982). Pyeloscopy in urothelial tumors. *Journal of Urology* **127**: 1088–9.

Vest, S.A. (1945). Conservative surgery in certain benign tumors of the ureter. *Journal of Urology* **53**: 97–121.

Von Eyben, F., Mattsson, W., Glifberg, I. and Lindholm, E.-E. (1979). Chemotherapy of advanced transitional cell carcinoma of the renal pelvis: report of 3 cases treated with vinblastine and chloroethyl-cyclohexyl-nitrosourea. *Journal of Urology* **121**: 367–8.

Wagle, D.G., Moore, R.H. and Murphy, G.P. (1974). Primary carcinoma of the renal pelvis. *Cancer* **33**: 1642–8.

Werth, D.S., Weigel, J.W. and Meburst, W.K. (1981). Primary neoplasms of the ureter. *Journal of Urology* **125**: 628–31.

Williams, C.B. and Mitchell, J.P. (1973a). Carcinoma of the renal pelvis: a review of 43 cases. *British Journal of Urology* **45**: 370–76.

Williams, C.B. and Mitchell, J.P. (1973b). Carcinoma of the ureter: a review of 54 cases. *British Journal of Urology* **45**: 377–87.

Zincke, H. and Neves, R.J. (1984). Feasibility of conservative surgery for transitional cell cancer of the upper urinary tract. *Urologic Clinics of North America* **11**: 717–24.

17

The management of bladder cancer: current practice and future prospects

Derek Raghavan

Introduction

In this volume, we have attempted to summarize and to assess the available data on the biology and treatment of urothelial cancer. Yet, for the clinician faced with specific problems in the management of this complex group of diseases, the final decision often remains difficult. How can one predict the likely behaviour of the disease in a particular instance? Which of the conflicting sets of data with regard to optimal treatment should be applied to a specific clinical problem? How can one resolve these differing opinions and biases?

Ultimately, the clinician must initiate a plan of management, based as rationally as possible. This chapter represents simply a personal overview—an attempt to resolve some of these issues, and to predict future trends in the management of urothelial malignancy.

Biology of urothelial cancer: applications to management

Urothelial cancer consists of a spectrum of diseases with diverse natural histories. When considered in the simplest fashion, the conventional morphological classifications provided by classical histopathology, including cell type, grade and stage, still remain the hallmarks of the decision-making process. In the great majority of experimental and clinical studies, transitional cell carcinoma (TCC) behaves differently from pure squamous carcinoma or adenocarcinoma; high-grade tumours are associated with a worse prognosis, as are those tumours of advanced stage. Eighty per cent of high-grade (III) tumours are associated with invasion at diagnosis; but why are the other 20 per cent only superficial? Invasive and superficial TCC seem often to be manifestly different diseases. Superficial tumours tend not to invade or metastasize in most cases; but paradoxically, it is the most superficial variant, carcinoma-in-situ (TIS), that is often associated with the worst prognosis.

Invasive TCC is usually found to be invasive at the first presentation (Chapters 2, 4 and 6). However, many of these tumours can be unpredictable, especially those with intermediate (grade-II) differentiation. Progression from grade I to II does not necessarily mandate an increase in the vigour of therapy, although it is often difficult to define which tumours will remain indolent. Thus one of the most important goals of the laboratory should be to define predictors of the natural history of urothelial cancer to facilitate and rationalize the choice of treatment (Raghavan *et al.*, 1986). As outlined in Chapter 1, attempts are being made to do this.

The experimental models reviewed in Chapter 1 have demonstrated substantial heterogeneity of tumours with apparently identical light morphology, with respect to ultrastructure, the expression of tumour markers, DNA content, natural history and response to treatment. The application of carcinogenic stimuli to apparently normal urothelial tissue can produce a marked spectrum of neoplastic changes, ranging from superficial and indolent disease to invasive, aggressive malignancy (Hicks and Wakefield, 1972). Although it is not yet known why such diversity can arise from common stimuli, an understanding of this phenomenon could yield insights into the basis of the heterogeneity of these tumours and thus could reveal predictors of their patterns of behaviour.

In xenograft studies and in tissue culture, we have demonstrated the range of differentiation that can be expressed in serial passage by sublines derived from common parent tumours (Chapter 1). Thus, a moderately differentiated TCC can yield foci of moderately differentiated tissue with variable staining for carcinoembryonic antigen and other tumour markers, diverse patterns of lectin binding, and a range of ploidy from $2n$ to $5n$. Such xenografts can show marked heterogeneity of response to treatment (see Chapter 1, Fig. 1.4 and 1.5). It is thus hardly surprising that the choice regarding the optimal management of patients with urothelial malignancy is often difficult and that reliable investigators can often draw markedly different conclusions regarding apparently similar treatment programmes (even when the same criteria of evaluation are applied).

From a clinical viewpoint, the contributions of the laboratory to the decision-making process have not yet been substantial. There are a number of potential predictors of response (see Table 17.1), but these are mostly not yet applicable for routine clinical use, either because of their complexity, the degree of technical difficulty, a lack of reproducibility, or the nature of the required sampling of tumour tissue.

However, as described in Chapter 2, the simple methodology for demonstrating the expression of blood group substances on the surface of bladder cancer cells can easily be applied in clinical practice and can thus influence treatment decisions. For example, the patient with a low-grade, superficial papillary TCC with expression of blood group substances can be treated endoscopically with less than a 20 per cent chance of developing invasion. By contrast, a similar tumour with deletion of blood group substances is at higher risk (greater than 50 per cent) of invasion or metastasis, and is thus a candidate for more aggressive treatment (Chapter 2). Of critical importance, if these innovations are to be used correctly, is the need for high-quality biopsy material, adequate sampling of the available tumour tissue, and standardization and accuracy of the methodology used.

Similarly, the use of other potential predictors, such as the measurement of EGF receptors (Neal *et al.*, 1985) or the assessment of tumour ploidy (Chapter 1) will require the availability of technology of only the highest standard—there is little justification for attempts at implementing new

Table 17.1 Possible prognostic factors in urothelial TCC

Index	Application
Light morphology	Routine
grade, stage	
TIS	
dysplasia	
papillary versus solid	
Ultrastructure	Routine/experimental
Tumour markers	
ABO/Lewis antigens	Routine ?
monoclonal reagents	Experimental
conventional (CEA, EMA, etc.)	Routine
EGF receptor	Experimental
lectin binding	Experimental
Expression of oncogenes/oncogene products	Experimental
Karyotype	Experimental
DNA flow cytometry	Experimental
Clonigenicity *in vitro*	Experimental
Ability to be xenografted	Experimental

techniques if the applied methods are inadequate to produce accurate and significant results.

In addition to the use of experimental methods to improve the clinician's ability to predict the natural history of a tumour, attempts have been made in the laboratory to predict the clinical response to treatment with radiotherapy or chemotherapy (Chapter 1), or to use models to assess the potential antitumour activity of novel cytotoxic or biological agents (Chapter 3; Courtenay *et al.*, 1978). As reviewed in Chapters 1 and 3, these models are flawed, and major limitations include the relatively low 'take' rates or plating efficiencies, allowing adequate testing of only a limited proportion of the specimens tested. The paucity of positive correlations is another function of the limited sensitivity and specificity of this approach with the available techniques.

Nevertheless, in some centres, methods such as the soft agar clonogenic assay have even been applied commercially, on the presumption that the data generated should, in some fashion, influence patient management. This stance is clearly premature, as reviewed by Selby *et al.* (1983). It is possible, however, that improvements in the techniques applied, such as the use of cell-adhesive matrices (Baker *et al.*, 1986) or conditioned culture media may allow *in vitro* assays to serve a useful clinical role.

Other approaches for the prediction of response to chemotherapy are currently under investigation. Mathematical models that predict mechanisms of drug resistance have been formulated. For example, the concept that drug resistance is a function of cell number and the spontaneous mutation rate (Goldie and Coldman, 1979) has resulted in a series of investigational programmes based on the early introduction of chemotherapy, or the use of rapidly alternating non-cross-resistant cytotoxic combination regimens. Although these have been applied hitherto to tumours with rapid growth fractions (e.g. small-cell undifferentiated lung cancer), it may well be that these options will provide useful future approaches to the treatment of invasive and metastatic bladder cancer.

In addition, the ability to predict the presence of pleiotropic drug resistance (Carlsen, Till and Ling, 1977) by measuring the expression of p-glycoprotein in tumour cells may assist in the selection of the most appropriate cytotoxic agents for intravesical and systemic use. The term 'pleiotropic resistance' refers to the development of insensitivity to several cytotoxic agents (e.g. vincristine, actinomycin, doxorubicin) after prior exposure to another antitumour antibiotic or plant alkaloid. This may have particular application in cases of resistance to regimens such as MVAC chemotherapy (Chapters 10, 12, 16) in patients who have failed to respond or relapsed after treatment with intravesical or systemic single agents.

An alternative mechanism of drug resistance has recently been shown to have a genetic basis—i.e. amplification of the gene coding for a specific target enzyme, thus producing increased mRNA copies and thus increased cellular levels of the protein. For example, it appears that methotrexate-resistant tumour cells may express an amplified gene for dihydrofolate reductase, which may be integrated with chromosomal DNA or may be located in extra-chromosomal DNA fragments known as double-minute chromosomes (Kaufman *et al.*, 1979). A wide variety of biochemical and pharmacological probes may ultimately provide clinically useful tools for the prediction of therapeutic efficacy (Curt *et al.*, 1984), which may have applications in the management of bladder cancer.

Important issues in the management of superficial bladder cancer

Two-thirds of patients with bladder cancer present with superficial disease—stages TIS, Ta or T1 (Chapters 2, 4, 6 and 7). In most instances, optimal management is relatively simple and does not bear great discussion here: there is a requirement for careful and meticulous endoscopic resection, with expert histological assessment of the resected material by a tumour pathologist, augmented by urinary cytological examination of high quality. The importance of the standard of the histological assessment cannot be emphasized too much—far too often, an inexperienced pathologist is unable to differentiate accurately between dysplasia, treatment-related changes, and carcinoma-in-situ, limiting the accuracy of endoscopic assessment by the most experienced urological surgeon. Similarly, there is great importance for adequate sampling and staging to be carried out, including assessment of the prostate gland (possibly by perineal biopsy) and the use of deep biopsies to exclude muscle invasion. There is little justification for a hasty endoscopic assessment without due attention to the possible sites of involvement and the search for evidence of increasing grade or stage of the disease.

Low grade, superficial tumours (grade-I, Ta/T1) are associated with a good prognosis, especially if they elaborate blood group antigens, and in the great majority of cases can be controlled endoscopically for many years. Paradoxically, it is the most superficial of these tumours, carcinoma-in-situ (confined, by definition, to the most superficial layer of the urothelium), that is associated with the worst prognosis. Between 50 and 75 per cent of patients with bladder tumours with associated TIS will develop invasive or metastatic cancer (Chapters 2, 4 and 7). The dilemma is posed by the 25 per cent of cases that remain indolent and superficial. Histologically, they cannot be distinguished from the more dangerous variants. Guides to likely invasion include multicentricity, extent of mucosal involvement, duration of the disease, presence or absence of associated solid or papillary disease, and previous treatment. The extent and localization of TIS can be difficult to assess endoscopically. However, the use of haematoporphyrin derivative (HPD), which localizes in dysplastic and neoplastic urothelium, and fluoresces under certain wavelengths of light (Benson *et al.*, 1982), can facilitate this in a difficult case.

As noted above, at first presentation, the optimal treatment of localized, superficial TCC is endoscopic resection. In the situation where there is multifocal disease, intravesical cytotoxic prophylaxis will reduce the rate of recurrence and will delay recurrence in those patients destined to suffer this problem. The role of intravesical cytotoxic chemotherapy is no longer an issue, having been proved in several randomized trials (Chapters 6 and 14). As yet, there are no convincing data to prove the superiority of any one cytotoxic agent over another for intravesical use (Chapters 6 and 14). Each of the commonly used agents (thiotepa, Epodyl, doxorubicin, mitomycin C and VM-26) yields complete response rates of 35–45 per cent and increases the relapse-free time interval. At the present time, there seems to be little point for the clinician to agonize over which agent should be used first—the relevant data are simply not yet available. Thiotepa and Epodyl have the advantage of low cost and a long track record of antitumour activity. However, thiotepa is an alkylating agent and thus, at least in theory, poses a carcinogenic hazard to the staff using it and possibly to the patient (Chabner, 1977; Kapadia and Krause, 1978; Selevan *et al.*, 1985). Of some concern has been the potentially dangerous habit of some urological surgeons to abandon the routine safety precautions recommended for the handling of all cytotoxic agents.

While discussing the potential hazards of intravesical chemotherapy, it is appropriate to re-emphasize two additional issues. Although cisplatin is one of the most active single agents against TCC, the EORTC has shown that it may be hazardous when used intravesically because of the risk of inducing anaphylaxis (Chapter 14). The mechanism for this is not known. The ready availability of several other active agents suggests that, at least for the present time, cisplatin should not be recommended for intravesical use.

One also should not lose sight of the fact that superficial TCC can become invasive and that the risk of this increases with increasing numbers of recurrences. Thus, the potential for curative cystectomy should not be lost through repeated unsuccessful attempts at intravesical or alternative treatment. In particular, the adverse prognosticators discussed above should be monitored. If cystectomy is considered in the situation where urinary cytology remains persistently abnormal, the upper tracts should be carefully reassessed for occult malignancy prior to the planned surgery, especially in the patient who has been an analgesic abuser (Chapter 16).

It is important to emphasize that there is no defined current 'best' treatment for intravesical use. Despite anecdotal data to suggest greater activity from the use of BCG, randomized trials supporting this view have not been completed. In the patient who is deemed unsuitable for cystectomy, any of the cytotoxic agents discussed above may have a role in the management of superficial disease. Where these drugs fail to show activity, alternatives such as photodynamic therapy (laser treatment) may have an important role to play. Although the choice of agents is of no great importance, it is clear that, where possible, patients should be treated according to established and evaluable protocols, preferably in controlled and/or randomized fashion, in order to allow the ultimate demonstration of the optimal approach to the management of superficial TCC. There is a great risk that this may not be possible if individual clinicians fail to accept this responsibility, channelling newly diagnosed cases into random and unevaluable treatment programmes. In this context, an excellent opportunity exists for the formal assessment of combination intravesical chemotherapy. Although the synchronous use of two or more cytotoxic drugs may not be practicable because of the risk of chemical interactions or incompatibility, it may be feasible to treat patients with rapid sequential chemotherapy, based either kinetically (attempting to schedule the drugs to achieve a synergistic effect on the basis of different actions at the level of the cell cycle) or empirically. To evaluate such an approach, it will be necessary to implement similar principles as for the investigation of intravenous regimens—i.e. phase-I studies to assess the toxicity and optimal dosage, phase-II trials to demonstrate the level of antitumour activity, and phase-III studies to assess possible superiority over conventional approaches in a randomized fashion. It may even be possible ultimately to select the most appropriate drugs for individual patients on the basis of one of the experimental assay systems discussed above.

Invasive bladder cancer: evolving trends in treatment

The prognosis for patients with T2–T4 clinically non-metastatic TCC has been poor, with 5-year survival figures in most published series of less than 40 per cent, whether treated by radiotherapy, cystectomy or a combination of both (Chapters 7, 8 and 15). As outlined in Chapters 5 and 11, the greater precision of non-invasive staging may now allow more appropriate selection of patients for aggressive local treatment. Thus the introduction of the CAT scan has facilitated the demonstration of small-volume metastases in the retroperitoneum, lung and liver, thus saving the patient from a cystectomy or radical radiotherapy that will fail because of a geographical 'miss' (incomplete treatment of the full extent of the tumour). Not surprisingly, therefore, one could anticipate the publication of surgical and radiotherapeutic series in the late 1980s that will show improved 5-year survival due only to improved methods of staging (with the exclusion from locally directed treatment programmes of patients with established metastases, and the possibility of more accurate radiotherapy planning to avoid incomplete coverage of the tumour volume) (see also Chapter 5).

As noted in Chapters 8, 13 and 15, several pilot studies of first-line or 'neoadjuvant' intravenous chemotherapy have been initiated in an attempt to improve the prognosis of these patients. Several of the preliminary reports suggest improved survival with the introduction of this approach. Whether this is a true effect of the chemotherapy or merely the result of greater precision of staging techniques and radiotherapy planning remains to be seen (Raghavan, 1988). Randomized trials, comparing this innovative approach with standard treatment, will have to show a survival benefit before neoadjuvant chemotherapy can be considered as 'state of the art' medicine, rather than as an investigational programme.

The issue remains as to what is the 'optimal' definitive treatment for invasive TCC. The ultimate decision depends upon several factors (see Table 17.2). In an era of increasing frequency of medical litigation and a more informed patient population, it has become even more important for the clinician to be able to explain in detail the benefits and hazards of each programme of management. Our current practice is to enter consenting patients with T_2–T_4, Nx, M_0 TCC into a randomized multicentre trial comparing radical radiotherapy versus first-line intravenous cisplatin plus radical radiotherapy (Chapter 15). The use of radical radiotherapy as the definitive treatment simply reflects current clinical practice in Australia. Similar randomized trials with cystectomy as the mainstay of treatment are in progress in the USA and Europe.

For the patient who does not wish to enter into a randomized trial (or who is ineligible to do so), an approximately equivalent chance of cure is offered by modern techniques of radiotherapy (with CAT scan-controlled planning) or by the current techniques of radical cystectomy. For the clinician who attempts to evaluate the available literature to decide on this issue, comparisons are often difficult to achieve accurately for several reasons:

1. The published data often represent heavily selected populations of patients, either with respect to entry criteria, details of evaluation or follow-up.

2. Comparisons of end-results often reflect surgical staging (in reports of

Table 17.2 Radiotherapy verus cystectomy for invasive transitional cell carcinoma: benefits and drawbacks

Index	Radiotherapy	Cystectomy
Patient's preference	+	+
Age	+	−
>70 yrs	?	+
≤70 yrs		
Presence of upper tract neoplasia	−	+
Multifocal disease	−?	+
Poor performance status/fitness	+	−
Prior radiotherapy	−	+
Prior extensive intravesical chemotherapy	−	+
Uncertain stage	−	+
Hydronephrosis/renal dysfunction	?	?
Stage T4	+*?	−*?
Side effects		−
risk of postop./sudden death	+	−
impotence	−?	+
cystitis, colitis	−	

+ Denotes *relative* indication for that treatment.
− Denotes *relative* contraindication for that treatment.
* Because of poor results with conventional treatment, *may* be suited to neoadjuvant programmes.

cystectomies) versus non-invasive investigation for patients treated with radiotherapy (which is likely to result in a higher proportion of understaged tumours).

3. There is often a tendency for the proponents of one treatment modality to compare their results with historical data from other techniques and to conclude that the apparent improved survival is due to their treatment, rather than to improved staging, etc.

4. There is no mechanism to ensure the publication of negative results, and thus the literature is biased by the availability of apparently positive trials. Simes (1986) has suggested the initiation of an international registry of clinical trials to resolve this problem.

5. Much of the published information with regard to the morbidity of treatment reflects inaccurate methods of data collection. For example, in retrospective reviews of medical records, an absence of documentation of a particular side effect is often interpreted to show that the side effect did not occur (rather than simply representing an error of recording). The use of methods to evaluate formally the quality of life in long-term survivors (Chapter 15) suggests the possibility of substantial underreporting of toxicity in standard medical records.

Ultimately, a mechanism will be required that will allow the direct comparison of modern radiotherapy versus the current techniques of cystectomy (including the nerve-sparing procedures and the use of continent ileostomies). It is unlikely that a randomized clinical trial could answer this question as it is difficult to conceive that patients would consent to be allocated randomly to radical radiotherapy or radical cystectomy, in view of the substantially different side effects of each treatment. An alternative mechanism could be offered by a collaborative clinical trial in which, after a common non-invasive staging protocol, patients with invasive TCC could undergo either radical radiotherapy or cystectomy, depending on institutional policy. Thus, clinicians within an individual participating institution would treat patients according to their predefined 'standard' practice, recording details of all patients seen, all patients treated, and all those excluded from the trial. Although flawed in design, such an approach would minimize the systematic errors that can beset non-randomized comparisons of two treatments. In order for such a trial to be effected, each institution would have to adopt a common protocol for the 'standard' treatment—e.g. common field size, fractionation, total dose and equipment for those centres practising radiotherapy; a common protocol of surgical technique (nerve sparing, extent of dissection, type of ileostomy) in the institutions using cystectomy. Until such a trial has been completed, it seems reasonable for the choice between cystectomy and radiotherapy to be made on the basis of the patient's perceptions and preferences, the experience of the individual clinician (or his institutional data) and the availability of equipment and facilities.

Several outstanding issues remain to be resolved in the management of invasive bladder cancer:

1. What is the optimal definitive treatment (radiotherapy, cystectomy or a combination)?

2. Does neoadjuvant chemotherapy confer a survival benefit?

3. What is the optimal approach to neoadjuvant chemotherapy with regard to drugs (single agents versus combination regimens; choice of drugs)?

4. What is the optimal scheduling of neoadjuvant chemotherapy (how many cycles)?

5. Is there a role for conventional adjuvant chemotherapy (after the completion of definitive treatment)?

6. Is there a role for hyperfractionation of radiotherapy (with multiple doses per day in order to reduce damage to the normal tissues)?

7. Do specific drugs synergize with radiotherapy (for example, cisplatin, doxorubicin)?

8. Should there be an individualization of treatment, with specific regimens for particular cases (e.g. the older patient, T4 tumours, females)?

It will only be through carefully designed, well-executed collaborative studies that some of these problems will be solved. With the increasing prevalence of small innovative studies carried out by isolated groups of clinicians or by individuals, there is reason to believe that progress in this area may be slow.

Recurrent and metastatic disease

The management of recurrent and metastatic TCC is a common problem. More than 50 per cent of patients with invasive tumours ultimately develop recurrence, either locally or at distant sites. Depending on the nature of the clinical practice, up to one-third of patients present initially with metastases.

In patients who fail after radical radiotherapy, there is a definite role for salvage cystectomy in those who are considered sufficiently fit to undergo the procedure; long-term survival can be achieved in these patients in 20–30 per cent of cases (Blandy *et al.*, 1980; Goodman *et al.*, 1981). The management of locoregional failure after radical cystectomy is more difficult. Further surgery is usually ineffective and radiotherapy has only a limited, palliative role. For many years, a variety of cytotoxic regimens have been used in this setting, but with little success.

More recently, the introduction of newer combinations of cisplatin, methotrexate, vinblastine with or without doxorubicin, the so-called MVAC or CMV regimens (Sternberg *et al.*, 1985; Harker *et al.*, 1985; Scher and Sternberg, 1985), have been reported to yield response rates of 60–70 per cent, with complete remission rates of 30–40 per cent (see Chapters 10–14). Although there may be cause for enthusiasm, previous experience with combination chemotherapy has shown that initial reports are often not able to be reproduced (Chapter 11). Interestingly, in this volume, similar sets of data have been interpreted somewhat differently, with Tonkin and Tannock expressing concern about the reproducibility of the results (Chapter 11), in contrast to the enthusiasm of Young and Garnick (Chapter 12).

Certain facts are clear. Single-agent or combination cytotoxic chemotherapy can achieve durable responses in 20–30 per cent of cases, with definite evidence of subjective and objective benefit in patients with recurrent or metastatic TCC. Factors such as selection criteria, exclusion of patients from treatment and/or reporting, and the methods of evaluating response, will alter the reported success rate in any series. Active drugs against TCC include doxorubicin, cisplatin, methotrexate, mitomycin C and possibly vinblastine (Chapters 10–14). The randomized trials of combination regimens versus single agents that have been completed to date (CAP versus cisplatin; methotrexate plus cisplatin versus cisplatin; cyclophosphamide plus cisplatin versus cisplatin) have yielded negative results with respect to a clinically significant survival benefit (Khandekar *et al.*, 1985; Hillcoat and Raghavan, 1986; Soloway *et al.*, 1983). TCC of the upper urinary tracts is also relatively sensitive to cytotoxic chemotherapy (Chapter 16).

Perhaps the most important priority at present is to define the true role of the CMV and MVAC regimens. A multicentre international trial, coordinated by the Eastern Cooperative Oncology Group (Study Chairman: Lawrence Einhorn) is currently evaluating the respective efficacy and toxicity of the MVAC regimen and single-agent cisplatin as follows:

Regimen A: cisplatin 70 mg/m^2 i.v. on day 1; repeat every 28 days.

Regimen B: methotrexate 30 mg/m^2 i.v. on day 1, day 15 and day 21;
　　　　　　cisplatin 70 mg/m^2 i.v. on day 2;
　　　　　　vinblastine 3 mg/m^2 i.v. on day 2, day 15 and day 21;
　　　　　　doxorubicin 30 mg/m^2 i.v. on day 2;
　　　　　　repeat cycle every 28 days.

Investigators from the United States, Canada and Australia are entering patients into this study, which will be of considerable importance in defining the true role of the newly introduced regimens.

If this study confirms a survival benefit for MVAC, it may be appropriate either to compare MVAC versus CMV with regard to efficacy and toxicity, or perhaps to accept the MVAC regimen as a standard, and to add other drugs (e.g. mitomycin C) in an effort to increase the cure rate.

However, it should be emphasized that, at the present time, it would be inappropriate to accept these newer combination regimens as any standard until this has been validated in randomized trials. The situation is *not* analogous to the use of the PVB regimen for germ cell tumours (Einhorn, 1981), where there was a sudden increase in cure rates with the introduction of cisplatin-containing combination regimens. Even if one believed the situations to be similar, it is worth noting that current studies in the management of testicular cancer are directed towards the amelioration of side effects (without loss of efficacy) by decreasing the doses or by omitting agents from established regimens (Levi *et al.*, 1986). Thus, in the management of recurrent and metastatic bladder cancer, it will also be important to identify subgroups that will require more aggressive treatment and others in which less intensive regimens are effective.

Non-transitional cell tumours of the bladder

The management of non-transitional cell cancers of the urothelium continues to present a particularly difficult problem. These tumours, including squamous cell carcinomas, adenocarcinomas, soft-tissue sarcomas and metastatic tumours, occur infrequently, and represent fewer than 8 per cent of urothelial malignancies (Rous, 1978; Rousselot *et al.*, 1978; Jones *et al.*, 1980; Jones *et al.*, 1980; Anderstrom *et al.*, 1983; Khoury and Gilloz, 1984).

Although uncommon in Western society, squamous carcinoma of the bladder occurs more frequently in North Africa and Asia, and in particular in regions where schistosomiasis is endemic (Ghoneim *et al.*, 1985; Khoury and Gilloz, 1984). Squamous carcinoma is also associated with denervation of the bladder. Adenocarcinoma, which consists of urachal and non-urachal variants, is associated with schistosomiasis, bladder extrophy and the non-functioning bladder (Kickham and Keegan, 1963; Anderstrom *et al.*, 1983; Nielsen and Nielsen, 1983; Johannson and Anderstrom, 1987).

Apart from the unusual aetiological associations, non-transitional cell tumours of the urothelium have a similar clinical presentation to that of TCC (Chapter 4). However, there is a greater predominance of females with adenocarcinoma (Anderstrom *et al.*, 1983). Furthermore, a much higher proportion of squamous and adenocarcinomas are invasive at first presentation (Rous, 1978; Rousselot *et al.*, 1978; Jones *et al.*, 1980; Jones *et al.*, 1980; Anderstrom *et al.*, 1983; Khoury and Gilloz, 1984; Johannson and Anderstrom, 1987).

Approaches to the diagnosis and management of these tumours are quite similar to those described for TCC (Chapters 4–7). The mainstay of treatment has been surgery—either partial or segmental cystectomy, especially for adenocarcinomas (Anderstrom *et al.*, 1983; Kakizoe *et al.*, 1983), or a more radical approach (Ghoneim *et al.*, 1979; Johannson and Anderstrom, 1987). There is little established evidence to support the use of preoperative radiotherapy for adenocarcinoma (Khoury and Gilloz, 1984), although Ghoneim *et al.* (1985) have suggested a survival benefit for patients with high-grade and advanced-stage tumours.

The role for radiotherapy in this context is not clear. Although invasive adenocarcinoma or squamous carcinoma may respond to radical radiotherapy, cure is uncommon. Similarly, the role for chemotherapy has not been defined. Most reports of systemic chemotherapy for squamous or adenocarcinoma have been disappointing, although occasional sustained responses have been documented; for example, the use of 5-fluorouracil, doxorubicin and mitomycin C for advanced urachal carcinomas (Logothetis *et al.*, 1985). Several agents have had limited activity against squamous carcinomas associated with schistosomiasis (Gad-el-Mawla *et al.*, 1978a,b, 1979), although the results in Western populations have been less encouraging (Jones *et al.*, 1980; Khoury and Gilloz, 1984). However, it should be noted that these tumours occur uncommonly, and there is a paucity of well-executed phase-II studies of cytotoxic chemotherapy. To date, insufficient patients with non-transitional cell tumours have been treated with the MVAC regimen to allow a response rate to be defined (C. Sternberg, personal communication).

The prognosis of non-transitional tumours of the urothelium is poor, probably owing to the large proportion of patients presenting with advanced and/or metastatic disease (Anderstrom *et al.*, 1983; Khoury and Gilloz, 1984). Five-year survival figures remain less than 30 per cent for patients with non-metastatic disease, whatever the treatment. The most promising avenue for progress in these tumours may be offered by improved methods for early diagnosis—the use of improved cytological and imaging techniques to screen high-risk populations. Whether the improved surgical techniques and the use of the newer combination cytotoxic regimens will improve the survival of patients with non-transitional tumours of the urothelium remains to be seen.

Future directions

Progress in the laboratory and in the clinical setting has resulted in a greater appreciation of the extent of functional heterogeneity of urothelial tumours. More sophisticated probes are now being applied at the molecular level, especially since the demonstration of the range of oncogenes expressed in bladder cancer (Chapter 1). More recently, clinical application of these molecular probes has been investigated—for example, the search for evidence of gene amplification or rearrangement of the c-H-*ras*-1 gene in superficial and invasive bladder cancer by Southern blot analysis (Malone *et al.*, 1985).

With an apparent plateau having been reached in the use of single cytotoxic agents for superficial and advanced TCC, there has been renewed interest in the evaluation of combination regimens, and more recently in the development of methods of immunological manipulation. In particular, the apparent efficacy of intravesical BCG in the treatment and prophylaxis of superficial disease has resulted in several innovative programmes. Inter-leukin-2 has been demonstrated to induce cytotoxic activity *in vitro* against melanoma cells in co-cultured lymphocytes (Hersey *et al.*, 1981). This has been applied clinically in a phase I–II study of intralesional injections of interleukin-2 into superficial urothelial tumours (Pizza *et al.*, 1984). More recently, it has been shown that intravesical administration of BCG results in the local production of interleukin-2, as demonstrated in urine collections (Ratcliffe *et al.*, 1986). Several phase I–II studies are currently in progress to assess the efficacy of systemic or intravesical administration of interferons in the management of urothelial cancer.

The use of photodynamic therapy, with a variety of laser light sources, is being refined, with a greater precision of dosage and scheduling (Benson, 1986). The limitations of this form of treatment have been reassessed, and attempts are being made to apply the laser to the treatment of invasive cancer.

New tools are being developed for the assessment of quality of life in patients undergoing treatment, and particularly in those who may not be cured (Chapters 9, 11 and 15), allowing the patient to participate to a greater extent in assessing the balance between quality and quantity of life (McNeil *et al.*, 1981). However, great caution will have to be exercised to avoid over-interpretation of the results from these preliminary studies with a resultant inaccurate or inappropriate impact on management.

Increasing attention is being devoted to an understanding of the causes and genesis of urothelial cancer, particularly with regard to occupation and lifestyle (Chapter 1). The recent demonstration of the carcinogenicity of passive smoking (in particular with respect to bronchogenic carcinoma) (Sandler *et al.*, 1985) may have important implications with regard to the development of bladder cancer, another smoking-related disease. A greater understanding of the causes of bladder cancer should allow the identifica-tion of high-risk populations, facilitating the introduction of more rational community screening programmes. Such programmes should now be feasible, with the introduction of sensitive and specific techniques, such as urinary cytology.

Conclusions

The management of transitional cell carcinoma of the urothelial tract is in a state of flux. The introduction of improved imaging and staging techniques may yield an improved survival rate for patients with TCC without any change in treatment techniques, simply by defining the extent of disease more accurately, thus facilitating more appropriate selection of treatment. This mandates that any apparent improvement in survival achieved from recently introduced methods of treatment be tested in a controlled fashion to avoid the phenomenon of stage migration.

For superficial disease, the increased accuracy of urinary cytology and other diagnostic methods, accompanied by a greater therapeutic armamentarium of cytotoxic and immunoactive agents, has allowed greater numbers of patients to achieve cure or control of their disease without the loss of their bladders. Yet with all of these advances, it behoves the clinician to remain vigilant for evidence of increasing aggression or invasion of the tumour, so as not to miss the opportunity of curative cystectomy.

The introduction of the MVAC and CMV combination cytotoxic regimens has once again raised the question of the relative merits of combination versus single agents. If confirmed, the preliminary data from the use of MVAC and CMV suggest that the management of recurrent and metastatic disease will be revolutionized. However, there are already disturbing reports that these regimens may be less effective than originally thought. Our own preliminary experience in treating TCC of the upper and lower tracts has yielded responses of relatively short duration, and accordingly we are participating in an international trial comparing the MVAC regimen against single-agent cisplatin.

Perhaps the most difficult area of therapeutic decision-making relates to invasive TCC. The conventional approaches to treatment (radiotherapy, cystectomy or combinations of both) have yielded 5-year survival rates of less than 50 per cent. There has been a recent wave of enthusiasm for the surgical innovations (nerve-sparing cystectomy, continent ileostomy, penile prostheses) and for the introduction of neoadjuvant chemotherapy. However, it is crucial that, whenever possible, patients with invasive non-metastatic TCC be entered into the available trials that aim to improve the results of treatment. There is no 'best available' treatment today. If we are to improve the state of our knowledge and our management, we must continue to question the methods that we use and the results that we achieve.

References

Anderstrom, C., Johansson, S.L. and Von Schultz, L. (1983). Primary adenocarcinoma of the urinary bladder: a clinicopathologic and prognostic study. *Cancer* **52**: 1273–80.

Baker, F.L., Spitzer, G., Ajani, J.A. *et al.* (1986). Drug and radiation sensitivity measurements of successful primary monolayer culturing of human tumor cells using cell-adhesive matrix and supplemented medium. *Cancer Research* **46**: 1263–74.

Benson, R.C. (1986). Integral photoradiation therapy of multifocal bladder tumours. *European Urology* **12** (Suppl. 1): 47–53.

Benson, R.C., Farrow, G.M., Kinsey, J.H., Cortese, D.A., Zincke, H. and Utz, D.C. (1982). Detection and localization of *in situ* carcinoma of the bladder with hematoporphyrin derivative. *Mayo Clinic Proceedings* **57**: 548–55.

Blandy, J.P., England, H.R., Evans, S.J.W. *et al.* (1980). T3 bladder cancer: the case for salvage cystectomy. *British Journal of Urology* **52**: 506–10.

Carlsen, S.A., Till, J.E. and Ling, V. (1977). Modulation of drug permeability in Chinese hamster ovary cells: possible role for phosphorylation of surface glycoproteins. *Biochemica Biophysica Acta* **467**: 238–50.

Chabner, B.A. (1977). Second neoplasm: a complication of cancer chemotherapy. *New England Journal of Medicine* **279**: 213–15.

Einhorn, L.H. (1981). Testicular cancer as a model for a curable neoplasm. *Cancer Research* **41**: 3275–80.

Gad-el-Mawla, N.M., Hamza, R., Cairns, J., Anderson, T. and Ziegler, J.L. (1978a). Phase II trial of methotrexate in carcinoma of the bladder. *Cancer Treatment Reports* **62**: 1075–6.

Gad-el-Mawla, N.M., Muggia, F.M., Hamza, M.R. *et al.* (1978b). Chemotherapeutic management of carcinoma of the Bilharzial bladder: a phase II trial with hexamethylmelamine and VM-26. *Cancer Treatment Reports* **62**: 993–6.

Gad-el-Mawla, N.M., Chevlen, E., Hamza, M.R. and Ziegler, J.L. (1979). Phase II trial of c-DDP (II) in cancer of the Bilharzial bladder. *Cancer Treatment Reports* **63**: 1577–8.

Ghoneim, M.A., Ashamallah, A.G., El-Hammady, S., Gaballah, M.A. and Soliman, E.S. (1979). Cystectomy for carcinoma of the Bilharzial bladder: 138 cases 5 years later. *British Journal of Urology* **51**: 541–4.

Ghoneim, M.A., Ashamallah, A.K., Awaad, M.K. and Whitmore, W.F. (1985). Randomized trial of cystectomy with or without radiotherapy for carcinoma of the Bilharzial bladder. *Journal of Urology* **134**: 266–8.

Goldie, J.H. and Coldman, A.J. (1979). A mathematical model for relating the drug sensitivity of tumors to their spontaneous mutation rate. *Cancer Treatment Reports* **63**: 1727–33.

Goodman, G.B., Hislop, T.G., Elwood, J.J. and Balfour, J. (1981). Conservation of bladder function in patients with invasive bladder cancer treated by definitive irradiation and selective cystectomy. *International Journal of Radiation Oncology, Biology and Physics* **7**: 569–73.

Harker, W.A., Meyers, F.J., Freiha, F.S., Palmer, J.M., Shortliffe, L.D., Hannigan, J.F., McWhirter, K.M. and Torti, F.M. (1985). Cisplatin, methotrexate and vinblastine (CMV): an effective chemotherapy regimen for metastatic transitional cell carcinoma of the urinary tract: a Northern California Oncology Group study. *Journal of Clinical Oncology* **3**: 1463–70.

Hersey, P., Bindon, C., Edwards, A., Murray, E., Phillips, G. and McCarthy, W.H. (1981). Induction of cytotoxic activity in human lymphocytes against antologous and allogeneic melanoma cells *in vitro* by culture with Interleukin-2. *International Journal of Cancer* **28**: 695–703.

Hicks, R.M. and Wakefield, J.St.J. (1972). Rapid induction of bladder cancer in rats with N-methyl-nitrosourea. *Chemical and Biological Interactions* **5**: 139.

Hillcoat, B.C. and Raghavan, D. (1986). A randomised comparison of cisplatinum (C) versus cisplatinum and methotrexate (C+M) in advanced bladder cancer. *Proceedings of the American Society of Clinical Oncology* **5**: abstract 426.

Johansson, S.L. and Anderstrom, C.R. (1987). Primary adenocarcinoma of the urinary bladder and urachus. In *Textbook for Uncommon Cancer*. Edited by Williams, C., Krikorian, J. and Raghavan, D. John Wiley, Chichester.

Johnson, D.E., Hodge, G.B., Fahdi, N. and Ayala, A. (1985). Urachal carcinoma. *Urology* **26**: 218–21.

Jones, M.A., Bloom, H.J., Williams, G., Trott, P.A. and Wallace, D.M. (1980). The management of squamous cell carcinoma of the bladder. *British Journal of Urology* **52**: 511–14.

Jones, W.A., Gibbons, R.P., Comea, R.J., Cummings, K.B. and Mason, J.T. (1980). Primary adenocarcinoma of bladder. *Urology* **15**: 119–22.

Kakizoe, T., Matsumoto, K., Andoh, M., Nishio, Y. and Kishi, K. (1983). Adenocarcinoma of urachus: report of 7 cases and review of the literature. *Urology* **21**: 360–66.

Kapadia, S.B. and Krause, J.R. (1978). Ovarian carcinoma terminating in acute nonlymphocytic leukaemia following alkylating agent therapy. *Cancer* **41**: 1676–9.

Kaufman, R.J., Brown, P.C. and Shimke, R.T. (1979). Amplified dihydrofolate reductase genes in unstably methotrexate-resistant cells is associated with double minute chromosomes. *Proceedings of the National Academy of Sciences* (USA) **76**: 5669–73.

Khandekar, J.D., Elson, P.J., De Wys, W.D., Slayton, R.E. and Harris, D.T. (1985). Comparative activity and toxicity of cis-diamine-dichloroplatinum (DDP) and a combination of doxorubicin, cyclophosphamide & DDP in disseminated transitional cell carcinomas of the urinary tract. *Journal of Clinical Oncology* **3**: 539–45.

Khoury, S. and Gilloz, A. (1984). Nontransitional cell carcinoma of the bladder in adults—Review. *Progress in Biological and Clinical Research* **162B**: 275–88.

Kickham, C.J. and Keegan, J.J. (1963). The bladder 'left behind'. *Journal of Urology* **89**: 689–91.

Levi, J., Raghavan, D., Harvey, V. *et al.* (1986). Deletion of bleomycin from therapy for good prognosis advanced testicular cancer: a prospective randomised study. *Proceedings of the American Society of Clinical Oncology* **5**: abstract 374.

Logothetis, C.J., Samuels, M.L. and Ogden, S. (1985). Chemotherapy for adenocarcinoma of the bladder and urachal origin: 5-fluorouracil, doxorubicin and mitomycin C. *Urology* **26**: 252–5.

Malone, P.R., Visvanathan, K.V., Ponder, B.A.J. and Summerhayes, I.C. (1985). Oncogenes and bladder cancer. *British Journal of Urology* **57**: 664–7.

McNeil, B.J., Weichselbaum, R. and Pauker, S.G. (1981). Tradeoffs between quality and quantity of life in laryngeal cancer. *The New England Journal of Medicine* **17**: 982–7.

Narayana, A.S., Loening, S., Weimar, G.W. and Culp, D.A. (1978). Sarcoma of the bladder and prostate. *Journal of Urology* **119**: 72–6.

Neal, D.E., Marsh, C., Bennett, M.K., Abel, P.D., Hall, R.R., Sainsbury, J.R.C. and Harris, A.C. (1985). Epidermal growth factor receptors in human bladder cancer: comparison of invasive and superficial tumours. *Lancet* **1**: 366–8.

Nielsen, K. and Nielsen, K.K. (1983). Adenocarcinoma in extrophy of the bladder: the last case in Scandinavia? *Journal of Urology* **130**: 1180–1182.

Pizza, G., Severesini, G., Menniti, D., De Vinci, C. and Corrado, F. (1984). Tumour regression after intra-lesional injection of interleukin-2 (Il-2) in bladder cancer—preliminary report. *International Journal of Cancer* **34**: 359–67.

Raghavan, D., Debruyne, F., Herr, H *et al.* (1986). Experimental models of bladder cancer: a critical review. *Progress in Clinical and Biological Research* **221**: 171–208.

Raghavan, D. (1988). Neoadjuvant chemotherapy for invasive bladder cancer. *British Journal of Urology* **61**: in press.

Ratliffe, T.C., Haaff, E.O. and Catalona, W.J. (1986). Interleukin-2 production during intravesical BCG therapy for bladder cancer. *Cancer Immunology and Immunopathology* **40**: 375–9.

Rous, S.N. (1978). Squamous cell carcinoma of the bladder. *Journal of Urology* **120**: 561–2.

Rousselot, F., Paoletti, G., Laroze, M. *et al.* (1981). Squamous cell carcinomas of the bladder: a study of twenty-one cases. *Annales d'Urologie* (Paris) **15**: 46–8.

Sandler, D.P., Wilcox, A.J. and Everson, R.B. (1985). Cumulative effects of lifetime passive smoking on cancer risk. *Lancet* **i**: 312–14.

Scher, H.I. and Sternberg, C.N. (1985). Chemotherapy of urologic malignancies. *Seminars in Urology* **3**: 239–80.

Selby, P., Buick, R.N. and Tannock, I. (1983). A critical appraisal of the 'human tumor stem cell assay'. *New England Journal of Medicine* **308**: 129–34.

Selevan, S.G., Lindbohm, M.L., Hornung, R.W. and Hemminki, K. (1985). A study of occupational exposure to anti-neoplastic drugs and fetal loss in nurses. *New England Journal of Medicine* **313**: 1173–8.

Simes, R.J. (1986). Publication bias: the case for an international registry of clinical trials. *Journal of Clinical Oncology* **4**: 1529–41.

Soloway, M.S., Einstein, A., Corder, M.P., Bonney, W., Prout, G.R. and Coombs, J. (1983). A comparison of cisplatin and the combination of cisplatin and cyclophosphamide in advanced urothelial cancer. *Cancer* **52**: 767–72.

Sternberg, C.N., Yagoda, A., Scher, H.I. *et al.* (1985). Preliminary results of MVAC (methotrexate, vinblastine, doxorubicin and cisplatin) for TCC of the urothelium. *Journal of Urology* **133**: 403–7.

Index

Bold type indicates key entries

electron microscopy   3ff
  carcinoma-*in-situ*   6
  carcinosarcomma   6
  dysplasia   6
  exfoliative cytology and   7
  intracytoplasmic lumina   5
  microvilli   5
  morphometry   5
  reversed polarity   5
  pseudosarcoma   6
  scanning   5
  transmission   4
  umbrella cells   6
EMA (*see* tumour markers,
    immunocytochemistry)
EORTC trials (*see also* clinical
    trials):   131, 277ff, 321
4′-epiadriamycin (*see* doxorubicin
    analogues)
epidemiology   1ff
  analgesic nephropathy   2, 287
  carcinogens   2ff
  coffee   1, 287, 301
  congenital anomalies   301
  dietary sweeteners   1
  dye industry   2, 301
  exhaust   1
  industrial exposure   1, 301
  phenacetin   2, 301
  renal pelvic tumours   70, 299
  rubber industry   2
  schistosomiasis   1, 327
  tobacco   1, 301
  ureteric tumours   299
epithelial membrane antigen (*see*
    tumour markers,
    immunocytochemistry)
Epodyl   80, 281, 321
ethoglucid (*see* Epodyl)
Etoposide (*see* podophyllotoxines)
European Organization for
    Research and Treatment of
    Cancer (*see* EORTC trials,
    clinical trials)
exfoliative cytology (*see* cytology)
experimental models (*see* models)

FANFT (*see* models, carcinogenesis)
field defect   3, 42, 53
first-line chemotherapy (*see*
    chemotherapy, neoadjuvant)
flow cytometry   10, 12, 53, 74, 318

  aneuploidy   12, 53
  carcinoma-in-situ   10
  cytogenetics and   12
  diploid   12
  DNA   10
  exfoliative cytology   10, 53
  grade and   12, 53
  prognosis   12
  stage and   12, 53
  tetraploidy   12
5-fluorouracil   64–5, 249, 313
functional pathology (*see*
    histopathology,
    immunocytochemistry)

geriatrics
  neoadjuvant programmes   182ff
  pharmacology   177ff
  physiology   174–6
  quality of life   185
  side effects   176, 180
  treatment   174ff
Goldie–Coldman hypothesis   319
grade   2, 44, 53, 71, 79, 287, 300,
    317

haematoporphyrin derivative   321
haematuria (*see* presentation)
  diagnostic service   73
HCG (*see* human chorionic
    gonadotrophin)
heterogeneity   2ff, 318
hexamethylmelamine   250
histogenesis   2
histopathology   2ff, 42ff, 75ff
  classification   2, 44, 75ff, 143ff,
    298ff
  dysplasia   3, 49, 120
  functional pathology   7, 53
  hyperplasia   49
  upper tract tumours   299ff
human chorionic gonadotrophin (*see*
    tumour markers,
    immunocytochemistry)
hydronephrosis (*see* urinary
    obstruction)
hyperbaric oxygen   82, 268
hyperplasia (*see* histopathology)

immunocytochemistry   7, 43, 55
  cell lines   24
  xenografts   27